Silent Myocardial Ischemia and Angina

Silent Myocardial Ischemia and Angina

Prevalence, Prognostic, and Therapeutic Significance

Edited by
Bramah N. Singh, M.D., D.Phil., F.R.C.P.
Chief of Cardiology, Veterans Administration Medical Center, West Los Angeles, California

Professor of Medicine, UCLA School of Medicine, Los Angeles, California

PERGAMON PRESS
New York ■ Oxford ■ Beijing ■ Frankfurt
São Paulo ■ Sydney ■ Tokyo ■ Toronto

Pergamon Press Offices:

U.S.A.	Pergamon Press, Maxwell House, Fairview Park, Elmsford, New York 10523, U.S.A.
U.K.	Pergamon Press, Headington Hill Hall, Oxford OX3 0BW, England
PEOPLE'S REPUBLIC OF CHINA	Pergamon Press, Qianmen Hotel, Beijing, People's Republic of China
FEDERAL REPUBLIC OF GERMANY	Pergamon Press, Hammerweg 6, D-6242 Kronberg, Federal Republic of Germany
BRAZIL	Pergamon Editora, Rua Eça de Queiros, 346, CEP 04011, São Paulo, Brazil
AUSTRALIA	Pergamon Press (Aust.) Pty., P.O. Box 544, Potts Point, NSW 2011, Australia
JAPAN	Pergamon Press, 8th Floor, Matsuoka Central Building, 1-7-1 Nishishinjuku, Shinjuku-ku, Tokyo 160, Japan
CANADA	Pergamon Press Canada, Suite 271, 253 College Street, Toronto, Ontario M5T 1R5, Canada

---

First printing 1988

Library of Congress Cataloging in Publication Data

Silent myocardial ischemia and angina.

Based on an international symposium held in Irvine, Calif. on Nov. 14-15, 1987, and sponsored by the Dept. of Continuing Education in Health Sciences (UCLA Extension), UCLA School of Medicine.
Includes bibliographies and index.
1. Silent myocardial ischemia--Congresses. 2. Angina pectoris--Congresses. I. Singh, B. N. (Bramah N.) II. University of California, Los Angeles. Dept. of Continuing Education in Health Sciences. [DNLM: 1. Coronary Disease--congresses. WG 300 S5824 1987]
RC685.S48S55 1988 616.1′23 88-25511
ISBN 0-08-036078-5

Printed in the United States of America

To the Memory of My Parents,
Shri Ram and Janki Singh

Contents

List of Contributors

B. GREG BROWN, M.D., Ph.D.

Professor of Medicine
Cardiology Division RG-22
University of Washington Hospital
Seattle, Washington 98195

PETER F. COHN, M.D.

Professor of Medicine
State University of New York
Health Sciences Center (T-17-020)
Stony Brook, New York 11794

TIMOTHY COX

University of Southern California
School of Medicine
2025 Zonal Ave.
Raulston Bldg., Room 100
Los Angeles, CA 90033

MICHAEL H. CRAWFORD, M.D.

Professor of Medicine
Department of Medicine/Cardiology,
University of Texas Health Science Center
7703 Floyd Curl Drive
San Antonio, Texas 78284

JOHN DEANFIELD, M.D.

The Hospital for Sick Children
Great Ormond Street
London WC1H 3JN, England

PRAKASH C. DEEDWANIA, M.D.

Clinical Professor of Medicine, UCSF
School of Medicine
VA Medical Center
2615 East Clinton Avenue
Fresno, California 93703

VINCENT DEQUATTRO, M.D.

Professor of Medicine
University of Southern California
School of Medicine
2025 Zonal Ave.
Raulston Bldg., Room 100
Los Angeles, CA 90033

JAIME FIGUERAS, M.D.

Unidad Coronaria
Ciudad Sanitaria Vall d'Hebron
Passeig Vall d'Hebron, s/n
Barcelona, Spain

SIDNEY O. GOTTLIEB, M.D.

Assistant Professor of Medicine
Division of Cardiology, B-1 South
Francis Scott Key Medical Center
The Johns Hopkins Medical Institutions
4940 Eastern Ave.
Baltimore, MD 21224

MARTIN A. JOSEPHSON, M.D.

Associate Professor of Medicine
UCLA School of Medicine
Cardiology Section 691/111E
VA Wadsworth Hospital,
Los Angeles, California 90073

WILLIAM B. KANNEL, M.D.

Professor of Medicine
Boston University Medical Center
Doctors Office Bldg.
720 Harrison Avenue
Suite 1105
Boston, Massachusetts 02118

SHINOBU KIMURA, M.D.

University of Southern California
School of Medicine
2025 Zonal Ave.
Raulston Bldg., Room 100
Los Angeles, CA 90033

DEBORA DE-PING LEE, M.D.

University of Southern California
School of Medicine
2025 Zonal Ave.
Raulston Bldg., Room 100
Los Angeles, CA 90033

ALBERTO MALLIANI, M.D.

Instituto Richerche Cardiovasculari
Via Bonfadini 214
20138 Milano, Italy

ATTILIO MASERI, M.D., F.R.C.P.

Sir John McMichael Professor of Cardiology
Royal Postgraduate Medical School
Hammersmith Hospital
Du Cane Road
London W12 OHS, England

FRENY VAGHAIWALLA MODY, M.D.

Assistant Professor of Medicine
UCLA School of Medicine
Cardiology Section 691/111E
VA Wadsworth Hospital
Los Angeles, California 90073

KOONLAWEE NADEMANEE, M.D.

Associate Professor of Medicine
UCLA School of Medicine
Cardiology Section 691/111E
VA Wadsworth Hospital
Los Angeles, California 90073

RICHARD W. NESTO, M.D.

Assistant Professor of Medicine,
Harvard Medical School
New England Deaconess Hospital
Department of Medicine
Section of Cardiology
185 Pilgrim Road
Boston, Massachusetts 02215

VIHN NGO, M.D.

University of Southern California
School of Medicine
2025 Zonal Ave.
Raulston Bldg., Room 100
Los Angeles, CA 90033

CARL J. PEPINE, M.D.

Professor of Medicine
Division of Cardiology
University of Florida
Box J-277 JHMHC
Gainesville, Florida 32610

THUY QUANG PHAM, M.D.

University of Southern California
School of Medicine
2025 Zonal Ave.
Raulston Bldg., Room 100
Los Angeles, CA 90033

SHAHBUDIN RAHIMTOOLA, M.D., F.R.C.P.

Professor of Medicine
USC School of Medicine
2025 Zonal Ave.
Los Angeles, California 90033.

KATHRYN RIGONAN, M.D.

University of Southern California
School of Medicine
2025 Zonal Ave.
Raulston Bldg., Room 100
Los Angeles, CA 90033

WILLIAM C. ROBERTS, M.D.

Pathology Branch
NHLB Institute
National Institutes of Health
Building 10A
Room 3E30
Bethesda, Maryland 20892

MICHAEL B. ROCCO, M.D.

Brigham and Women's Hospital
Cardiovascular Division
75 Francis Street
Boston, Massachusetts 02115

BIMLENDRA SHARMA, M.D.

Professor of Medicine
University of Arkansas for Medical Sciences
Department of Cardiology
4301 W. Markham
Slot 532
Little Rock, AR 72205

WILLIAM E. SHELL, M.D.

Associate Clinical Professor of Medicine
UCLA School of Medicine
435 North Roxbury Drive
Suite 300
Beverly Hills, California 90210

ANDREW P. SELWYN, M.D.

Associate Professor of Medicine
Harvard School of Medicine and
Brigham and Women's Hospital
75 Francis St.
Boston, Massachusetts

BRAMAH N. SINGH, M.D., D.Phil, F.R.C.P.

Professor of Medicine
UCLA School of Medicine
Cardiology Section 691/111E
VA Wadsworth Medical Center
West Los Angeles, California 90073

BUDGE H. SMITH, M.D.

Department of Medicine
Cardiology Division RG-22
University of Washington Hospital
Seattle, Washington 98195

CAROLE A. WARNES, M.D.

Division of Cardiovascular Medicine
Department of Medicine
Mayo Clinic
Rochester, MN

SALIM YUSUF, M.D., D.Phil, M.R.C.P.

NHLBI
Federal Building
Clinical Trials Branch
National Institutes of Health
7550 Wisconsin Avenue
Room 604
Bethesda, Maryland 20892

Preface

Silent myocardial ischemia was recently demonstrated to be a common "manifestation" of ischemic heart disease. However, its precise clinical significance is still unclear, and it remains the subject of much debate. The focal point of controversy centers on the issue of the prognostic importance of silent myocardial ischemia, particularly of episodes documented by continuous ECG monitoring in hospitalized as well as in ambulatory patients. It is reasonable to assume that controlled clinical trials to determine whether reduction or elimination of silent ischemic episodes can be achieved by therapeutic modalities can only be undertaken once it has been confirmed that episodes that persist after medical therapy do constitute an undoubted incremental prognostic index of adverse outcome in myocardial ischemic syndromes over and above that revealed by conventional approaches.

The purpose of this monograph on a growing subject is to present a current perspective on the pathophysiologic mechanisms, prevalence, prognostic significance, and therapeutic implications of the phenomenon of silent myocardial ischemia. The contributors to this are investigators and clinicians actively involved in studying myocardial ischemia. It is hoped that the information presented will be of value not only to investigators interested in directions for future research in silent ischemia, but also to clinicians for their current practice in the evaluation and treatment of coronary artery disease.

I am most grateful to the contributors for their efforts in providing the manuscripts in a timely fashion. I would also like to acknowledge my special thanks to Ruth Hayden and her staff at Conference Management Associates for their invaluable help with all aspects of this monograph. Finally, my thanks are due to Lawrence Kimble and Francesca Frederick for their secretarial assistance and Roger Dunn and his staff at Pergamon Press for their help and guidance in the preparation of this volume.

Bramah N. Singh
Los Angeles, California

PART A

Pathophysiology

CHAPTER 1

Silent Myocardial Ischemia

Historical Development of the Concept and Scope of the Clinical Problem

Bramah N. Singh MD, DPhil

Since it has become possible to record the electrical correlates of the human heart beat, there has been an increasing appreciation that aberrations of cardiac rhythm and conduction can occur without symptoms. Indeed, the largest numbers of these disorders in an individual patient are silent. The issue clearly became an exceedingly important clinical question in the early 1960s with the introduction of ambulatory ECG recordings as a clinical tool. For example, numerous studies were undertaken to determine the prevalence of premature ventricular contractions; subsequently, it became evident that these contractions were ubiquitous. They were found to occur in healthy subjects, but their frequency and complexity tended to increase with age and cardiac disease. It is now clearly established that premature ventricular contractions have little or no effect on prognosis in healthy subjects,[1] but they are prognostically of greatest significance in patients with severe heart disease with marked reduction in ventricular function.[2] They are clinically silent, yet we now know that their occurrence in patients with heart disease and severely decreased ventricular ejection fraction may increase three- to fivefold the incidence of sudden death. This gives the investigator the opportunity to test the hypothesis that suppression of such "malignant" premature ventricular contractions may prolong survival. Definitive answers are still lacking, but control trials are in progress.

Holter monitoring in various ischemic myocardial syndromes recently revealed that most episodes of transient myocardial ischemia also are clinically silent. This "discovery" has raised a number of clinically relevant questions. What is the exact prevalence of silent myocardial ischemia? Does it differ from symptomatic myocardial ischemia? Does it have the same significance as silent ischemia revealed by provocative exercise stress testing? Above all, does silent myocardial ischemia have an independent prognostic significance? For example, does it play a significant role in the development of myocardial infarction, ventricular dysfunction, arrhythmias, and sudden death? Perhaps of even greater importance, is it amenable to pharmacologic and nonpharmacologic suppression, and what degree of reduction in silent myocardial ischemia might be necessary to favorably alter the clinical outcome?

This chapter will provide a brief historical and current perspective of this developing subject as a preamble to an international symposium that was held to specifically examine some of these issues.

WHAT IS SILENT MYOCARDIAL ISCHEMIA?

Silent myocardial ischemia is present when unequivocal biochemical, hemodynamic, perfusion, functional, and ECG abnormalities indicative of an imbalance in myocardial oxygen demand and supply develop in the absence of angina or equivalent symptoms. It is clearly desirable to distinguish asymptomatic coronary artery disease from silent myocardial ischemia. Asymptomatic coronary artery disease provides the substrate for the development of silent myocardial ischemia, which may become manifest as the "activity" of the disease changes or the major determinants of oxygen consumption are altered. For example, a patient with significant triple-vessel coronary disease may demonstrate no myocardial ischemia during continuous ambulatory ECG monitoring if the disease is not active. Conversely, under the stress of a strenuous exercise treadmill test, compelling ECG evidence of myocardial ischemia may develop in this patient *without angina or its equivalents*. However, in the absence of other confirmatory evidence of coronary disease in an individual patient the significance of positive ECG changes on the treadmill test as an isolated phenomenon will be difficult to define. The available data suggest however that silent ischemia in patients with known coronary artery disease may be identified by provocative stress tests or continuous ECG or even hemodynamic monitoring. Through these approaches in different subsets of patients with ischemic heart disease, silent or symptomatic myocardial ischemia clearly may occur spontaneously or it may be revealed by appropriate stress tests (Table 1.1). The recognition of silent myocardial ischemia is facilitated by a knowledge of the measurable correlates of myocardial ischemia.

MEASURABLE CORRELATES OF MYOCARDIAL ISCHEMIA: HEMODYNAMIC AND FUNCTIONAL CONFIRMATION OF SILENT EPISODES

When a coronary artery or its branch in an experimental animal is occluded, certain reversible electrophysiologic, metabolic, inotropic, and hemodynamic alterations ensue.[3,4] The ECG changes are characterized by T-wave augmentation, ST-segment elevations and depressions, R-wave augmentation, accelerated heart rate, and increased systemic blood pressure. Preceding these changes are depression in the indexes of myocardial contractility, diminution in ventricular compliance, elevation of ventricular filling pressures, and a reduction in cardiac index. Accompanying these alterations is an increase in lactate concentrations in the venous effluent from the ischemic region, another hallmark of myocardial ischemia.[5] This pattern of abnormalities also occurs when ischemia develops spontaneously in man. Indeed, the term

Table 1.1. Subsets of Patients with Silent Myocardial Ischemia

I. Completely asymptomatic subjects
   A. Those with risk factors for coronary disease.
   B. Those without risk factors for coronary disease.
II. Patients with manifest coronary artery disease.
   • Prinzmetal's angina
   • Unstable angina
   • Chronic stable angina
   • Postmyocardial infarction
   • Postmyocardial revascularization

"ischemic cascade"[6] may be applied to the sum total of temporal changes in the various parameters that accompany a transient episode of myocardial ischemia.

Of particular interest are the hemodynamic observations that deal with the accurate determination of the temporal sequence of changes in the major determinants of myocardial oxygen consumption. These provide an insight into the nature of individual episodes of transient ischemia in patients with coronary artery disease (see Chapter 5). The pattern of hemodynamic alterations in symptomatic and asymptomatic ischemic episodes in a patient with a history of rest angina is shown in Figure 1.1. Many features are immediately apparent. The earliest hemodynamic change is an elevation in pulmonary systolic and diastolic pressure or in left ventricular end-diastolic pressure.[7–9] Many issues are pertinent herein. Most of these episodes of ischemia documented in various formal studies of hemodynamics are *not* preceded by major increases in heart rate or systemic arterial or right heart pressure. However, these indexes do increase as does the intensity of ischemia as ECG abnormalities progress. Particularly important are the changes in heart rate and blood pressure that increase apparently *in response* to the onset of ischemia itself. These changes reach a peak before regression towards the baseline begins. The observed crescendo-decrescendo pattern of hemodynamic alterations that are associated with a similar pattern of ECG abnormalities appears to be a hallmark of myocardial ischemia.[10] Undoubtedly, a similar sequence of changes is likely in the metabolic and biochemical parameters that accompany episodes of myocardial ischemia. Recently, recognition of this characteristic cascade of changes, in particular those in heart rate (Figure 1.2), ST segment of the ECG, and pulmonary diastolic pressure (Figure 1.3), has facilitated the identification of transient episodes of ischemia with a high degree of confidence. The hemodynamic features of myocardial ischemia, symptomatic or silent, are essentially identical. They tend to validate the ECG alterations that accompany myocardial ischemia. Further validation of the approach stems from the observation that ischemic patterns noted on Holter recordings resemble those occurring during the treadmill stress test[10,11] in patients with known coronary artery disease (to be described). These observations have formed the basis for the increasing use of ECG monitoring as a noninvasive approach to the detection of silent myocardial ischemia in both hospitalized as well as ambulatory patients undertaking daily activities in their natural environment. However, ECG monitoring antedated the hemodynamic validation. This may have been the source of earlier concerns regarding the reliability of Holter recordings[12] to detect silent myocardial ischemia, because the lack of standardized criteria for ischemia can frequently lead to false-positive test results.

DEVELOPMENT OF SILENT MYOCARDIAL ISCHEMIA AS AN ELECTROCARDIOGRAPHIC ENTITY

Although as early as 1961 Holter[13] described the association of ST-segment deviation and angina in a patient undergoing continuous ECG monitoring, there was little confidence in the technique for monitoring ischemia in ambulatory patients. The major concerns were the poor low-frequency response of recording devices and the lack of reproducibility of ST-segment deviations.[14] Sporadic reports nonetheless indicated that ischemic ST-segment deviations could be detected by ambulatory ECG monitoring.[15,16] The use of Holter monitoring in detecting disorders of cardiac rhythm and myocardial ischemia gained momentum with increasing refinements in recorders and analysis systems over the next 10 years.[17] The earliest systematic observations to focus on the possibility of silent myocardial ischemia in ambulant subjects as a clinical entity in angina were those of Stern and Tzivoni[18,19] in 1974. They obtained Holter recordings in patients with coronary artery disease during the course of their daily activities. They found episodes of ST-segment deviation that were not associated with angina but which in every other way resembled those of angina. These

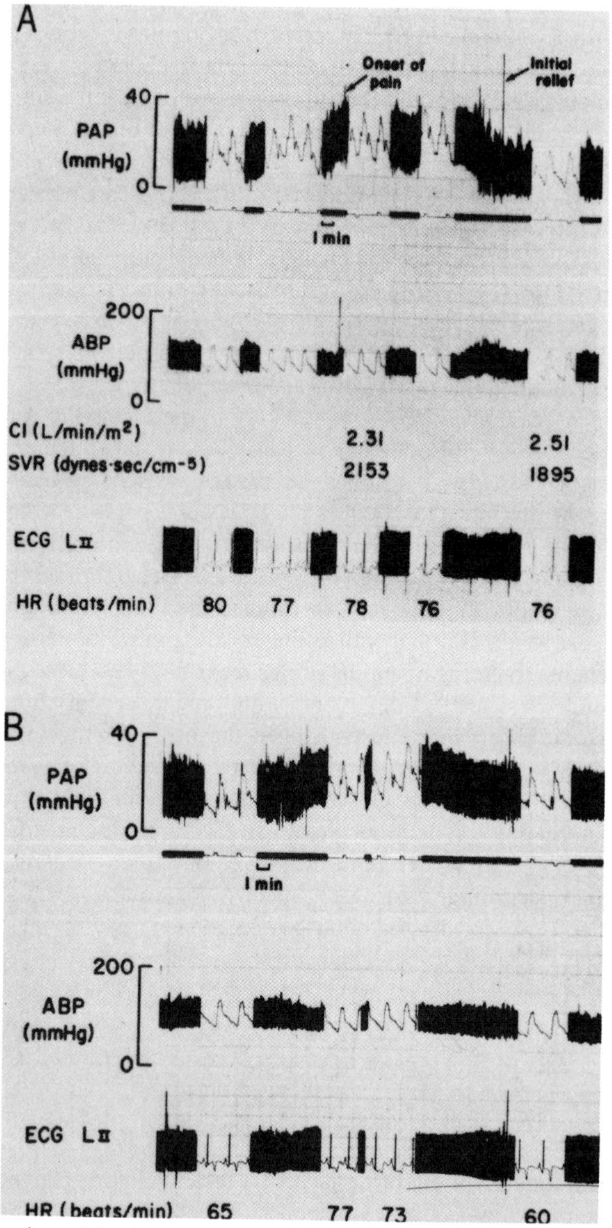

FIGURE 1.1. Comparison of the temporal sequence and of the magnitude and duration of changes in heart rate, arterial blood pressure (ABP), and pulmonary artery pressure (PAP) in a symptomatic (**A**) and an asymptomatic episode (**B**) of myocardial ischemia in the same patient with rest angina. Note the overall similarities between the two episodes, with a longer duration of changes in the symptomatic episode. (Based on data from Figueras et al.[8])

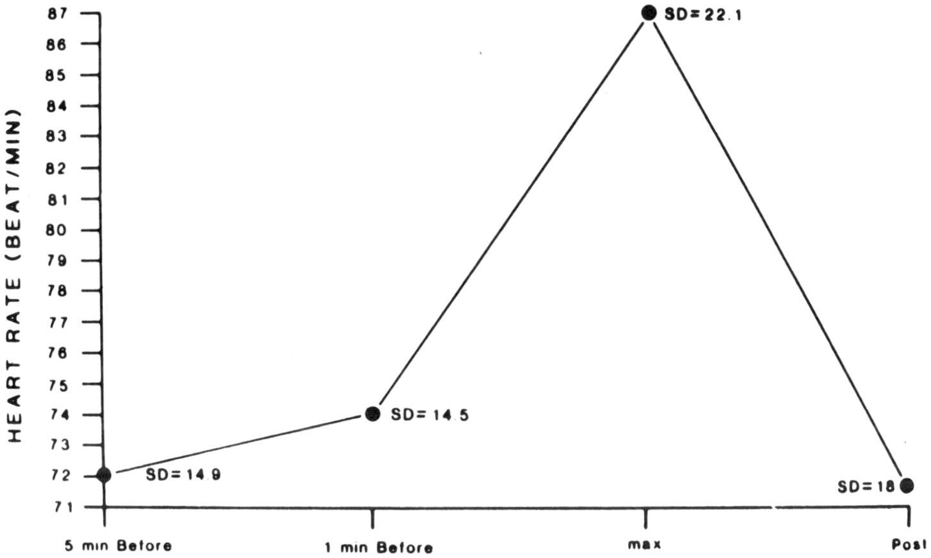

FIGURE 1.2. Temporal sequence of heart rate changes 5 and 1 minute preceding the onset of ischemia, during ischemia (maximum), and at the termination of the episode. The data represent mean and standard deviations (SD). In only 10 percent of the episodes were there significant increases in heart rate at the onset of ischemia when compared with the baseline value (5 minutes before the onset of ischemia). Note the crescendo-decrescendo pattern of heart rate changes during an episode of ischemia. (From Nademanee et al;[9] reproduced with the permission of the authors and the *American Journal of Cardiology*.)

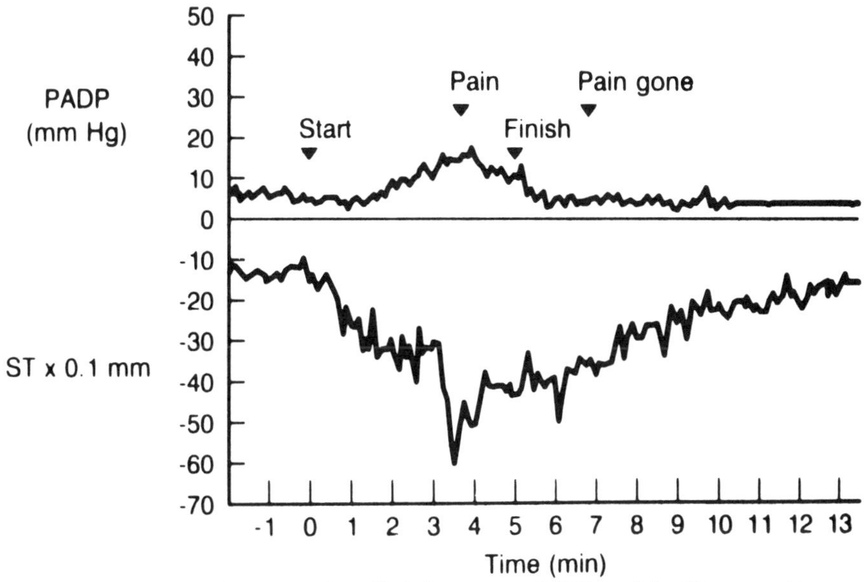

FIGURE 1.3. Changes in pulmonary artery diastolic pressure (PADP) and the ST segment in a patient with coronary artery disease who performed treadmill exercise (modified Bruce protocol) for 5 minutes. Note again the crescendo-decrescendo pattern of the temporal sequence of change in the parameters recorded during an episode of myocardial ischemia. (Reproduced with permission from Levy RD, Shapiro LM, Wright C, et al: Hemodynamic response to myocardial ischemia during unrestricted activity, exercise testing and atrial pacing assessed by ambulatory pulmonary artery pressure monitoring. *Br Heart J* 1986;56:1218.)

episodes did not occur in normal subjects. Attention to painless ST-segment deviations in patients with angina pectoris was also drawn by Allen et al[20] in 1976 and a year later by Schang and Pepine[21] who demonstrated that the episodes of silent myocardial ischemia in patients with effort angina not only were frequent, but also were reduced or eliminated by the administration of sublingual nitroglycerin. In the last 7 to 8 years interest in the detection and quantification of silent myocardial ischemia by Holter monitoring in various myocardial ischemic syndromes has burgeoned. Overall data indicate that if criteria are stringently predetermined especially in relation to changes in heart rate (Figure 1.4), the occurrence of painless as well as painful episodes of ischemia can be detected reasonably accurately by ambulatory ECG recordings.

There have been considerable refinements in the technique of Holter recording in general in the last 10 years.[22–26] Amplitude as well as frequency[23,25,27] modulated systems are now available. Analysis systems also vary from completely automated

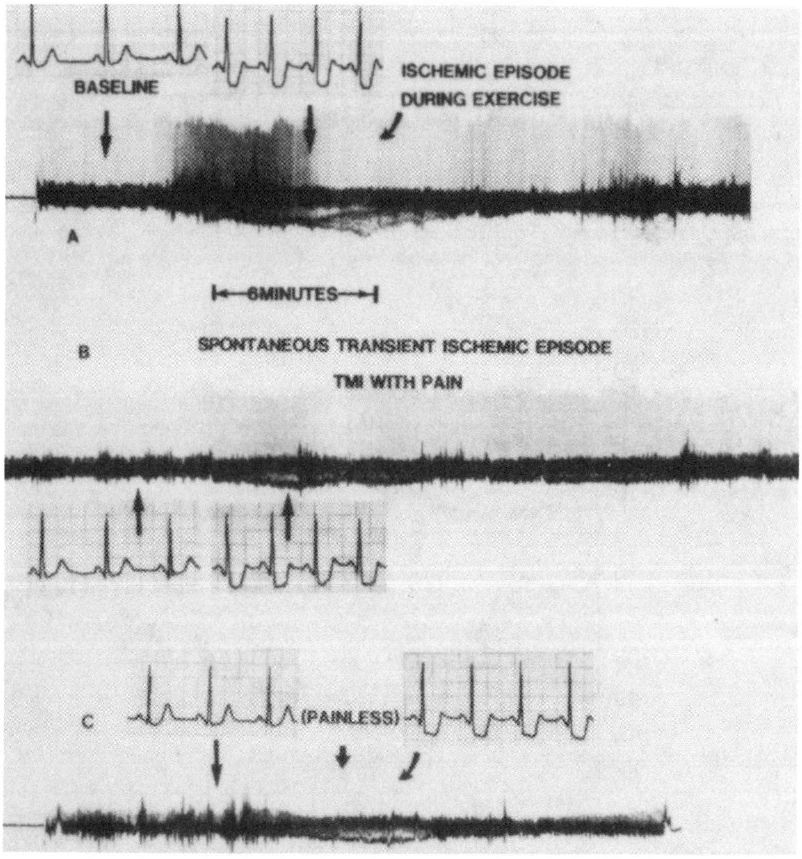

FIGURE 1.4. Examples of myocardial ischemic episodes from compact analog analysis of Holter recordings in chronic stable angina. TMI = transient myocardial ischemia. The *upper panel* shows changes in heart rate and the ST segment during treadmill exercise. The *middle panel* shows pain-associated episode of ischemia occurring spontaneously; it is similar to that on exercise, but the heart rate at peak ST-segment change is slower. The *lower panel* shows an episode of painless ischemia. All episodes demonstrate the crescendo-descrescendo pattern of ECG abnormality characteristic of myocardial ischemia. (Singh et al.,[10] 1985; reproduced with the permission of the authors and the *American Journal of Cardiology*.)

approaches to those with varying degrees of operator interactions. ST-segment deviations can also be recorded and analyzed by solid-state systems.[28] Except for the somewhat cumbersome complete disclosure methods using analog signals,[27,29] there are still problems in the accuracy and validation of the numerous systems available to detect ST-segment alterations in myocardial ischemic syndromes by ambulatory ECG recordings. Nevertheless, an extensive data base has developed on the detection, prevalence, and quantification of the frequency and duration of myocardial ischemia, symptomatic and asymptomatic, in chronic stable angina, unstable angina, and Prinzmetal's angina. Furthermore, much insight has been gained from studies about the nature of silent versus symptomatic episodes. This will be discussed at length in different parts of this monograph. Some features (Table 1.2) are germane here and will be discussed briefly.

Overall data[6,10,26,30–35] from studies in patients with rest angina, unstable angina, and chronic stable angina subjected to serial Holter recordings reveal a number of significant findings. First, they show that over two thirds of myocardial ischemic episodes in these subsets of patients with coronary artery disease are clinically silent. Second, over 80 to 90 percent of the episodes of ischemia were not preceded by significant increases in heart rate. The findings are in line with results of Berndt et al[36] who reported that the rate-pressure product was significantly lower at the onset of spontaneous ischemia than at anginal threshold during atrial pacing in patients with coronary artery disease with unstable angina. Deanfield et al[35] showed that the peak heart rate is lower in spontaneous episodes than in those induced by exercise in patients with chronic stable angina. Third, the distribution of ischemic episodes over a 24-hour period in chronic stable angina exhibits a distinct circadian rhythmicity, with few episodes between midnight and 6 AM and the largest number between 6 AM and midday.[37–39] Fourth, increasing data now suggest that the highest incidence of silent ischemia occurs in patients with the most symptomatic and anatomically severe coronary artery disease.

DETECTION OF SILENT MYOCARDIAL ISCHEMIA BY AN EXERCISE STRESS TEST

It has long been recognized that the presence of significant coronary artery disease can be established with a high degree of sensitivity and specificity by exercise stress testing in an asymptomatic population with a high prevalence of the disease.[40] In patients with electrocardiographically positive tests for ischemia, other objective indexes such as scintigraphic perfusion defects[41] and segmental wall motion abnormalities[42] are usually present. It is also known that during exercise in patients

Table 1.2. Characteristics of Silent Myocardial Ischemia Detected by Ambulatory ECG Recordings

1. Characteristic pattern of associated heart rate and blood pressure changes.
2. Marked variation in duration of individual episodes.
3. Considerable temporal variability.
4. Exhibition of circadian periodicity in chronic stable angina.
5. Rarely demonstrable in healthy subjects.
6. Most frequent occurrence in patients with known and severe coronary artery disease.
7. Amenable to reduction by pharmacologic as well as invasive treatment modalites.
8. Of possible prognostic significance at least in certain subsets of patients with coronary artery disease.
9. Prognostic significance probably similar to that of symptomatic ischemia.

with coronary artery disease, ischemic ST-segment changes may precede the onset of angina which, in many patients, may fail to develop even at peak levels of stress. For example, Amsterdam et al[43] in a study involving 92 patients with angiographically documented coronary artery disease (Figure 1.5) found greater than 1-mm ST-segment depression alone or in association with delayed angina in 39 patients (42%). Lindsey and Cohn[44] studied 122 patients with angiographically documented coronary artery disease with an exercise stress that found that in 44 no pain developed during the stress test. The data agree with the analysis of Rozanski and Berman[45] who found in a review of 13 studies that approximately 30% of transient ischemic ST-segment depressions during exercise testing occurred without angina in patients with documented coronary artery disease. The extent of coronary artery disease as evaluated angiographically was similar in the group with pain and in those without pain. The data emphasized that in patients with known coronary artery disease, symptomatic as well as silent myocardial ischemia is likely to have the same clinical significance.

In this context, data from the Coronary Artery Surgery Study (CASS) evaluating 2,982 patients are of particular interest. The 1,583 patients with coronary artery disease (≥70%) were analyzed on the basis of the presence of ischemic ST-segment depression (≥1 mm) and the occurrence of anginal symptoms.[46] The cumulative 7-year survival rates (Figure 1.6) in the three groups of patients (with chest pain only,

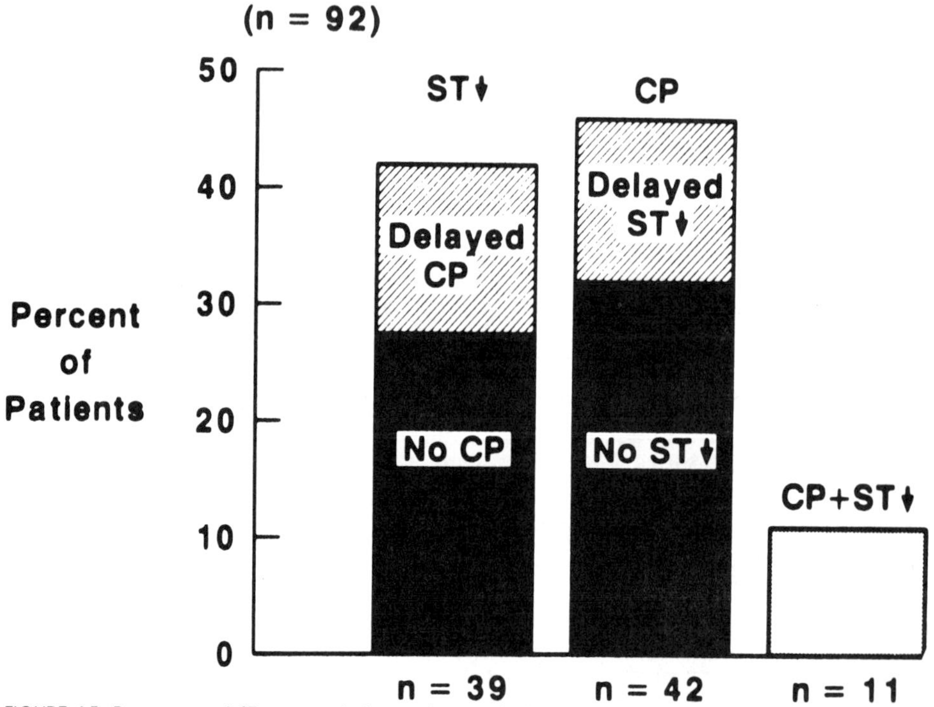

FIGURE 1.5. Response of ST-segment depression and chest pain to treadmill exercise in patients with angiographic demonstration of coronary artery disease. *Left,* ST indicates patients with ischemic ST-segment depression without angina (no CP) or with delayed (≥1 minute) angina (CP); *middle,* patients with angina (CP) and no ischemic ST-segment depression (no ST↓) or delayed (≥1 minute) ST-segment depression; *right,* patients with simultaneous angina (CP) and ischemic ST-segment depression (ST↓). (Reproduced with permission of Amsterdam et al[43] and the *American Journal of Cardiology.*)

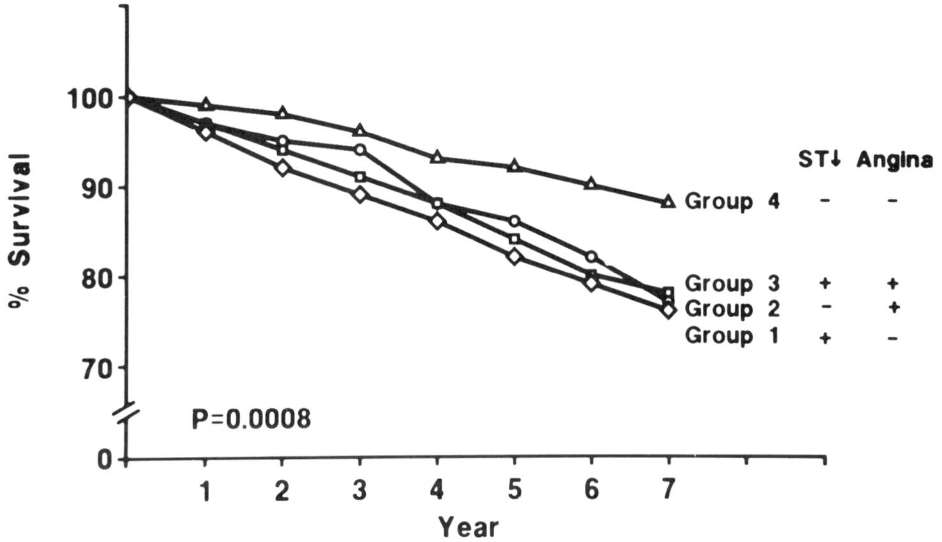

FIGURE 1.6. Seven-year cumulative survivial rates for 1,583 patients with coronary artery disease in the CASS registry. Survival rates were similar for patients with ischemic ST-segment depression, angina, or both and were significantly higher for patients who had neither. (Reproduced with permission of Weiner, Ryan, McCabe, et al[46] and the *American Journal of Cardiology*.)

ST-segment depression only, or both) were nearly identical (about 77%). In contrast, the figure was higher in patients without ischemic ST-segment depression or angina (88%). Among patients with silent ischemia during exercise stress testing, survival was related to the severity of coronary artery disease. The findings of the CASS study have been supported by those of Falcone et al[47] who compared the outcome of 209 patients with silent myocardial ischemia during exercise testing with that of 269 patients with both ischemic ST-segment depression and angina. The mortality rate at 5 years was similar among the two groups, emphasizing that patients with known coronary artery disease and myocardial ischemia (demonstrated by exercise stress testing) have the same prognosis, whether the myocardial ischemia is silent or symptomatic.

Numerous recent studies[11,48–50] have attempted to determine the relation between ischemia demonstrated by exercise treadmill testing and that documented on 24-hour Holter recordings. This overall issue is discussed elsewhere (see Chapter 12) in this volume. Emerging data suggest that Holter monitoring as a screen test to detect coronary artery disease has a lower sensitivity and lower predictive accuracy than does the exercise treadmill test. The occurrence and frequency of silent myocardial ischemia on Holter recordings in totally asymptomatic middle-aged or elderly men with or without risk factors of coronary artery disease are unknown; however, they are likely to be low.

That objective evidence of myocardial ischemia by stress testing combined with radionuclide techniques can also be obtained in completely asymptomatic persons with coronary artery disease is now increasingly recognized.[42] However, without angiographic confirmation and in the absence of pain, it may be difficult to be entirely certain whether positive ECG evidence of ischemia is always indicative of significant coronary artery disease. Nevertheless, early recognition of ischemia in these patients is important, because it might allow the identification of asymptomatic subjects with "silent" coronary artery disease whose initial presentation is either acute myocardial infarction or sudden cardiac death. Exercise testing in middle-aged men between 40 and 60 years suggests a 5 percent incidence of essentially silent coronary artery disease (see Chapter 7), an incidence that probably doubles after the age of 60 years. There is evidence that asymptomatic patients with unequivocally positive stress tests may not necessarily have multivessel coronary artery disease, but as a group they have an increased risk of developing the manifestations of ischemic heart disease in the future.[51,52] The important question is whether among such individuals it might be possible to identify, by Holter monitoring, those with silent myocardial ischemia who are particularly prone to a serious morbid coronary event. At present, there is little systematic and controlled data on this important clinical issue.

THERAPEUTIC IMPLICATIONS

A number of important findings have recently emerged from various investigations into the prevalence of silent myocardial ischemia in patients with symptomatic and asymptomatic coronary artery disease. Silent myocardial ischemia, detected by either exercise stress testing or ambulatory Holter recordings, is a common phenomenon in patients with known coronary artery disease. In symptomatic patients, silent ischemic episodes considerably outnumber the symptomatic ones. The occurrence of silent myocardial ischemia in such patients has raised some clinically important issues. It is clearly important to determine if this silent ischemia should be treated in the same way as symptomatic ischemia. Data on ischemia revealed by stress testing suggest that the prognosis of patients with silent and symptomatic ischemia is similar. Thus, treatment strategies should allow for the extent of ischemia rather than the associated symptoms. In silent ischemia documented on Holter recordings in patients with various ischemic syndromes the issue is less clear, in part because the prognostic significance of silent episodes of ischemia detected by ambulatory ECG monitoring is not entirely certain. However, as will be discussed elsewhere in this volume (see Chapter 13), silent episodes that persist after the symptomatic ones have been eliminated by medical therapy in unstable angina are associated with an adverse prognosis. Whether this finding also holds for all other ischemic syndromes is uncertain. Similarly, it is not known whether in unstable angina in which the prognostic significance of persistent silent ischemic episodes is established, controlled studies are lacking to resolve the hypothesis that a significant reduction or elimination of silent ischemia will be associated with reduced mortality and morbidity. Such studies will be needed to vindicate the role of ambulatory ECG monitoring in silent myocardial ischemia as an endpoint of therapy in ischemic heart disease.

The available data indicate that silent myocardial ischemia is a significant entity in patients with known coronary artery disease as well as in those who are completely asymptomatic. Its detection and prevalence and the identification of patients in whom it occurs are of great clinical significance. Aspects of this growing facet of ischemic heart disease are the focus of this monograph.

Acknowledgment: We are indebted to Lawrence Kimble for secretarial assistance and to Medical Media of the Wadsworth Veterans Administration Hospital for illustrations and photography. The original work reported herein was supported by the Medical Research Services of the Veterans Administration and the American Heart Association, the Greater Los Angeles Affiliate.

REFERENCES

1. Kennedy HL, Whitlock JA, Sprague, RS et al: Long-term follow-up of asymptomatic healthy subjects with frequent and complex ventricular ectopy. *N Engl J Med* 1985;312:193–197.
2. Ruberman W, Weinblatt E, Goldberg JD, Frank CW, Chaudhary BS, Shapiro S: Ventricular premature complexes and sudden death after myocardial infarction. *Circulation* 1981;64(2):297–305.
3. Hess ML, Barnhart GR, Crute S, Komwatana P, Krause S, Greenfield LJ: Mechanical and biochemical effects of transient myocardial ischemia. *J Surg Res* 1979;26:175–1984.
4. Heyndricks GR, Millard RW, McRitchie RJ, Maroko PR, Vatner SF: Regional myocardial functional artery occlusions in conscious dogs. *J Clin Invest* 1975;56:978–985.
5. Braasch W, Gudbjarnason S, Puri PS, Ravens KG, Bing RJ: Early changes in energy metabolism in the myocardium following acute coronary artery occlusion in anesthetized dogs. *Circ Res* 1968;23:429–438.
6. Nesto RW, Kowalchut GJ: The ischemic cascade: Temporal sequence of hemodynamic, electrocardiographic and symptomatic expressions of ischemia. *Am J Cardiol* 1987;57:23C–30C.
7. Maseri A. Pathogenetic mechanisms of angina pectoris: Expanding views. *Br Heart J* 1980;43:648–660.
8. Figueras J, Singh BN, Ganz W, Charuzi Y, Swan HJC: Mechanism of rest and nocturnal angina: Observations during continuous hemodynamic and electrocardiographic monitoring. *Circulation* 1979;59:955–966.
9. Nademanee K, Intarachot V, Josephson MA, Singh BN: Characteristics and clinical significance of silent myocardial ischemia in unstable angina. *Am J Cardiol* 1986;58:26B–33B.
10. Singh BN, Nademanee K, Figueras J, Josephson MA: Hemodynamic and electrocardiographic correlates of symptomatic and silent myocardial ischemia: Pathophysiologic and therapeutic implications. *Am J Cardiol* 1986;38:3B–10B.
11. Tzivoni D, Gavish A, Benhorin J, Keren A, Stern S: Myocardial ischemia during daily activities and stress. *Am J Cardiol* 1982;58:47B–5B.
12. Armstrong WF, Jordan JW, Morris SN, McHenry PL: Prevalence and magnitude of ST-segment and T-wave abnormalities in normal men during continuous ambulatory electrocardiography. *Am J Cardiol* 1982;49:1638–1642.
13. Holter N: New method for heart studies with continuous electrocardiography of active subjects. *Science* 1962;134:1214–1220.
14. Hinkle L, Meyer J, Stevens M, Carver ST: Tape recordings of the ECG of active man. *Circulation* 1987;36:752–757.
15. Norland CC, Semler HJ: Angina pectoris and arrhythmias documented by cardiac telemetry. *J Am Med Sci* 1964;190:115–120.
16. Corday E, Bazika V, Long TW, Papelbaum S, Gold H, Bernstein H: Detection of phantom arrhythmias and evanescent electrocardiographic abnormalities. *J Am Med Sci* 1965;133:417–421.
17. Stern S, Tzivoni D: The reliability of the Holter-Avionics system in reproducing the ST-T segment. *Am Heart J* 1972;84:427–432.
18. Stern S, Tzivoni D: Early detection of silent ischaemic heart disease by 24-hour electrocardiographic monitoring of active subjects. *Br Heart J* 1974;36:481–485.
19. Stern S, Tzivoni D: Early detection of silent ischemic heart disease by 24-hour electrocardiographic monitoring, as validated by coronary arteriography. *Circulation* 1975;52:1045–1050.
20. Allen RD, Gettes LS, Phalan C, Avington D: Painless ST-segment depression in patients with angina pectoris. *Chest* 1976;69:467–473.
21. Schang SJ, Pepine CJ: Transient asymptomatic ST segment depression during daily activity. *Am J Cardiol* 1977;39:297–302.
22. Morganroth J: Ambulatory Holter electrocardiography: Choice of technologies and clinical uses. *Ann Int Med* 1985;102:73–81.
23. Bala Subramanian V, Lahiri A, Green HL, Stott FD, Raftery EB: Ambulatory ST-seg-

ment monitoring: Problems, pitfalls, solutions and clinical applications. *Br Heart J* 1980;44:419–425.

24. Subramanian BV: Clinical and research application of ambulatory Holter ST-segment and heart rate monitoring. *Am J Cardiol* 1986;58:11B–20B.
25. Bragg-Remschel BD, Anderson CM, Winkle RA: Frequency-response characteristics of ambulatory ECG monitoring systems and their implications for ST-segment analysis. *Am Heart J* 1982;103:20–31.
26. Nademanee K, Singh BN, Guerrero J, Hendrickson JA, Intarachot V, Baky S: Accurate rapid compact analog method for the quantification of frequency and duration of myocardial ischemia by semi-automated analysis of 24 hour Holter ECG recordings. *Am Heart J* 1982;103:802–813.
27. Shook TL, Bolke W, Kotilainen PW, Hubelbank M, Selwyn AP, Stone PH: Comparison of amplitude-modulated and frequency-modulated ambulatory techniques for recording ischemic electrocardiographic changes. *Am J Cardiol* 1987;60:895–900.
28. Levin RI, Cohen D, Frisbie W, Selwyn AP, Barry J, Deanfield JE, Keeler B, Campbell DQ: Potential for realtime processing of the continuously monitored electrocardiogram in the detection, quantification and intervention of silent myocardial ischemia. *Cardiol Clin* 1986;4:735–744.
29. Biagini A, Antonelli R, Michelassi C, Corpeggiani C, Mazzei MG, Riva ALC, Chierchia S, L'Abbate A, Maseri A: Analisi di tracuati Holter in forma analogica compattata per il riconoscimento di episodi ischemia miocardica transitoria. *G Ital Cardiol* 1980;10:668–676.
30. Wolf E, Tzivoni D, Stern S: Comparison of exercise stress tests and 24-hour ambulatory electrocardiographic monitoring of ST-T changes. *Br Heart J* 1980;86:501–506.
31. Biagini A, Mazzei MG, Carpeggiani C, Testa R, Antonelli R, Michelassi C, L'Abbate A, Maseri A: Vasospastic ischemic mechanism of frequent asymptomatic transient ST-T changes during continuous electrocardiographic monitoring in selected unstable angina patients. *Am Heart J* 1980;103:13–19.
32. Chierchia S, Brunelli C, Simonetti I, Lazzari M, Maseri A: Sequence of events in angina at rest: Primary reduction in coronary flow. *Circulation* 1980;61:759–764.
33. Cocco G, Brown G. Strozzi C, Leishman B, Chu B, Rochat N: Asymptomatic myocardial ischaemia in patients with stable and typical angina pectoris. *Clin Cardiol* 1982;5:403–408.
34. Cecchi A, Dovellini EV, Morchi F, Pucci P, Santo-oro GM, Fazzini PF: Silent myocardial ischemia during ambulatory electrocardiographic monitoring in patients with effort angina. *J Am Coll Cardiol* 1983;1:934–939.
35. Deanfield JE, Museri A, Selwyn AP, Ribesito P, Chierchia S, Krikler S: Myocardial ischaemia during daily life in patients with stable angina: Its relation to symptoms and heart rate changes. *Lancet* 1983;2:753–758.
36. Berndt TB, Fitzgerald J, Harrison DC, Schroeder JS: Hemodynamic changes at the onset of spontaneous versus pacing-induced angina. *Am J Cardiol* 1977;39:784–790.
37. Nademenee K, Intarachot V, Josephson MA, Singh BN: Circadian variation in occurrence of transient overt and silent myocardial ischemia in chronic stable angina and comparison with Prinzmetal angina in men. *Am J Cardiol* 1987;60:494–498.
38. Rocco MB, Nabel EG, Selwyn AP: Circadian rhythms and coronary artery disease. *Am J Cardiol* 1987;59:13C–17C.
39. Rocco MB, Barry J, Campbell S, Nabel E, Cook EF, Goldman L, Selwyn AP: Circadian variation of transient myocardial ischemia in patients with coronary artery disease. *Circulation* 1987;75:395–400.
40. Ellestad MH, Allen W, Wan MCK, Kemp Gl: Maximal stress testing for cardiovascular evaluation. *Circulation* 1969;39:517–522.
41. Gibson RS, Beller GA, Keiser DL: Prevalence and clinical significance of painless ST-segment depression during early post infarction exercise testing. *Circulation* 1987;75:1136–1142.
42. Bonow RD, Kent KM, Rosing DR, Lau KKG, Lakatos E, Boner JS, Bacharach SL, Green MV, Epstein SE: Exercise induced ischemia in mildly symptomatic patients with coronary artery disease and preserved left ventricular function: Identification of subgroups at risk of death during medical therapy. *N Engl J Med* 1984;331:1339–1344.

43. Amsterdam EA, Martschinske R, Laslett LJ, Rutledge JC, Vera Z: Symptomatic and silent myocardial ischemia during exercise testing in coronary arterial disease. *Am J Cardiol* 1986;58:43B–46B.
44. Lindsey HE, Cohn PF: "Silent" myocardial ischemia during and after exercise testing in patients with coronary artery disease. *Am Heart J* 1978;95:441–445.
45. Rozanski A, Berman DS: Silent myocardial ischemia: Pathophysiology, frequency of occurrence and approaches toward detection. *Am Heart J* 1987;114:615–626.
46. Weiner DA, Ryan TJ, McCabe CH, et al: Significance of silent myocardial ischemia during exercise testing in coronary artery disease. *Am J Cardiol* 1987;59:725–729.
47. Falcone C, DeSevi S, Porna E, et al: Clinical significance of exercise-induced silent myocardial ischemia in patients with coronary artery disease. *J Am Coll Cardiol* 1987;9:295–299.
48. Campbell S, Barry J, Rocco MB, et al: Features of the exercise test that reflect ischemic heart disease activity out of hospital. *Circulation* 1986;74:72–80.
49. Nademanee K, Intrachot V, Piontek M, Mody Vaghaiwalla F, Josephson MA, Singh BN: Relationship of myocardial ischemia detected by compact Holter analog technique to that induced by ETT. *Circulation* 1984;70(Suppl II):451.
50. Mody FV, Nademanee K, Intarachot V, et al: Severity of silent myocardial ischemia on ambulatory ECG monitoring in patients with stable angina pectoris: Relation to prognostic determinants during exercise stress testing and coronary angiography. (in press to *J Am Coll Cardiol,* 1988.)
51. Epstein SE: Implications of probability analysis on the strategy used for the non-invasive detection of coronary artery disease. *Am J Cardiol* 1980;46:491–499.
52. Froelicher VF, Maron D: Exercise testing and ancillary techniques to screen for coronary heart disease. *Prog Cardiovasc Dis* 1981;14:261–275.

CHAPTER 2

Regulation of Myocardial Perfusion in Ischemic Heart Disease

Role of Dynamic Coronary Stenosis

B. Greg Brown, MD, PhD and Budge H. Smith, MD

Ambulatory ECG monitoring during daily activity in selected patients with known coronary disease and a positive exercise ST-segment response has shown that ischemic ST shifts are common.[1–5] These ECG ST shifts are symptomatic in only 20 to 30 percent of the episodes, and they usually occur between the hours of 5 AM and 12 PM and of 5 PM and 8 PM.[4] In patients with angina as well as asymptomatic episodes, pain is associated with a greater duration and magnitude of ST-segment depression.[5] Although ST-segment depression may occur in "normal" men[6] and therefore has been challenged as a reliable sign of ischemia, Deanfield et al[7] conclude that more than 30 seconds of ST-segment depression on frequency-modulated Holter tapes can be ascribed confidently to ischemia. Patients with painless ST-segment depression during exercise have associated radionuclide evidence of ischemic global and regional myocardial dysfunction.[8] Although a selection bias may exist, to date most patients with silent ST-segment shifts have significant atherosclerotic coronary narrowing. The prognosis and proper treatment of the silent ischemia syndrome probably relate to the severity of the underlying coronary artery disease (CAD) and left ventricular (LV) dysfunction, but it is currently the subject of active investigation.[9]

In this report, ischemia may be either *silent* or *symptomatic,* occurring in one of three common clinical settings. The first is *spontaneous,* without apparent exertional provocation. Mental effort falls into this category. The second category is *exertional,* as with painless ST-segment shift on exercise treadmill test (ETT), and the third is *unstable,* usually occurring on intensive care unit (ICU) admission for unstable angina. We will discuss briefly some of the existing data supporting proposed mechanisms for the silent ischemia syndrome.

CORONARY PERFUSION IN SPONTANEOUS ISCHEMIA

Clinical Observations

The traditional view that angina in CAD is due to increased regional O_2 demand during fixed obstruction to coronary flow has been revised in the last two decades. In patients admitted to the ICU with angina at rest,[10,11] hemodynamic and ECG monitoring demonstrate that 70 to 85 percent of spontaneous ST-segment shifts are asymptomatic. Left ventricular function abnormalities and increased extraction of O_2 from coronary sinus blood[10] during these episodes suggest that the ST-segment changes reflect true ischemia, albeit commonly "silent." In most cases (65%) ischemia is preceded by small increases in heart rate,[4] but seldom by more than 15 beats per minute and uncommonly by an increase in LV systolic pressure or LV dp/dt, all indices of myocardial oxygen demand. In a given patient, heart rate is significantly lower at the onset of silent ST-segment depression at rest than at the onset of asymptomatic exertional ECG changes.[4] It thus appears that slight increases in metabolic demand commonly precede spontaneous ischemia, but rarely of a magnitude that would explain ischemia; and episodes may occur under conditions of constant metabolic demand. Episodes of spontaneous ischemia[12] and those silent episodes provoked by mental effort[13] and cigarette smoking[14] are accompanied by transient abnormalities of regional thallium uptake.

The foregoing evidence suggests that spontaneous ischemia, both silent and with pain, is commonly mediated by a transient reduction in regional perfusion by vessels with significant atherosclerotic narrowing. In a given patient, episodes of silent ischemia and of angina appear to be qualitatively similar and presumably have a common mechanism.

Regulation of Subendocardial Perfusion in Coronary Artery Disease

Coronary flow is controlled at the arteriolar level in patients without CAD. About 90 percent of the vascular resistance normally resides at the level of the small vessels, which are capable of dilation to a fourfold flow increase. The energy (pressure) used to force flow across the arteriolar bed is, by definition, the product of flow (Q) and the vascular resistance (R_a), which is constantly adjusted in response to metabolic demands and sympathetic vasomotor tone. With coronary stenosis there is an additional flow resistor in series at the level of the epicardial vessel. Coronary *stenosis* pressure loss in millimeters of mercury, is approximated[15] as $4Q^2/A_{min}{}^2$, where Q is stenosis flow in milliliters per second, and A_{min} is the minimum lumen area at the site of stenosis, in square millimeters. Thus, the pressure remaining to perfuse the myocardium (P_{COR}) after blood is forced through the stenosis is, in simplified terms:

$$P_{COR} = \frac{P_{Ao}}{1 + 4Q/(A^2_{min} \cdot R_a)}$$

This approximate expression tells us that for a given aortic pressure (P_{Ao}), the myocardial perfusion pressure (P_{COR}, distal to the stenosis) is adversely affected by an increase in coronary flow and by a decrease in arteriolar resistance or a constriction in stenosis lumen area. For example, when the lumen area in a proximal LAD stenosis is 0.42 mm^2 (corresponding to 76% diameter stenosis of a 3.0-mm artery) and flow is maintained at a normal level of 1.1 ml/s[16] by a moderately dilated arteriolar resistance of 50 mm Hg/ml per second sec, one-third of the aortic pressure is dissipated in forcing blood through the stenosis and only 55 mm Hg remains to perfuse the subendocardium. Wyatt et al[17] showed that at this level of coronary pressure, subendocardial perfusion becomes inadequate and regional contractile function deteriorates. McMahon, et al[18] showed that isolated 78 percent lesions of the LAD in man cause subendocardial infarction. By contrast, a 72 percent stenosis, with a lumen area of 0.55 mm^2, will result in an *adequate* P_{COR} of 65 mm Hg. Thus, small changes in lumen area in a significant coronary lesion can cause profound effects on the adequacy of subendocardial perfusion, not only because of the increase in stenosis resistance, but also because of the compensatory arteriolar vasodilation necessary to maintain constant flow.

Transient Reduction in Stenosis Lumen Area

There are three transient mechanisms that operate to compromise stenosis lumen area, reducing subendocardial perfusion and thus provoking ischemia: (1) active coronary stenosis constriction; (2) intraluminal thrombus formation; and (3) passive partial collapse of the compliant stenosis due to reduced distending pressure.[19,20] These three mechanisms and their various dynamic combinations are prime suspects in the etiology of spontaneous ischemia in the clinical setting.

Morphologic Determinants of Stenosis Vasomotion:
The histologic section in Figure 2.1 is from a documented vasospastic arterial segment removed at surgery from a patient with Prinzmetal's angina.[21] The lumen is severely compromised by a large, typical atheroma. The arc of relatively normal arterial wall partially surrounding the residual lumen provides the anatomic basis for stenosis vasomotion. Neurohumoral and pharmacologic agents capable of inducing constriction or dilation of the normal coronary vascular smooth muscle will have a

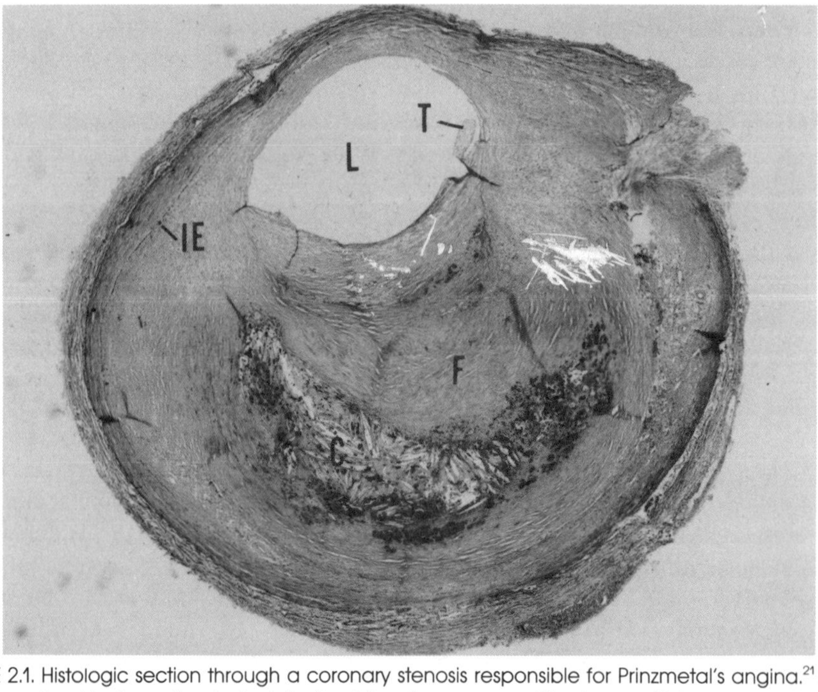

FIGURE 2.1. Histologic section through a coronary stenosis responsible for Prinzmetal's angina.[21] Segment was fixed in formalin at physiologic distending pressure. The lumen (L) is compromised by an eccentric atheroma, but is partially surrounded by an arc of nearly normal arterial wall. IE is the internal elastic membrane; T is a tag of intraluminal thrombus; F is fibrosis; and C is cholesterol crystals.

comparable effect on lesions with this morphology. Figure 2.2 demonstrates that three fourths of all significant lesions fall into this category. Thus, vasomotion is a common property of stenosis in man.[22]

Alpha-Adrenergic Coronary Constriction:
Sympathetic fibers innervate the epicardial coronary vessels;[23] exercise or isometric handgrip or mental concentration releases catecholamines into the circulation.[24] These observations provide the physiologic basis for alpha-mediated coronary constriction. Similarly, bicycle exercise has been found to constrict coronary lesions.[25] As illustrated in Figure 2.3, normal coronary arteries in man constrict during alpha-adrenergic stimulation (epinephrine plus propranolol, isometric handgrip) despite an increase in arterial pressure. By this reasoning, these agents would also be expected to constrict most coronary lesions, as in Figure 2.4. This right coronary arteriogram of a patient with both rest and exertional angina shows handgrip-induced constriction of the stenosis lumen. In 11 such patients, handgrip caused a 24 percent increase in systemic blood pressure, a 9 percent increase in heart rate, and an ischemic increase in pulmonary capillary wedge pressure (PCW) from 13 to 24 mm Hg. Although 8 of these 11 had an ischemic rise in PCW, only 3 had handgrip-induced angina. Infusion of a tiny amount (12.5 μg/min) of nitroglycerin directly into the diseased left coronary artery during a repeat handgrip resulted in net stenosis dilation without alteration of the expected systemic blood pressure and heart rate responses. Yet the PCW actually fell from 13 to 10 mm Hg during this second handgrip with nitroglycerin.[26] This clinical experiment separates the direct stenosis effects of sympathetic activation from the systemic hemodynamic effects. Stenosis constriction appears to be the principal determinant of ischemia.

The similarity of hemodynamic response to sympathetic activation and the changes

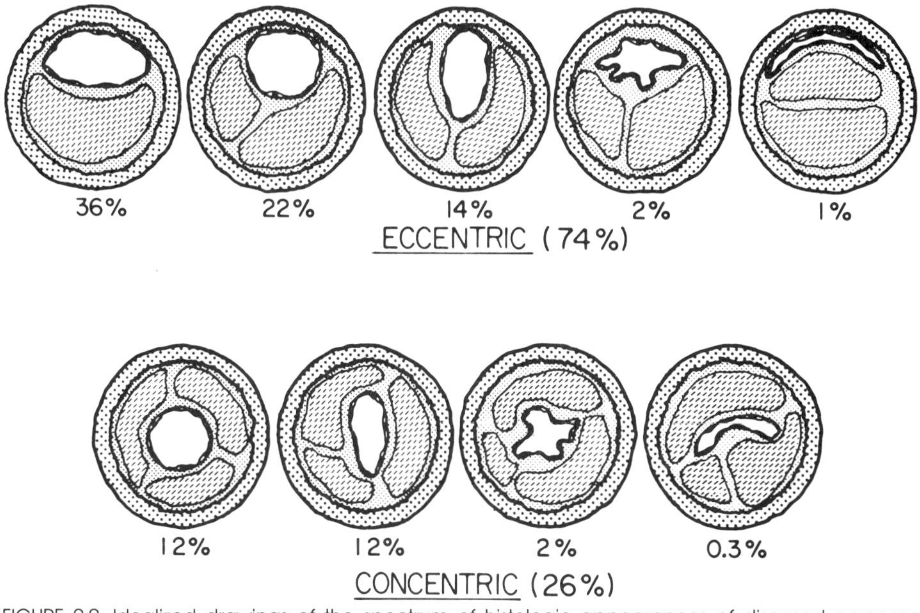

FIGURE 2.2. Idealized drawings of the spectrum of histologic appearances of diseased coronary arteries. Approximately three fourths of all significantly obstructed vessels demonstrated the potential for active vasomotion because at least 16 percent of the residual lumen is normal wall. (Adapted with permission from Freudenberg H, Lichtlen PR: *Z Kardiol* 1981;70:863.)

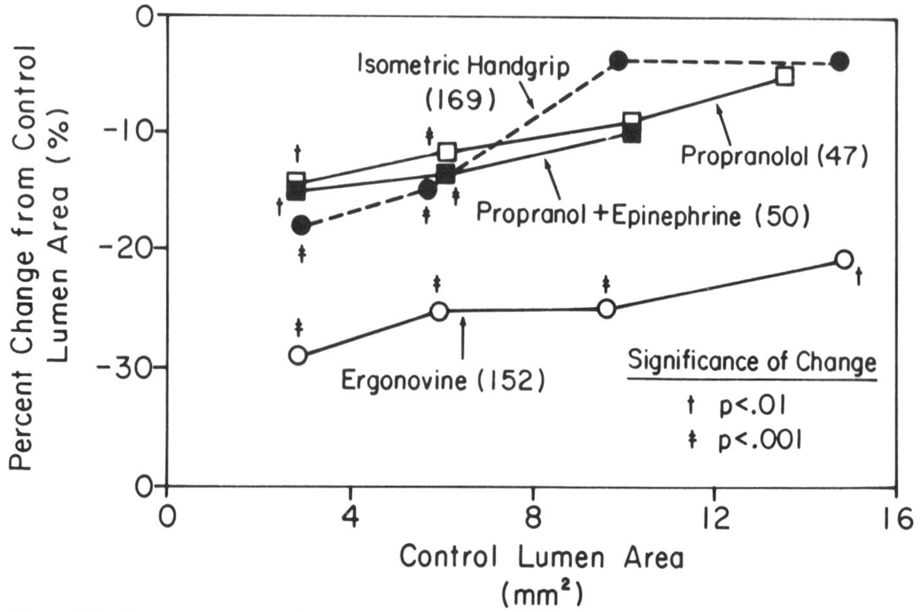

FIGURE 2.3. Mean constriction of normal coronary lumen area in response to sympathetically mediated vasoactive stimuli, and to the serotonergic receptor agonist ergonovine maleate. Numbers in parentheses indicate number of coronary segments measured.

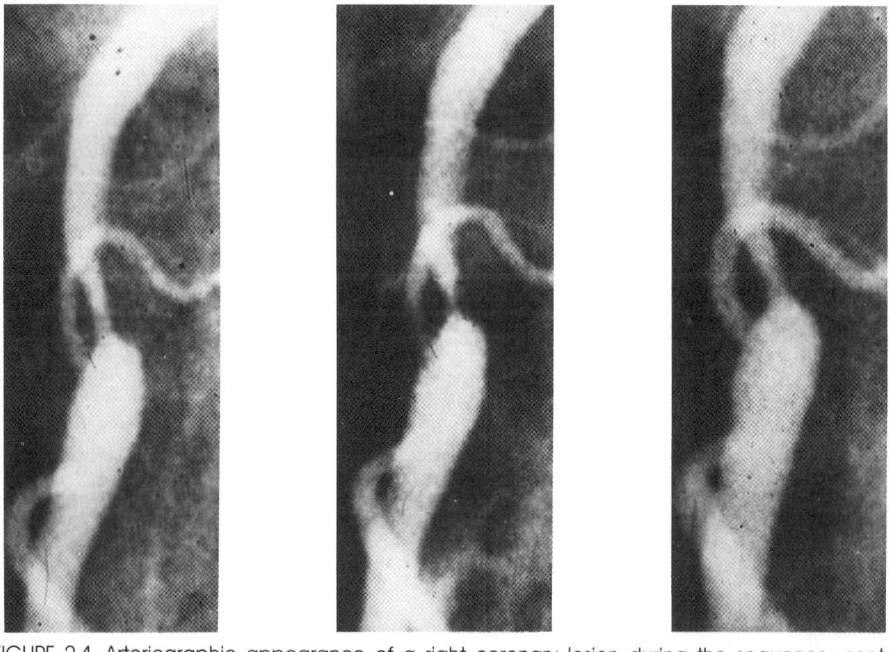

FIGURE 2.4. Arteriographic appearance of a right coronary lesion during the sequence: control (*left*), isometric handgrip (*center*), then isometric handgrip with simultaneous infusion of 50 μg of nitroglycerin (*right*) into the right coronary artery over 4 minutes. Both the normal and the diseased portions of these arteries constrict with handgrip and dilate with handgrip plus nitroglycerin.

observed during spontaneous ischemia further implicate sympathetically mediated constriction of coronary lesions as a cause of the silent ischemia syndrome. Although the dramatic coronary constriction associated with classical "spasm" is probably not mediated by the more modest alpha-adrenergic constriction,[26,27] the variation in angina threshold during emotional stress, exposure to cold,[28] and the cold pressor test[29] is almost certainly linked to this mechanism.

Stenosis Hyperactivity in Spontaneous Angina:

Clinically, angina is of three general sorts: (1) spontaneous episodes of pain, but with a normal exercise response; (2) mixed angina, with both spontaneous and effort-induced pain; and (3) effort-only angina. Isometric handgrip for 4 to 5 minutes at 25 percent of maximum grip was performed at catheterization in 34 patients, none of whom had variant angina. Seven had rest angina only, with ECG changes of subendocardial ischemia; 16 had mixed angina; and 11 had exertional pain only with abnormal results on the exercise stress test. All lesions were measured from a control arteriogram and again from an arteriogram taken at the end of the sustained handgrip. As before, handgrip provoked a significant constriction in normal and diseased epicardial coronary segments despite an increase in blood pressure. Lumen caliber response to handgrip was measured in all mild (<50%) and significant (≥50%) lesions in these 34 patients. The data are presented in Figure 2.5. There was no difference among the three clinical angina categories in the response of normal segments or mild lesions to the handgrip stress (approximately 35% increase in estimated stenosis flow resistance). However, as Figure 2.5 shows, significant lesions were quite vaso-

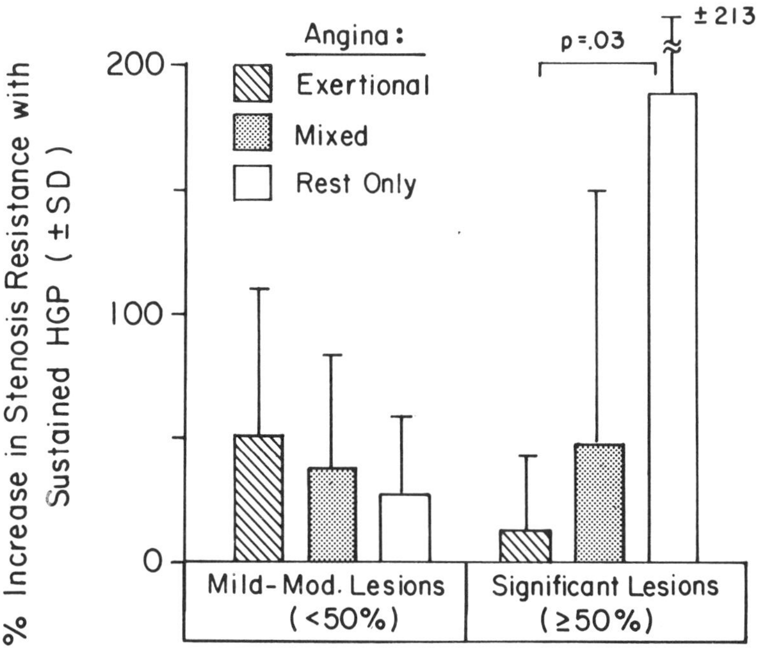

FIGURE 2.5. Predicted change in flow resistance in mild (<50% diameter reduction) and significant (>50%) coronary lesions. Although the response of mild lesions to handgrip did not distinguish among the three clinical angina types (rest, exertional, and mixed), significant lesions were significantly more vasoactive among patients with rest-only angina than among those with exertional-only angina (p <0.03).

active in patients with only rest angina (188% resistance increase) and were relatively fixed in those with only exertional angina (14% increase).[21] Thus, patients with rest angina are likely to have at least one significant lesion with a marked vasoconstrictor response to handgrip. Furthermore, the tendency to rest angina is associated with focal hyperreactivity of an identifiable lesion, but not of the entire epicardial arterial tree.

Acetylcholine-Mediated Coronary Constriction:

Experimentally, acetylcholine (ACh) dilates arteries by releasing a vasorelaxant substance (EDRF) from endothelial cells. In the absence of endothelial cells, ACh constricts arteries.[30] There is clinical evidence that ACh can cause profound coronary constriction in patients with atherosclerosis.[31] Our experience with direct intracoronary infusion of small amounts of ACh is also consistent with this finding. As illustrated in Figures 2.6 and 2.7, ACh was a moderate arterial constrictor in a 54-year-old patient with atypical chest pain and apparently normal arteries, and a dramatic constrictor in the diffusely diseased marginal branch of the post-coronary artery

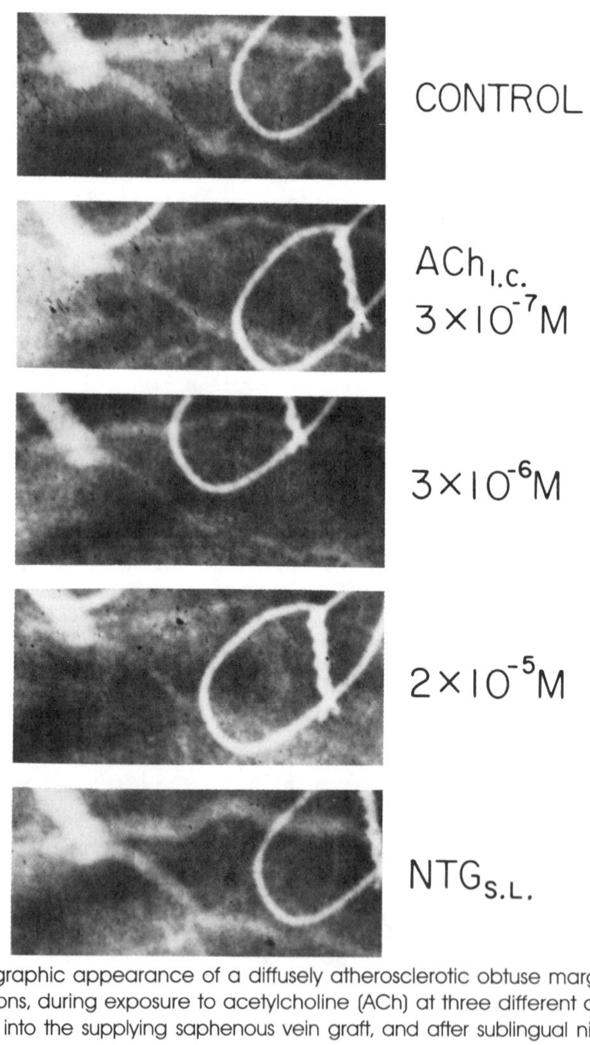

FIGURE 2.6. Arteriographic appearance of a diffusely atherosclerotic obtuse marginal branch during control conditions, during exposure to acetylcholine (ACh) at three different concentrations by continuous infusion into the supplying saphenous vein graft, and after sublingual nitroglycerin (NTG).

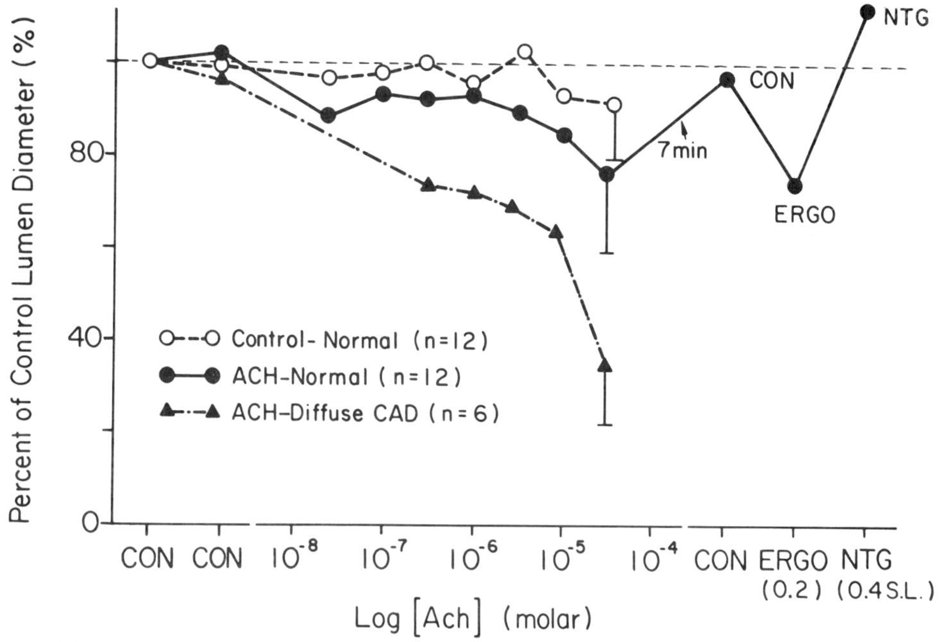

FIGURE 2.7. Effect on lumen diameter of exposure to different concentrations of acetylcholine (ACh) at six points in the obtuse marginal branch of a patient with severe coronary atherosclerosis (see Figure 2.6), at 12 points in the normal-appearing left anterior descending artery of a patient with noncardiac atypical angina, and at 12 points in a nonexposed normal left circumflex artery in the same patient.

bypass graft patient in Figure 2.6. Figure 2.7 demonstrates dose-dependent constriction of the coronary arteries in both patients. Parasympathetic trigger mechanisms have been implicated in coronary spasm, because methylcholine has been shown to provoke it and atropine to block it.[32,33]

Serotonergic Coronary Constriction:
Ergonovine maleate is the most potent clinically used constrictor of the epicardial arteries.[34] Although ergonovine has alpha-adrenergic activity, its vasoconstrictor response appears to be mediated principally by the serotonergic receptor.[35,36] Although ergonovine is not a naturally occurring substance, its analog, serotonin, is released from platelets at sites of atherosclerosis. However, roles for the serotonergic receptor[37] and for platelet vasoactive substances (serotonin and thromboxane A_2)[38] in clinical coronary vasomotion have yet to be demonstrated.

Thrombus Formation in Transient Coronary Obstruction:
An increasingly popular hypothesis holds that the dynamic interplay between formation and dispersion (or embolization) of thrombus in arterial stenosis accounts for the lability of subendocardial perfusion in unstable angina. Forrester et al,[39] using the angioscope, report that intraluminal thrombus, adherent to the plaque, is a consistent finding in unstable angina. The presence of thrombin, and its growth, in a patient with recurrent unstable angina is illustrated angiographically in Figure 2.8.[40] Lewis et al[41] report a 51 percent reduction in myocardial infarction and death in patients with unstable angina treated with a daily aspirin tablet. However, because the frequency of attacks of unstable angina was not reduced by aspirin in this study,

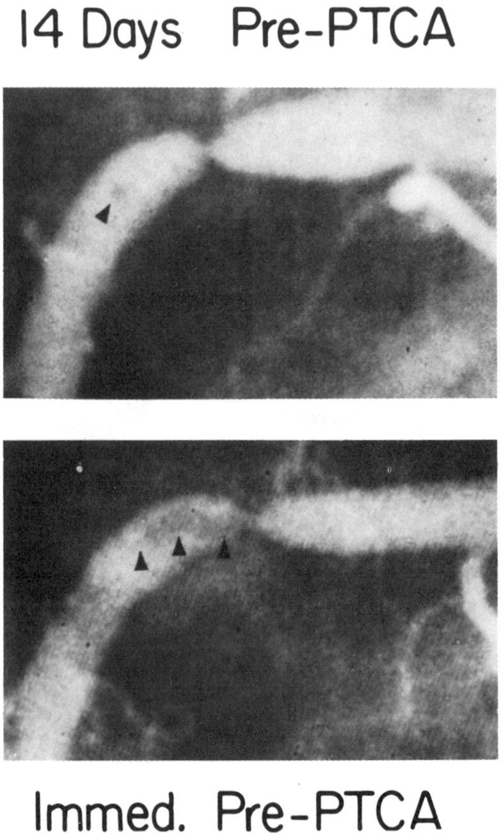

FIGURE 2.8. Arteriographic appearance of a right coronary lesion in a patient initially treated medically for unstable angina (severe episodes of spontaneous rest pain) and then treated with angioplasty (PTCA) for recurrent unstable angina 14 days later. A small intraluminal radiolucent thrombus (*arrow*) seen on the initial arteriogram (*top*, 14 days before PTCA) which has grown on the second (*arrows*) (*bottom*, immediately before PTCA).

it may be argued that the mechanism underlying transient, reversible ischemia in this syndrome is unaltered by a drug that suppresses platelet aggregation, thrombus growth, the release of platelet vasoactive substances, and vascular prostacyclin production.

SUMMARY

Episodes of silent myocardial ischemia virtually always occur in significant coronary atherosclerosis. They appear to be qualitatively similar, but somewhat less severe, in physiologic mechanisms and hemodynamic effects, to their symptomatic counterparts. Episodes of spontaneous ischemia are commonly associated with a small increase in heart rate, but seldom a major increase in O_2 demand. Instead, the precipitating mechanism is a transient reduction in regional perfusion, apparently due to a transient reduction in coronary lumen area at a site of significant atherosclerotic narrowing. Such lumen constriction occurs in certain morphologic, thrombogenic, and neurohumoral settings. Histologically, about three fourths of all significant coronary lesions are eccentric, so that the stenosis lumen is partly circumscribed by an arc of normal mural smooth muscle, which can respond normally to vasoconstrictor (or vasodilator) stimuli. Coronary smooth muscle can be constricted by a variety of agents, including alpha-adrenergic and serotonergic receptor agonists, histamine,[42] acetylcholine, and certain agents released from adherent intraluminal thrombus. Furthermore, growth of thrombus in the lesion may worsen flow obstruction. We believe that all of these mechanisms operate in the clinical spectrum of silent ischemia, as they do in that of angina.

Acknowledgment: This work was supported in part by USPHS grants HL 13517 and HL 19451, and by Established Investigator Award 79–116 from the American Heart Association (Dr. Brown).

REFERENCES

1. Stern S, Tzivoni D: Early detection of silent ischemic heart disease by 24-hour electrocardiographic monitoring of active subjects. *Br Heart J* 1974;36:481–486.
2. Schang SJ, Pepine CJ: Transient asymptomatic ST depression during daily activity. *Am J Cardiol* 1977;39:396–402.
3. Selwyn AP, Fox KM, Eves M, Oakley D, Dergie H, Shillingford J: Myocardial ischemia in patients with frequent angina pectoris. *Br Med J* 1978;2:1594–1596.
4. Campbell S, Barry J, Rebecca GS, Rocco MB, Nabel EG, Wayne RR, Selwyn AP: Active transient myocardial ischemia during daily life in asymptomatic patients with positive exercise tests and coronary artery disease. *Am J Cardiol* 1986;57:1010–1016.
5. Cecci AC, Dovellini EV, Marchi F, Pucci P, Santoro G, Fazzini F: Silent myocardial ischemia during ambulatory electrocardiographic monitoring in patients with effort angina. *J Am Coll Cardiol* 1983;1:934–939.
6. Armstrong WF, Jorden JW, Morris SN, McHenry PL: Prevalence and magnitude of ST-segment and T-wave abnormalities in normal men during continuous ambulatory electrocardiography. *Am J Cardiol* 1982;49:1638–1642.
7. Deanfield JE, Shea M, Ribiero P, de Landsheere CM, Wilson RA, Horlock P, Selwyn AP: Transient ST-segment depression as a marker of myocardial ischemia during daily life. *Am J Cardiol* 1984;54:1195–1200.
8. Cohn PF, Brown ES, Wynne J, Holman BL, Atkins HL: Global and regional left ventricular ejection fraction abnormalities during exercise in patients with silent myocardial ischemia. *J Am Coll Cardiol* 1983;1:931–933.
9. Cohn PF: Prognosis and treatment of asymptomatic coronary artery disease. *J Am Coll Cardiol* 1983;1:959–964.
10. Chierchia S, Lazzori M. Freedman B, Brunelli C, Maseri A: Impairment of myocardial perfusion and function during painless myocardial ischemia. *J Am Coll Cardiol* 1983;1:924–930.
11. Figueras J, Singh BN, Ganz W: Mechanisms of rest and nocturnal angina: Observations during continuous hemodynamic and electrocardiographic monitoring. *Circulation* 1979;59:955–968.
12. Robertson D, Robertson RM, Nies A, Oates JA, Friesinger GC: Variant angina pectoris: Investigation of indexes of sympathetic nervous system function. *Am J Cardiol* 1979;43:1080–1085.
13. Deanfield JE, Shea M, Kensett M, Horlock P, Wilson RA, de Landsheere CM, Selwyn AP: Silent myocardial ischemia due to mental stress. *Lancet* 1984;1:1001–1005.
14. Deanfield JE, Shea MJ, Wilson RA, Horlock P, de Landsheere CM, Selwyn AP: Direct effects of smoking on the heart: Silent ischemic disturbances of coronary flow. *Am J Cardiol* 1986;57:1005–1009.
15. Brown BG, Bolson EL, Dodge HT: Dynamic mechanisms in human coronary stenosis. *Circulation* 1984;70:917–922.
16. Ganz W, Tamura K, Marcus HS, Donoso R, Yoshida S, Swan HJC: Measurement of coronary sinus blood flow by continuous thermodilution in man. *Circulation* 1971;54:181.
17. Wyatt HC, Forrester JS, Tyberg JV, Goldner S, Logan SE, Parmley WW, Swan HJC: Effect of graded reduction in regional coronary perfusion on regional and total cardiac function. *Am J Cardiol* 1975;36:185.
18. McMahon MM, Brown BG, Cukingnan R, Rolett EL, Bolson E, Frimer M, Dodge HT:

Quantitative coronary arteriography: Measurement of the "critical" stenosis in patients with unstable angina and single-vessel disease without collaterals. *Circulation* 1979;60:106.
19. Schwartz JS, Carlyle PF, Cohn JN: Effect of dilation of the distal coronary bed on flow and resistance in severely stenotic coronary arteries in the dog. *Am J Cardiol* 1979;43:219.
20. Santamore WP, Walinsky P: Altered coronary flow responses to vasoactive drugs in the presence of coronary artery stenosis in the dog. *Am J Cardiol* 1980;45:276.
21. Brown BG: Coronary vasospasm: Observations linking the clinical spectrum of ischemic heart disease to the dynamic pathology of coronary atherosclerosis. *Arch Int Med* 1981;141:716–722.
22. Brown BG, Bolson EL, Peterson RB, Pierce CD, Dodge HT: The mechanisms of nitroglycerin action: Stenosis vasodilation as a major component of the drug response. *Circulation* 1981;64:1089–1097.
23. Denn MJ, Stone HL: Autonomic innervation of dog coronary arteries. *J Appl Physiol* 1976;41:30.
24. Stratton JR, Ritchie JL, Halter JB, Hamilton GW: Comparative catecholamine and hemodynamic responses to handgrip, cold pressor, and bicycle exercise testing in normal subjects. *J Am Coll Cardiol* 1983;2:93.
25. Gage JE, Hess OM, Murakami T, Ritter M, Grimm J, Krayenbuehl HP: Vasoconstriction of stenotic coronary arteries during dynamic exercise in patients with classic angina pectoris: Reversibility by nitroglycerin. *Circulation* 1986;73:865–876.
26. Brown BG, Lee AB, Bolson EL, Dodge HT: Reflex constriction of significant coronary stenosis as a mechanism contributing to ischemic left ventricular dysfunction during isometric exercise. *Circulation* 1984;70:18–24.
27. Chierchia S, Davies G, Berkenboom G, Crea F, Crean P, Maseri A: Alpha-adrenergic receptors and coronary spasm; an elusive link. *Circulation* 1984;69:8–14.
28. Epstein SE, Stamfer M, Beiser GD, et al: Effects of a reduction in environmental temperature on the circulatory response to exercise in men. *N Engl J Med* 1969;280:7–11.
29. Mudge GH Jr, Grossman W, Mills RM Jr, et al: Reflex increase in coronary vascular resistance in patients with ischemic heart disease. *N Engl J Med* 1976;295:1333–1337.
30. Furchgott RF: Role of endothelium in responses of vascular smooth muscle. *Circ Res* 1983;53:557–573.
31. Ludmer PL, Selwyn AP, Shook TL, Wayne RR, Mudge GH, Alexander RW, Ganz P: Paradoxical vasoconstriction induced by acetylcholine in atherosclerotic coronary arteries. *N Engl J Med* 1986;315:1046–1051.
32. Endo M, Hirosawa K, Kaneko N, Hase K, Inoue Y, Konno S: Prinzmetal's variant angina: Coronary arteriogram and left ventriculogram during angina attack induced by methacholine. *N Engl J Med* 1976;294:252–255.
33. Yasue H, Touyama M, Shimamoto M, Kato H, Tanaka S, Akiyama F: Role of autonomic nervous system in the pathogenesis of Prinzmetal's variant form of angina. *Circulation* 1974;50:534–539.
34. Henzaler FA, Proudfit SL, Razavi M, et al: Ergonovine maleate provocative test for coronary arterial spasm. *Am J Cardiol* 1978;41:631–640.
35. Holtz J, Held W, Sommer O, Kühne G, Bassenge E: Ergonovine-induced constrictions of epicardial arteries in conscious dogs: α-adenoceptors are not involved. *Basic Res Cardiol* 1982;77:278.
36. Brazenon RM, Angus JA: Ergometrine contracts isolated canine coronary arteries by a serotonergic mechanisms: No role for alpha adrenoceptors. *J Pharmacol Exp Ther* 1981;218:530.
37. Freidman SB, Chierchia S. Rodriguez-Plaza L, Bugiardini R, Smith G, Maseri A: Ergonovine-induced myocardial ischemia: No role for serotonergic receptors? *Circulation* 1984;70:178–183.
38. Chierchia S, de Caterina R, Crew F, Patrono C, Maseri A: Failure of thromboxane A_2 blockade to prevent attacks of vasospastic angina. *Circulation* 1982;66:702.
39. Forrester JS, Litvack F, Grundfest W, Hickey A: A perspective of coronary disease seen through the arteries of living man. *Circulation* 1987;75:505–513.
40. Brown BG, Bolson EL, Dodge HT: Percutaneous transluminal coronary angioplasty and subsequent restenosis: Quantitative and qualitative methodology for their assessment. *Am J Cardiol* 1987;60:348–388.

41. Lewis DH, Davis JW, Archibald DG, et al: Protective effects of aspirin against acute myocardial infarction and death in men with unstable angina. *N Engl J Med* 1983;309:396.
42. Ginsberg R, Bristow MR, Kantrowitz N, Bain DS, Harrison DC: Histamine provocation of clinical coronary artery spasm: Implications concerning pathogenesis of variant angina pectoris. *Am Heart J* 1981;102:819.

CHAPTER 3

Pathogenesis of Myocardial Ischemia

Current Concepts

Attilio Maseri, MD, Graham Davies, MD, and David Hackett, MB

Acute myocardial ischemia is a syndrome that can be caused by a variety of pathogenetic mechanisms resulting from different etiologic factors, mostly related to alterations in epicardial coronary vessels but occasionally in resistive coronary vessels.[1,2] The latter aspect is less well known and will not be discussed in this presentation.

At a first approximation, coronary atherosclerosis appears to be the most common denominator in ischemic syndromes. This discovery has led to rapid and progressive improvement in diagnostic and therapeutic procedures over the last 20 years.[3] This remarkable rate of progress is bound to reach a plateau unless we begin to focus on the differences rather than the similarities between ischemic mechanisms. It may therefore be useful to examine more closely the relation between atherosclerotic plaque and ischemic syndromes.

Although chronic obstruction to blood flow at the level of the epicardial coronary arteries is by far the most common cause of myocardial ischemia that occurs during effort, the mechanisms by which it causes ischemia appear to be multiple and complex.[4–6] Atherosclerotic plaques are usually traceable to a variable chronic background from which a variety of acute stimuli precipitate the onset of myocardial ischemia.

In turn, obstructive plaques may be the result of lipid deposition or thrombus organization in variable combinations, or both. They may be composed of lipids, fibrous tissue, or both, and they may narrow the lumen concentrically or only one segment of the wall. The resulting stenosis may be fixed or pliable and may be subject to the influence of distending intravascular pressure and smooth muscle tone. Evidence is accumulating to suggest that the nature of the stimuli that can cause myocardial ischemia depends on both the severity and the features of atherosclerotic plaques, particularly on their "stability" or "instability."

SEVERITY OF OBSTRUCTION CREATED BY PLAQUES AND SUBSEQUENT IMPAIRMENT OF FLOW

Theoretic calculations based on fluid mechanic equations indicate that the relation between transstenotic resistance and the degree of stenosis is highly nonlinear. Resistance begins to increase appreciably only when stenoses exceed the internal diameter reduction by 50 percent, but then it rises steeply. For example, resistance almost triples as the stenosis increases from 80 to 90 percent. The resistance to flow is mainly determined by the minimal residual artery lumen relative to control conditions and to a smaller extent by the length of the stenosis or the presence of another stenosis of similar severity in series. Resistance also increases as flow increases for the same degree of coronary stenosis because of turbulence, especially in the presence of irregularities in the lumen. This implies that the transstenotic pressure gradient increases dramatically with the severity of the stenosis and the increase in flow.[7]

These theoretic considerations are an oversimplication of the actual effects of the stenosis, as in vivo flow is pulsatile and the caliber of a stenosis may change in systole and diastole. Epicardial arteries have a considerable systolic capacitance that will be modified distal to the stenosis as a result of decreased distending pressure and pulsatility. However, many animal experiments confirm that a great reduction in vessel lumen is needed to reduce resting coronary flow, even when the inaccuracy of estimating the degree of stenosis is taken into account. Only reductions in internal diameter of 50 to 70 percent begin to impair peak reactive hyperemia and only reductions of 75 to 85 percent reduce resting flow.[7] Animal experiments suggest that collateral flow becomes established as soon as a transstenotic pressure gradient develops; however, collateral development subsequent to the establishment of the pressure gradient is variable for reasons not yet clear. Thus, only stenoses of 50 to 70 percent not subject to transient changes in the lumen as a result of a local increase in vasomotor tone or to intraluminal plugging by platelets or thrombosis and not compensated for by collaterals, are likely responsible for effort angina.

GEOMETRIC RELATION BETWEEN PLAQUE AND CORONARY LUMEN

Plaques may involve either the whole circumference of the vessel wall, with the residual lumen being placed centrally (concentric stenosis), or only one segment of the vessel wall, with the residual lumen displaced to one side of the midline (eccentric stenosis). Eccentric stenoses are more likely to vary in degree with vasomotor tone. The degree of alteration in cross-sectional area that can be achieved will depend on the amount of smooth muscle contraction and the compliance of the vessel wall. Calculations based on a 10 percent shortening, thought to be within the normal range of physiologic variations in vasomotor tone, show that for a plaque occupying 75 percent of the lumen (approximately 50% reduction in diameter), flow could be significantly impaired.[8] Spasm of smooth muscle, as seen in variant angina, could result in a much greater degree of shortening and alter flow through segments with much lesser degrees of fixed stenosis. The possibility of variations in caliber caused by changes in vasomotor tone is less likely for concentric plaques because of both the "splinting" effect of the thick intima and the loss of media.[9,10] Although some individuals have no eccentric high-grade stenoses, others have only eccentric lesions.

Eccentric lesions are more common at lower grades of stenosis. In a postmortem study 75 percent of stenoses were eccentric.[11] Finally, the lumen of the stenotic segment may be regularly tapering and smooth or irregular with anfractuosities that favor turbulence and platelet deposition.

COMPOSITION OF PLAQUES

Plaques also vary in their lipid content. At one extreme are plaques that are entirely fibrous; at the other extreme are plaques that contain a pool of lipids, mainly cholesterol encapsulated within the intima. Most individuals have varying proportions of plaque types, but some have all fibrous or all lipid-rich plaques. Proliferation of vasa vasorum is also a feature of most plaques,[12] and inflammatory cellular infiltration of variable degree in the adventitia is not uncommon. This variability of plaque types might underlie a spectrum of clinical behavior.

The etiology of the process that results in this variety of plaques is probably variable. At postmortem examination in many patients with a history of stable angina, even in the absence of old infarction, one or more segments of the coronary lumen contained several newly formed vascular channels consistent with a previous episode of occlusive thrombosis that underwent organization and subsequent recanalization. Organization of thrombus at the site of plaque fissures may also contribute to plaque growth, but fibrous organization will in time obliterate all evidence of its origin.[13] Recent analysis of 60 consecutive patients with a first myocardial infarction who underwent intracoronary thrombolysis indicates that 20 percent of infarct-related arteries have only residual stenoses smaller than 50 percent, and 60 percent have stenoses between 50 and 75 percent.[14] These findings are in sharp contrast to those in patients who did not undergo thrombolysis and who presented with a much greater severity of residual coronary obstruction in the infarct-related artery.[15]

Thrombosis therefore appears to be a frequent and important component of a considerable proportion of severely obstructive plaques, particularly in patients who have had coronary artery occlusion.

"STABLE" AND "UNSTABLE" PLAQUES

Mural thrombosis has been associated with unstable angina on both angiography and angioscopy in life.[4,13,16] Pathologic studies confirm that distal microemboli consisting predominantly of platelets occur in association with multifocal microscopic foci of necrosis in the myocardium supplied by that artery. Patients who at autopsy are noted to have had a regional transmural infarct have a high incidence of an occluded artery; 75 percent of these occlusive thrombi occur over fissured plaques in which there is a large intraplaque thrombotic element as well as the thrombus within the lumen.[17,18] Histologic studies of "control" subjects who died of a noncardiac cause show that plaque fissures are by no means confined to the heart of patients in whom ischemic disease caused death. Plaque fissuring can therefore be seen not as a process that inevitably leads to intraluminal thrombosis but as an intermittent stimulus for the formation of thrombosis in all subjects with advanced atheroma.[5] The formation of thrombi in the intima may lead to an increase in plaque size, and therefore plaque fissuring could represent an important cause of episodic increases in the degree of stenosis. It seems reasonable to assume that plaque fissure must not be rare in patients with diffuse coronary disease; yet unstable angina and coronary occlusion are rare events in the life of a coronary patient. Factors that determine whether thrombosis within the lumen occurs in response to an episode of plaque fissuring must therefore be considered.

A major factor is likely to be the size of the fissure; large tears that extrude free cholesterol into the lumen may well be followed by thrombosis. However, the degree of thrombotic or fibrinolytic activity at the time and the local vasoconstrictor response may also influence the development of thrombosis. Undoubtedly factors other than plaque fissure must be invoked in cases in which no fissure can be found. Chronic high-grade stenoses per se cannot explain sudden occlusion in the absence of precipitating events. Reduction in flow locally caused by local or distal vascular spasm may favor thrombosis.

A peculiar alteration in the coronary artery vessel wall is responsible for the hyperreactivity to constrictor stimuli resulting in spasm as observed in variant angina.[19] The nature of this alteration is still obscure.

It may therefore be conceptually useful to subdivide plaques into "stable" and "unstable" with reference to their tendency or lack thereof to undergo acute changes capable of producing sudden occlusion of the lumen. These changes may be due to thrombosis, occlusive spasm, or a combination of these events. "Unstable" plaques may be seen as those with fissures that have intense tendency to thrombosis or a tendency to hyperrespond to constrictor stimuli or both. "Stable" plaques may be seen as resulting in either fixed stenosis or stenosis that can be modulated by "physiologic" changes of vasomotor tone, but without any tendency to develop fissure or sudden episodes of complete occlusion.

ISCHEMIC STIMULI

In a stable plaque that produces critical coronary artery stenosis, the most common ischemic stimulus is a sudden, excessive increase of myocardial O_2 consumption.

For stable plaques that cause a fixed reduction in coronary lumen, this ischemic stimulus is the only one that can produce ischemia when the stenosis is sufficiently severe and not adequately compensated for by collaterals and when the increase in myocardial O_2 consumption supplied by the stenosed vessel exceeds the possible increase in coronary blood supply. When the smooth muscle coat is preserved and the vessel wall has remained sufficiently pliable at the site of a stable plaque, local changes in vasomotor tone can vary the severity of the stenosis and therefore influence the ischemic threshold when myocardial O_2 consumption increases and occasionally can even impair flow at rest. Ambulatory Holter monitoring indicates that this feature of chronic stable angina is relatively common.

For unstable plaques the ischemic stimulus is represented by thrombus formation either alone or in combination with vasoconstriction. Thrombus formation must be seen as a very dynamic process, because lysis and fragmentation with distal embolization appear to be common. Spasm as seen in variant angina represents another form of unstable plaque but most probably of a different etiology. It is not yet certain, however, whether in variant angina the local vascular alteration responsible for the hyperreactivity to constrictor stimuli is necessarily associated with plaque.

CONCLUSIONS

The provisional subdivision of plaques into stable and unstable ones finds its clinical correlation in the syndromes of stable and unstable angina. It may stimulate interest in identifying the characteristics and pathogenesis of these two aspects of plaque, which would have important diagnostic and therapeutic implications.

Although irregular stenoses detected on angiography are usually associated with unstable plaques, it must be recognized that they acquire this feature only after they become unstable. At present it is not possible to identify them before, as the features of stability and instability are not necessarily related to the severity of the stenosis they create. Moreover, with plaques showing irregular contours it is difficult to determine if they are heading towards a new period of stability or towards total vessel occlusion. A clearer understanding of these puzzling aspects will result in more appropriate forms of diagnosis and treatment.

REFERENCES

1. Opherk D, Zebe H, Weihe E, Mall G, Durr C, Gravert B, Mehmel HC, Schwarz F, Kubler W: Reduced coronary dilatory capacity and ultrastructural changes of the myocardium in patients with angina pectoris but normal coronary arteriograms. *Circulation* 1981;63:817–825.
2. Cannon RO III, Watson RM, Rosing DR, Epstein SE: Angina caused by reduced vasodilator reserve of the small coronary arteries. *J Am Coll Cardiol* 1983;1:359–373.
3. Maseri A, Chierchia S, L'Abbate A: Pathogenetic mechanisms underlying the clinical events associated with atherosclerotic heart disease. *Circulation* 1980;62(Suppl V):V3–13.
4. Ambrose JA, Winers SL, Arora RR, et al: Angiographic evolution of coronary artery morphology in unstable angina. *J Am Coll Cardiol* 1986;7:472–488.
5. Maseri A, Chierchia S, Davies G: Pathophysiology of coronary occlusion in acute infarction. *Circulation* 1986;73:233–239.
6. Maseri A: The role of coronary artery spasm in symptomatic and silent myocardial ischemia. 1986 Louis Bishop Lecture. *J Am Coll Cardiol* 1987;9:249–262.
7. Klocke FJ: Measurements of coronary blood flow and degree of stenosis: Current clinical implications and continuing uncertainties. *J Am Coll Cardiol* 1983;1:31–41.
8. MacAlpin RN: Contribution of dynamic vascular wall thickening to luminal narrowing during coronary arterial constriction. *Circulation* 1977;61:296–301.
9. Isner JM, Donaldson RF, Fortin AH, Tischler A, Clarke RH: Attenuation of the media of coronary arteries in advanced atherosclerosis. *Am J Cardiol* 1986;58:937–939.
10. Lichtlen PR, Rafflenbeul WM, Freudenberg H: Pathoanatomy and function of coronary obstructions leading to unstable angina pectoris–anatomical and angiographic studies, in Hugenholtz PM, Goldman BS (eds): *Unstable Angina*. Stuttgart, Schattauer, 1985, pp 81–94.
11. Vlodaver Z, Edwards JE: Pathology of coronary atherosclerosis. *Prog Cardiovasc Dis* 1971;14:256–259.
12. Barger AC, Beeuwkes R, Lainey LL, Silverman KJ: Hypothesis: Vasa vasorum and neovascularization of human coronary arteries: A possible role in the pathophysiology of atherosclerosis. *N Engl J Med* 1984;310:175–177.
13. Davies MJ, Thomas AC, Knapman PA, Hangartner JR: Intramyocardial platelet aggregation in patients with unstable angina suffering ischemic cardiac death. *Circulation* 1986;73:418–427.
14. Hackett D, Davies G, Chierchia S, Maseri A: Severity of pre-existing coronary stenoses in patients with first myocardial infarction. In press *Br Med J*.
15. Bertrand M, Lefebvre J, Laisne C, Rousseau M, Carre A, Lekieffre J: Coronary arteriography in acute transmural myocardial infarction. *Am Heart J* 1979;97:61–69.
16. Kranjec I, Delaye J, Bidier B, Delahaye F, Grand A: Angiographic morphology and

intraluminal coronary artery thrombus in patients with angina pectoris: Clinical correlations. *Eur Heart J* 1987;8:100–106.

17. Davies MJ, Thomas T: The pathological basis and microanatomy of occlusive thrombus formation in human coronary arteries. *Phil Trans R Soc Lond (Biol)* 1981;294:225–229.
18. Falk E: Plaque rupture with severe pre-existing stenosis precipitating coronary thrombosis: Characteristics of coronary atherosclerotic plaques underlying fatal occlusive thrombi. *Br Heart J* 1983;50:127–134.
19. Kaski JC, Crea F, Meran D, Rodriguez L, Araujo L, Chierchia S, Davies G, Maseri A: Local coronary supersensitivity to diverse vasoconstrictor stimuli in variant angina. *Circulation* 1986;74:1255–1265.

CHAPTER 4

The Link Between Transient Myocardial Ischemia and Pain

Alberto Malliani, MD

Physiologists know that sensation is an abstraction, not a replication of the real world. Clinicians should be aware that real pain more than an abstraction is only a possibility, and yet it is a cardinal symptom of myocardial ischemia.[1]

What follows concerns the new experimental pathopathologic knowledge that amply supports the growing clinical evidence of painless myocardial ischemia[2] with its possible prognostic relevance[3] as a clinical entity.[4] Yet, a few notes should be addressed to better contrast what is new to what can be defined as old.

THE TRADITIONAL INTERPRETATION

This view, based on a complex set of highly heterogeneous notions, is responsible for having convinced entire generations of physicians that acute myocardial ischemia, as a rule, leads to pain and that this symptom constitutes a reliable warning signal.

The Afferent Pathway

The concept that the afferent fibers in the cardiac sympathetic nerves were the only essential pathway for the transmission of cardiac pain arose from observations in both humans and experimental animals. In man, thoracic sympathectomy or section of higher thoracic dorsal roots was capable of relieving anginal pain,[5] whereas thoracic sympathectomy could abolish behavioral reactions accompanying coronary occlusion in acute experiments,[6,7] observations that were consistent with Langley's statement that "most of the afferent fibers, which on electrical stimulation give rise to pain, pass by the sympathetic strands and not by the vagus."[8] Generally, Langley's opinion was that the sympathetic nervous system was pure outflow. The afferent nerve fibers contained within it were considered without reflex function, merely subserving nociception and somatic in nature as they had their cell bodies located in the dorsal spinal ganglia together with somatic neurons.[8]

From this conceptual matrix originated the holistic view according to which pain of somatic and visceral origin was due to the "direct stimulation of a common system of pain nerves."[9]

The Adequate Stimulus:
When Sherrington[10] individuated in the "nocuous" event, threatening the integrity of a tissue, the stimulus capable, by definition, of triggering nociception, he furnished more a key for predicting all types of nociception. For instance, in the case of the heart, it became known in the same period that "in acute endocarditis, pain is rarely present, and ulceration of valves or of the wall may proceed to a most extreme degree without any sensory disturbance."[11] This is to say that for the heart an ambiguous relation between damage and pain has long been known to exist.

In the 1930s the problem of the adequate stimulus for cardiac pain was sharply focused in experimental terms. On the side of chemical stimuli the foreground was occupied by Lewis's[12] appealing proposal of a "factor P" capable of inducing nociception and accumulating in the tissue spaces when a muscle is exercising under ischemic conditions. However, at the same time,[13] evidence was also available on the adequacy of a pure mechanical stimulus to elicit pain from the heart.[14,15] Although the problem was far from being solved, Lewis's prestige transformed his hypothesis into a common belief, and the abnormal accumulation of chemical substances became the nub of the traditional view of how an adequate stimulus is engendered in the ischemic myocardium.

"Intensity" or "Specificity"? The general problem concerning the afferent code transmitting nociception has assumed, through the years, the best of two main hypotheses proposing, respectively, "intensity" or "specificity."[14,15]

The "intensity" mechanism,[16] the most obvious and probably the first to be formulated, assumes that pain results from excessive stimulation of receptive structures. Alternatively, pain may be conceived as a "specific" sensation[17] that is the product of the excitation of a well-defined nociceptive apparatus, the functional characteristic of which makes it responsible only for a limited class of events, the "nocuous" stimuli that threaten the integrity of a tissue.

According to these premises it should be clear that the "specificity" theory was also in the epicenter of the traditional interpretation of cardiac pain. Indeed, the assignment of the afferent sympathetic path to the exclusive transmission of pain coincided with the most committed conceptualization of a specific nociceptive channel, not only in the usual terms of a peculiar contingent of small diameter afferent fibers,[17] but also as the whole sensory input contained in an ensemble of nerves. Hence, the sympathetic sensory endings within the heart were "specific" nociceptors.

Do Cardiac-Specific Nociceptors Exist?

This question can be explored experimentally. Peripheral sensors purely nociceptive in function should have no background discharge[17] as a consequence of their high threshold which renders them unresponsive to normal events and excitable only with strong stimuli, likely to be noxious. Thus, the *recruitment* of their "silent" fibers by a peripheral stimulus could represent an unambiguous signal to the centers. It is well known, for instance, that on the somatic side there is a population of afferent fibers, innervating the skin, which have receptors that seem to fit the criteria for nociceptors:[17] no background discharge and recruitment only with strong mechanical or thermal stimuli.[18]

Recently, an intense electrophysiologic investigation[19–22] was carried out into the properties of either the small myelinated or the unmyelinated ventricular sympathetic afferent fibers (ie, the afferent fibers that are more likely to convey cardiac nociception). These fibers were found to possess a mechanosensitivity that makes them tonically active and responsive to normal hemodynamic events (Figure 4.1). Coronary occlusion[20] or intracoronary administration of bradykinin (ie, possible algesic stimulus) markedly increased their tonic impulse activity, but recruitment of silent afferent fibers could not be appreciated[21,23] (Figure 4.2). It was concluded that the "intensity" mechanism appeared the most likely candidate to account for the properties of the neural substrate subserving cardiac nociception.[13,22,24] Hence, ventricular sympathetic sensory endings are not "specific" nociceptors, but are low-threshold polymodal receptors.[22,24]

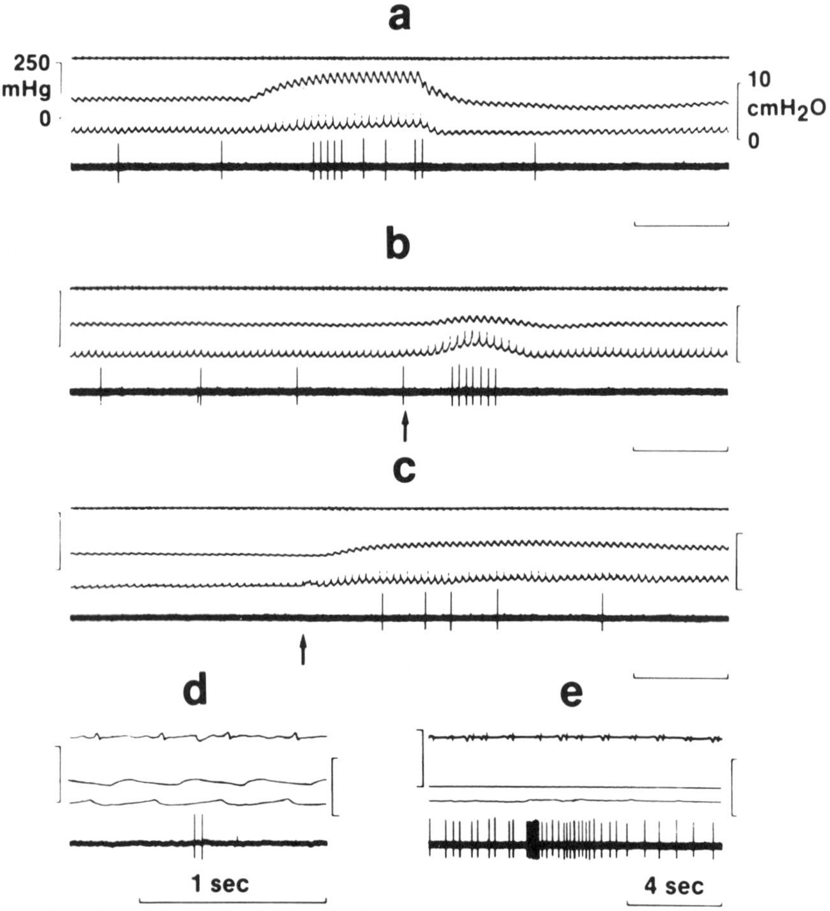

FIGURE 4.1. Activity of an afferent sympathetic nonmyelinated nerve fiber with its receptive field located in the left ventricle. Tracings represent, from *top to bottom,* the ECG, systemic arterial pressure, right atrial pressure, and nervous activity (all tracings are cathode-ray oscilloscope recordings). (*a*) Occlusion of the descending thoracic aorta (indicated by the increase in arterial pressure); (*b*) intravenous injection of 5 ml of warm saline solution, beginning at the *arrow;* (*c*) occlusion of the inferior vena cava released at the *arrow;* (*d*) electrical stimulation of the left inferior cardiac nerve activating the afferent fiber; the biphasic first deflexion is the action potential of the fiber. The approximate length of the fiber was 3.8 cm. The conduction velocity calculated for this fiber was 0.92 m/s. (*e*) mechanical probing of an area of the external surface of the left ventricle, performed on the nonbeating heart, after bleeding the animal to death; note the after-discharge typical of group-C fibers. (From Casati et al,[20] with the permission of the authors and the *Journal of Physiology.*)

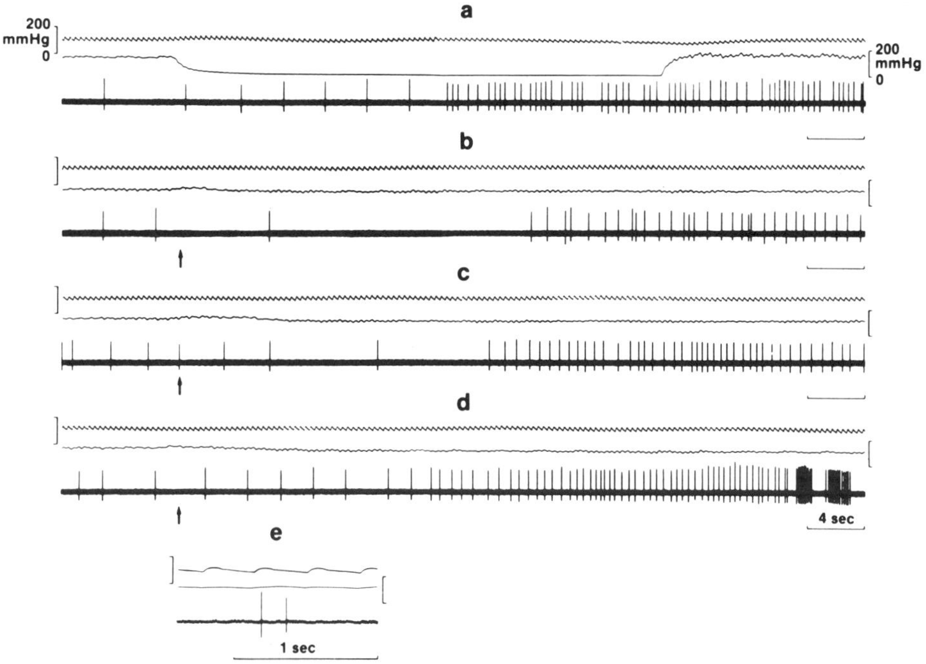

FIGURE 4.2. Activity of an afferent sympathetic nonmyelinated nerve fiber with a left ventricular sensory field. Tracings represent, from the *top to bottom,* systemic arterial pressure, coronary perfusion pressure, and nerve impulse activity (cathode-ray oscilloscope recordings). (*a*) Interruption of the left main coronary artery perfusion; (*b*) intracoronary administration, beginning at the *arrow,* of bradykinin, 5 ng/kg; (*c*) intracoronary administration of bradykinin, 30 ng/kg; (*d*) electrical stimulation of the left inferior cardiac nerve activating the afferent fiber; the biphasic first deflection is the artifact of the stimulus, and the second biphasic deflection is the action potential of the fiber. The approximate length of the nerve was 8 cm. The conduction velocity calculated for this fiber was 0.45 m/s; (*e*) mechanical probing, marked by a *bar,* of an area of the after-discharge. (From Lombardi et al,[21] with the permission of the authors and the publishers of *Circulation Research.*)

Experimental Models and Adequacy of the Stimulus

Pain is a conscious experience that can be explored only indirectly with experimental models; accordingly, different opinions on peripheral nociceptive mechanisms are often the result of different models.

In animals lightly anesthetized or recovering from anesthesia, it is easy to obtain behavioral reactions by applying stimuli likely to be noxious to the heart.[7,8] Decades ago Sutton and Leuth[6] observed that traction on a ligature placed around a coronary artery could elicit "evidence of severe pain" after a few seconds; this latency suggested the mechanical nature of the stimulus. In chronic conditions, when an implanted occluder is used, pain reactions seem absent for the initial 2 minutes of occlusion,[25,26] whereas in some cases they can supervene during prolonged occlusion.[25] Clearly, in all these cases it is difficult to quantify how "noxious" the stimulus is.

The nonapeptide bradykinin was likely to provide a remarkable tool for the experimental analysis of this subject, as it was considered the most powerful algogenic substance possible to be quantified when used as a stimulus.

Indeed, the initial observations by Guzman et al[27] appeared sound and easy to interpret when they reported that the intracoronary injections of bradykinin very effectively produced overt pain reactions in dogs recovering from recent surgery.

However, we recently analyzed the reflex hemodynamic effects of the chemical stimulation with bradykinin of the cardiac sensory innervation in conscious dogs after full recovery from the operation necessary for their instrumentation.[28]

In these animals the injections of bradykinin in either the left anterior descending or circumflex coronary artery consistently produced a marked gradual increase in systemic arterial pressure and heart rate as well as left ventricular pressure and dP/dt (Figure 4.3). These changes were never accompanied by pain reaction as expressed by agitation and sound. The amount of bradykinin injected into the cannulated coronary artery ranged from 10 (the threshold dose for the response) to 3 ng/kg. When the large dose was used, however, the direct vasodilatory effects of the drugs prevailed, and hypotension and tachycardia were observed, again in the absence of pain reactions. A similar pressor response in the absence of pain reactions was also seen when bradykinin was injected into the pericardial sac.[28]

The importance of recovery from anesthesia and recent surgery in explaining the apparent discrepancy with the findings by Guzman et al[27] was demonstrated by experiments performed soon after surgery, when recovery of the animals was still incomplete. The injections of bradykinin into the coronary bed of nine animals during the first week after surgery provoked either an early pressor (Figure 4.4) or depressor (Figure 4.5) response that became the usual constant pressor response at a time of complete recovery from surgery. Moreover, of the nine dogs, three exhibited vocalization and agitation, suggesting a pain reaction in response to the bradykinin injections given during the first week after surgery (Figure 4.4 and 4.5). This reaction was no longer present when the animals were tested later at a time of complete recovery.

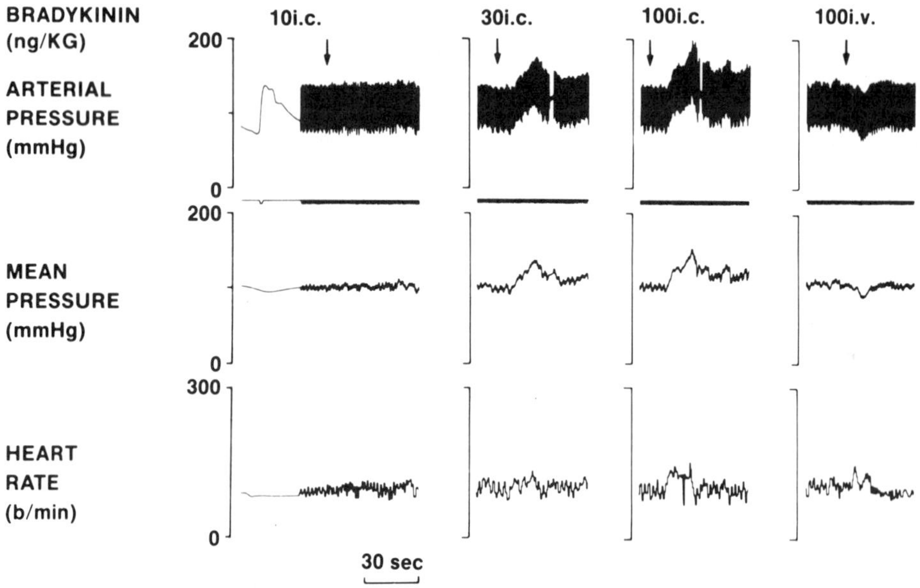

FIGURE 4.3. Progressive pressor responses to graded injections of freshly prepared bradykinin into the cannulated circumflex coronary artery of an unanesthetized conscious dog. Note that hypotension and tachycardia are produced by intravenous injections (100 ng/kg, *right panel*). (From Pagani et al,[28] with the permission of the authors and *Circulation Research*.)

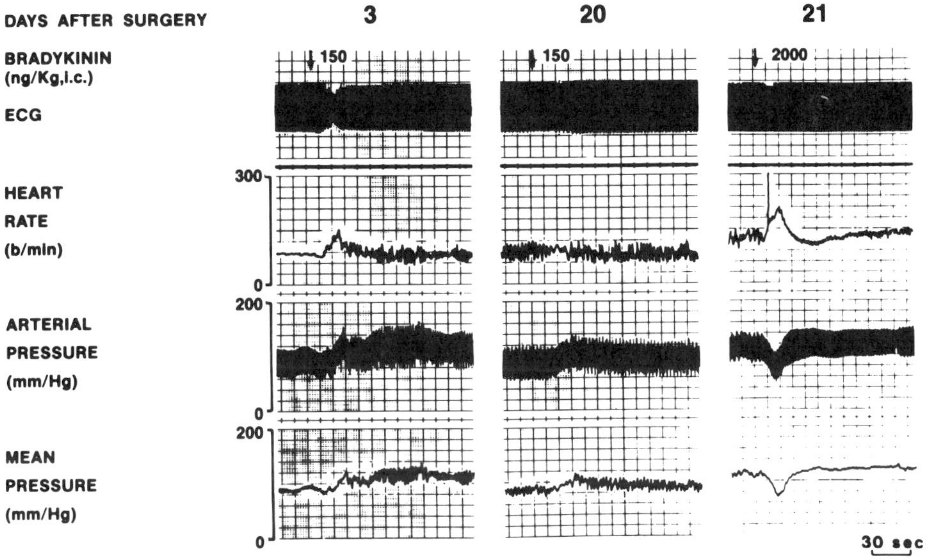

FIGURE 4.4. Hemodynamic effects of stimulation of cardiac sensory innervation with bradykinin injected into the left circumflex coronary artery of an unanesthetized dog shortly after surgery (3 days, *left panel*). Bradykinin 150 ng/kg induced a reflex increase in heart rate and arterial pressure together with a pain reaction, characterized by vocalization, agitation, and struggling, as shown by the motion artifacts or the ECG tracing. The same dose, administered after full recovery from surgery (20 days, *middle panel*), induced a marked pressor response in the absence of pain. Large doses of bradykinin (2,000 ng/kg, *right panel*) did not cause a pain reaction when administered after full recovery; in this case the direct vasodilator effect of the drug initially prevails, producing hypertension and tachycardia. (From Malliani et al,[24] with the permission of the authors and of Churchill Livingstone, Edinburgh.)

An absence of pain was also reported[29] in relation to intracoronary injections of veratridine, a nonphysiologic compound likely to directly stimulate[30] the nerve fibers and undoubtedly capable of activating both vagal[31,32] and sympathetic afferent fibers.[33]

The observation that in appropriate experimental conditions an excitation of the cardiac sensory supply, likely to be massive, did not elicit pain appears as a total defeat for the "specificity" theory, at least if nociceptors were postulated to be exquisitely sensitive to bradykinin.[23] Conversely, the "intensity" theory also does not explain in simple terms the lack of induction of pain.

As a working hypothesis, we propose a modified version of the intensity mechanism. Cardiac pain would result from the extreme excitation of a spatially restricted population of afferent sympathetic fibers.[22,24] Accordingly, coronary occlusion, performed for more than 2 minutes in chronically instrumented dogs seems to be a maneuver more effective than intracoronary injection of bradykinin to elicit overt signs of pain. This difference might be due to the fact that during coronary occlusion, excitation of the afferent sympathetic fibers is probably not only relevant, a condition that surely is also duplicated with bradykinin, but also characterized by marked spatial heterogeneity, as the mechanical and chemical components of the stimulus are likely to be different at the center or at the internal and external boundaries of the ischemic region. Thus, the afferent neural code resulting from this complex event could be of an intense spatiotemporal characterization.

A fortuitous observation in a chronically diseased dog after full recovery from

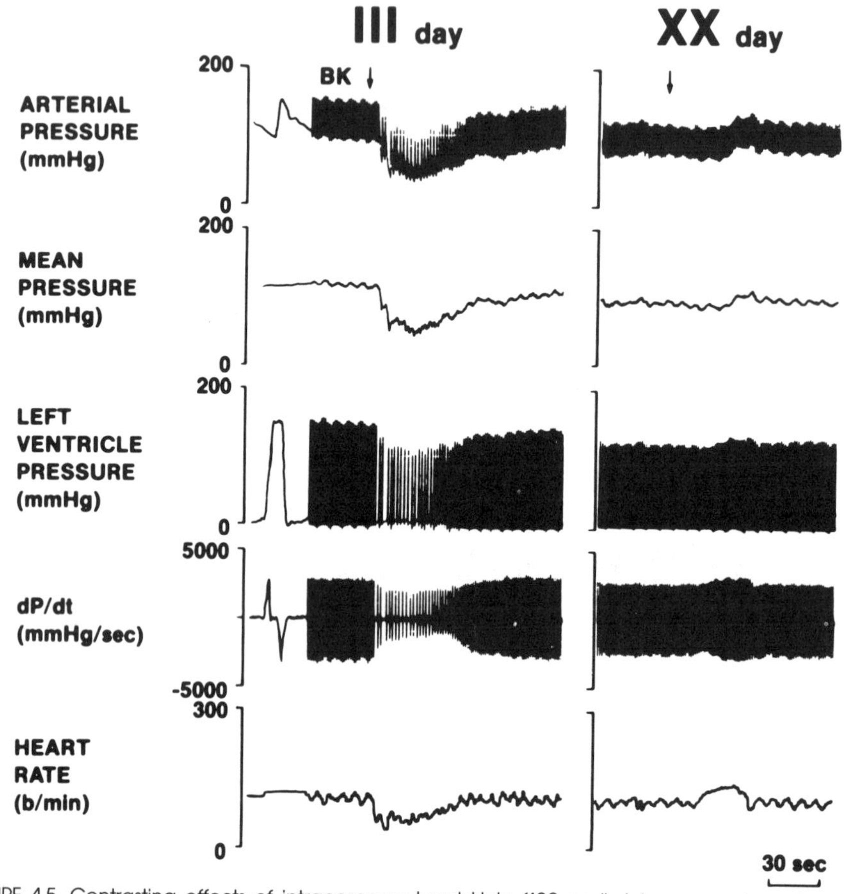

FIGURE 4.5. Contrasting effects of intracoronary bradykinin (100 ng/kg) in a conscious dog when examined early (*left panel*) and late after surgery (*right panel*). Note that although a depressor response was obtained on the third day postoperatively, reversion to a pressor response occurred on complete recovery from surgery (20th day postoperatively). (From Pagani et al,[28] with the permission of the authors and *Circulation Research*.)

surgery seemed to corroborate this point of view. In the course of one of these experiments,[28] the coronary cannula had slipped out of the lumen and was lying, as revealed by autopsy, just outside the wall of the vessel, below the adventitia. This peculiar position maintained by the cannula determined that each minute injection of liquid distended a very limited portion of this highly innervated tissue; and the animal constantly displayed overt pain reactions even when only saline solution was injected[34] (Figure 4.6).

One experiment should not be the basis for a theory, but it is well known that experimental serendipity has often offered new perspectives on a problem. The implications of this hypothesis may be relevant. A spatially restricted mechanical abnormality localized in the myocardium or in the abundantly innervated coronary arteries could lead to pain more efficiently than would a more widely distributed myocardial ischemia with its chemical components. Thus, coronary spasm may be a highly effective stimulus, whereas restricted coronary denervation accompanying bypass interventions could produce strategic interruption of afferent fibers.

According to this hypothesis, when activation of the cardiac sympathetic afferent fibers is widely and homogeneously distributed, as in intracoronary injections of

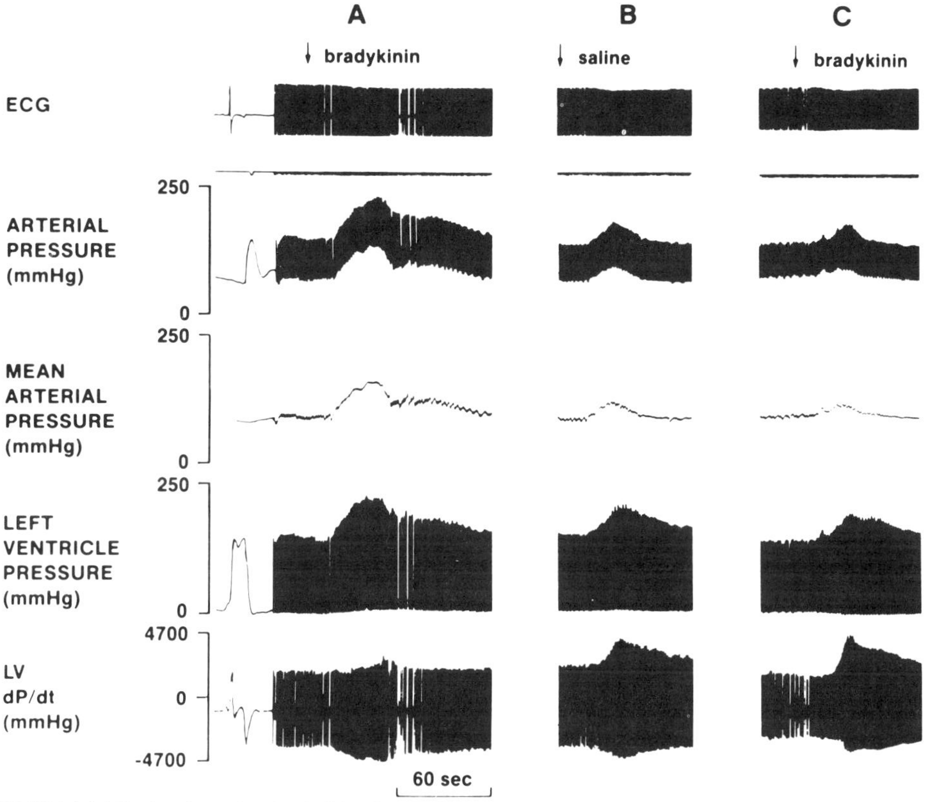

FIGURE 4.6. Effects of mechanical distentions of the adventitia of the left circumflex coronary artery produced in a conscious dog by subadventitial injections of either bradykinin or saline solution. Similar pain reactions (vocalization and agitation) were observed even if the pressor response was blunted by alpha-adrenergic receptor blockade with phentolamine (1 mg/kg between *A* and *B* and again between *B* and *C*) given intravenously into the left ventricle. (From Malliani et al,[34] with the permission of the authors and Elsevier Science Publications, Amsterdam.)

bradykinin, or more currently during a marked increase in arterial pressure,[22] central inhibitory modulations[35] would prevent the onset of pain. Conversely, recent thoracic surgery, by inducing localized somatic afferent barrage, could decisively contribute, through mechanisms of convergence at the spinal level,[36] to the genesis of the peculiar algogenic code.

Finally, the contribution by vagal afferent fibers to the mechanisms of cardiac nociception should be considered with caution and further explored. Indeed, anginal pain referred to the jaw, head, and neck, more frequent after sympathectomy (the phenomenon of "migration of pain"),[37] may indicate an additional central site, besides the spinal cord, where the mechanisms for referred pain would be activated, in this case by cardiac vagal afferent fibers. Moreover, even when nociception is transmitted through afferent sympathetic fibers, an important modulatory role in threshold and characteristics of pain may be exerted by vagal afferents.[38]

THE ELUSIVE LINK

In recent years, it has been well documented that in patients exhibiting spontaneous and reversible ECG changes typical of episodes of transient myocardial ischemia, the hemodynamic profile of the crises can appear substantially similar whether or not they are accompanied by pain.[39–43] Careful analysis revealed that several factors are likely to be implicated in the genesis of pain, such as duration of the episode or severity of ischemia. For instance, ischemic crises were usually painless when shorter than 3 minutes and associated with increases in left ventricular filling pressure less than 7 mm Hg.[44] However, above these values the onset of pain was unpredictable. In brief, duration and severity of ischemia appeared necessary but not sufficient in themselves. Be that as it may, the temporal sequence of ischemic episodes sometimes more than one per hour, about 70 percent of which are unaccompanied by pain, seems to furnish a most intriguing clinical puzzle.

The "elusive link"[1] between transient myocardial ischemia and pain is likely to reflect an interaction of multiple factors of various nature; each being largely unknown it should not be too scandalous if the result is so unpredictable as to appear stochastic.

This chapter is intended to be based on concrete experimental and clinical observations, contradictory though they might be, rather than on more reassuring general views. Taking as a model transient myocardial ischemic episodes, I wish to emphasize that I am not equating anginal pain (for which mechanical factors could be operative) with pain in the course of myocardial infarction, when accumulation of chemical substances and direct destruction of nerve fibers could provide different conditions for nociception.

With these conditions in mind, I suggest the following scheme on variables possibly included in the pathogenesis of anginal pain:

Pain as a multifactorial quantity

1. *The peripheral stimulus:* Herein lies the mystery of the effective nociceptive peripheral code. This level obviously includes the complications introduced by peripheral neuropathies.[45]
2. *The spinal modulatory factors:* Here converge neural mechanisms capable of either accentuating[36,46] or reducing nociception. The latter would comprise transcutaneous electrical nerve stimulation[47] or dorsal column stimulation[48] and excitation of cardiac vagal afferents,[38] the latter likely to be coactivated during the same normal or abnormal cardiac events exciting sympathetic afferents.[49] Here also are located the endogenous peptides,[50] a new legion of candidates that might mediate pathophysiologic mechanisms for pain.

   Some of the new trends in pain research[51] center on these two levels: peripheral input and spinal cord integration. As no spinal pathway has been found to carry exclusively visceral sensation but rather convergent information from the soma and the viscera, it is likely that the processing of either input could exert a reciprocal influence on the other. On the same grounds, some of the new findings on somatic nociception could be relevant to the mechanisms of visceral pain.

   For instance, it was shown that afferent nonmyelinated fibers from somatic deep tissues differ from C-afferent fibers innervating the skin in that they trigger a long duration of increase of excitability in spinal cells.[52] This heterosynaptic facilitation could enable neurones normally responding only to noxious stimuli to transmit information from low threshold inputs as well. This phenomenon seems to last for many minutes, and a whole spectrum of central changes in stimulus-response relations can result from activation of nonmyelinated fibers of different origin.[53]

As to the possible interpretations of these various changes, it is interesting that the chemistry of deep nonmyelinated fibers is partly different from that of C-fibers innervating the skin.[54] In addition, it has been reported recently that brief stimulations of nonmyelinated muscle afferents can induce long-lasting increases in the cutaneous receptive fields of C-afferent fibers; moreover, in some instances, units that originally responded only to noxious cutaneous mechanical stimulation began to respond to low threshold stimuli as well.[55]

Modulatory mechanisms generally should be envisaged as occurring at times comprised between milliseconds and months,[51] which suggests that no unique explanation is likely to be found.

3. *Central factors:* At the very least, these comprise cognition, attention, situational context, and psychologic distress.[56]

It is in the complexity of this frame that we should evaluate interesting findings such as the facilitatory role of tachyarrhythmias on the occurrence of pain during ischemic episodes.[57] Arrhythmias could represent an additional mechanical stimulus or, for instance, a further element of psychologic distress. On similar grounds, the subjective threshold for pain[58,59] could depend on various mechanisms; however, although this individual characteristic somewhat explains the asymptomatic patient, it provides no clue as to the most frequent events which are the asymptomatic episodes versus the symptomatic ones.

Again in this complexity, we should consider that angioplasty in humans, a sort of acute experimental ischemia, induces pain only in a variable manner of balloon occlusions.[60]

As an example of oversimplifications that are not likely to resolve the issue, I refer to the recent report by Sylven et al[61] claiming that a pain similar to that of angina pectoris can be provoked by intravenous injection of adenosine in healthy volunteers. In another report by Barnes et al[62] who more appropriately studied cardiovascular and airway function, adenosine produced abdominal pain and nausea.

THE CONTINUUM

From the heart, as probably from most other organs, a flow of tonic information reaches the centers. Normal and abnormal events produce reflexes (Figure 4.7). For example, neural mechanisms involved in cardiovascular regulation are likely to be not only a link between normal and abnormal but also a solid ground for the novel certainty that health and disease are both innervated entities.[63]

During episodes of transient myocardial ischemia, increased afferent activity reaches the centers through cardiac vagal[49] and sympathetic fibers.[22] Accordingly, neural reflexes can be predominantly of an inhibitory[49] excitatory[22,64,65] nature.

In clinics, most episodes of transient myocardial ischemia, as revealed on Holter monitoring, are characterized by ST-segment depression paralleled by a simultaneous increase in heart rate; this pattern is not influenced by the presence or absence of pain.[66] As it is known that the ischemic episodes are most frequently accompanied by an increase in arterial pressure,[67,68] the increase in heart rate should depend not on a baroreceptive mechanism but rather on a pressor reflex from the heart.[22,64]

It is of interest that power spectral analysis of heart rate and arterial pressure variabilities seems to offer some markers of sympathetic and vagal efferent activities and of sympathovagal interaction in man and in conscious dogs.[69] Hence, it seems

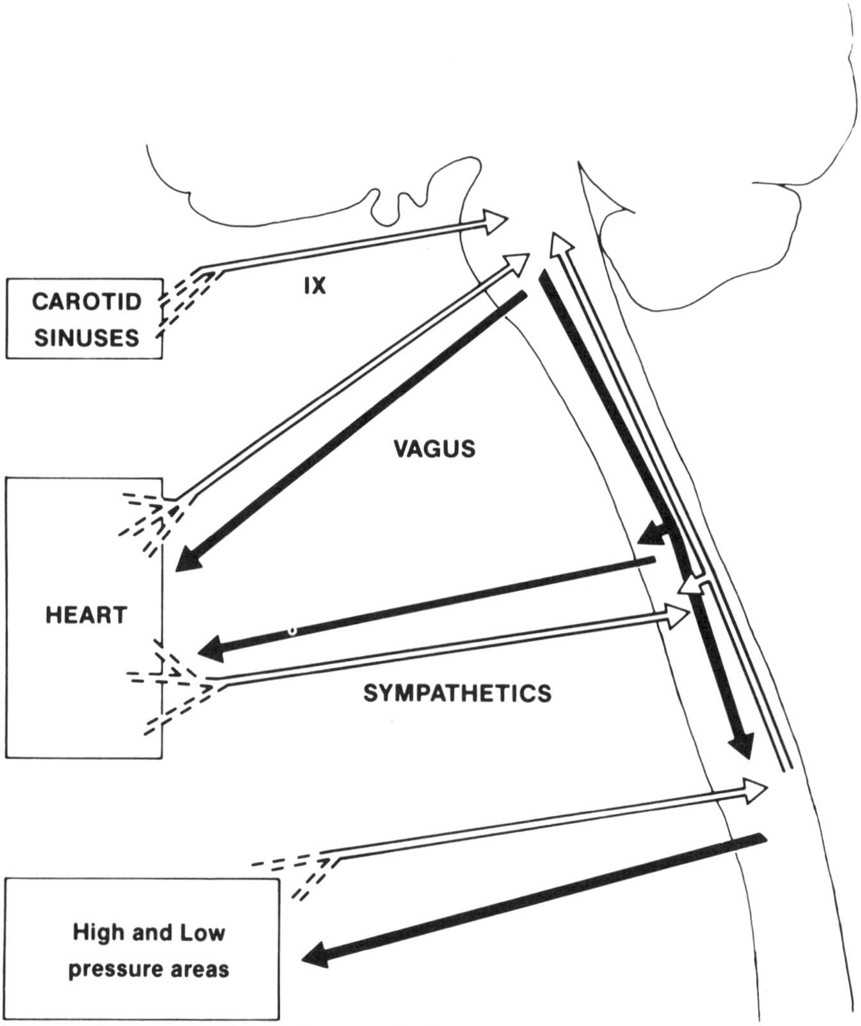

FIGURE 4.7. Schema of cardiovascular sympathetic innervation conceived as an input-output system interacting with supraspinal nervous mechanisms. (From Malliani,[22] with the permission of *Review of Physiology, Biochemistry and Pharmacology.*)

possible to monitor the buildup of sympathetic afferent activity as reflected, on the efferent side, not only by hemodynamic changes but also by these sensitive markers represented by rhythms. This approach could provide clues to the circumstance facilitating the breakthrough of pain.

REFERENCES

1. Malliani A: The elusive link between transient myocardial ischemia and pain. *Circulation* 1986;73:201–204.
2. Cohn PF: *Silent Myocardial Ischemia and Infarction*. New York, Marcel Dekker, 1986.
3. Nademanee K, Intarachot V, Josephson MA, Rieders D, Vaghaiwalla Mody F, Singh BN: Prognostic significance of silent myocardial ischemia in patients with unstable angina. *J Am Coll Cardiol* 1987;10:1–9.
4. Singh BN (ed): A Symposium: Detection, Quantification, and Clinical Significance of Silent Myocardial Ischemia in Coronary Artery Disease. *Am J Cardiol* 1986;58:1B–57B.

5. White, JC: Cardiac pain. Anatomic pathways and physiologic mechanisms. *Circulation* 1957;16:644–655.
6. Sutton DC, Lueth HC: Experimental production of pain on excitation of the heart and great vessels. *Arch Intern Med* 1930;45:827–867.
7. Brown AM: Excitation of afferent cardiac sympathetic nerve fibers during myocardial ischemia. *J Physiol* 1967;190:35–53.
8. Langley JN: The autonomic nervous system. *Brain* 1903;26:1–26.
9. Lewis T, Kellgren JH: Observations relating to referred pain, viscero-motor reflexes and other associated phenomena. *Clin Sci* 1939;4:47–71.
10. Sherrington CS: *The Integrative Action of the Nervous System,* New Haven, Yale University Press, 1906.
11. Osler, W: The Lumleian Lectures on "Angina Pectoris" (Lecture (II). *Lancet* 1910;1:839–843.
12. Lewis T: Pain in muscular ischemia—Its relation to anginal pain. *Arch Intern Med* 1932;49:713–727.
13. Martin SJ, Gorham LW: Cardiac pain. An experimental study with reference to the tension factor. *Arch Intern Med* 1938;62:840–844.
14. Malliani A, Lombardi F: Consideration of the fundamental mechanisms eliciting cardiac pain. *Am Heart J* 1982;103:575–578.
15. Malliani A: Pathophysiology of ischemic cardiac pain, in Arnim TV, Maseri A (eds): *Silent Ischemia.* New York, Springer-Verlag, 1987, pp 19–24.
16. Goody W: On the nature of pain. *Brain* 1957;80:118–131.
17. Perl ER: Is pain a specific sensation? *J Psychiatr Res* 1971;8:273.
18. Burgess PR, Perl ER: Cutaneous mechanoreceptors and nociceptors, in Iggo A (ed): *Handbook of Sensory Physiology,* Somatosensory System. Berlin, Springer-Verlag, 1973, vol 2, pp 29–78.
19. Malliani A, Recordati G, Schwartz PJ: Nervous activity of afferent cardiac sympathetic fibers with atrial and ventricular endings. *J Physiol* 1973;229:457–469.
20. Casati R, Lombardi F, Malliani A: Afferent sympathetic unmyelinated fibers with left ventricular endings in cats. *J Physiol* 1979;292:135–148.
21. Lombardi F, Della Bella P, Casati R, Malliani A: Effects of intracoronary administration of bradykinin on the impulse activity of afferent sympathetic unmyelinated fibers with left ventricular endings in the cat. *Circ Res* 1981;48:69–75.
22. Malliani A: Cardiovascular sympathetic afferent fibers. *Rev Physiol Biochem Pharmacol* 1982;94:11–74.
23. Baker DG, Coleridge HM, Coleridge JCG, Nerdrum T: Search for a cardiac nociceptor: Stimulation by bradykinin of sympathetic afferent nerve endings in the heart of the cat. *J Physiol* 1980;306:519–536.
24. Malliani A, Pagani M, Lombardi F: Visceral versus somatic mechanisms, in Wall PD, Melzack R (eds): *Textbook of Pain,* Edinburgh, Scotland, Churchill Livingstone, 1984, pp. 100–109.
25. Theroux P, Ross J, Franklin D, Kemper WS, Sasayama S: Regional myocardial function in the conscious dog during acute coronary occlusion and responses to morphine, propranolol, nitroglycerin and lidocaine. *Circulation* 1976;53:302–314.
26. Pagani M, Baig H, Sherman A, Manders WT, Quinn P, Franklin D, Vatner SF: Technique for measurement of pressure-dimension relations in the aorta and great arteries of conscious unanesthetized animals. *Am J Physiol* 1978;235:H610–H617.
27. Guzman F, Braun C, Lim RKS: Visceral pain and the pseudo-effective response to intra-arterial injection of bradykinin and other algesic agents. *Arch Int Pharmacodyn* 1962;136:353–359.
28. Pagani M, Pizzinelli P, Furlan R, Guzzetti S, Rimoldi O, Sandrone G, Malliani A: Analysis of the pressor sympathetic reflex produced by intracoronary injections of bradykinin in conscious dogs. *Circ Res* 1985;56:175–182.
29. Barron KW, Bishop VS: Reflex cardiovascular changes with veratridine in the conscious dog. *Am J Physiol* 1982;242:H810–H817.
30. Paintal AS: Action of drugs on sensory nerve endings. *Ann Rev Pharmacol* 1971;11:231–240.
31. Von Bezold A, Hirt L: Ueber die physiologischen Wirkungen des essigsauren Veratrins. *Untersuch Physiol Lab Wuerzburg* 1867;1:73–156.

32. Thoren P: Role of the cardiac vagal c-fibers in cardiovascular control. *Rev Physiol Biochem Pharmacol* 1979;86:1–94.
33. Malliani A, Peterson DF, Bishop VS, Brown AM: Spinal sympathetic cardiocardiac reflexes. *Circ Res* 1972;30:158–166.
34. Malliani A, Lombardi F, Pagani M: Sensory innervation of the heart in visceral sensations, in Cervero F, Morrison JFB (eds): *Progress in Brain Research,* Amsterdam, Elsevier Science Publ., 1986, vol 67, pp 39–48.
35. Wall PD, Melzack R (eds): *Textbook of Pain,* Edinburgh, Churchill Livingstone, 1984.
36. Forman RD, Ohata CA: Effects of coronary artery occlusion on thoracic spinal neurons receiving viscerosomatic inputs. *Am J Physiol* 1980;238:H667–H674.
37. Lindgren I, Olivecrona H: Surgical treatment of angina pectoris. *J Neurosurg* 1947;4:19–39.
38. Foreman RD: Spinothalamic tract and cardiac afferents, in Lown B, Malliani A, Prosdocimi M (eds): *Neural Mechanisms and Cardiovascular Disease; Fidia Research Series.* Heidelberg, Springer-Verlag, Liviana Press, 1986, vol 5, pp 169–181.
39. Guazzi M, Polese A, Fiorentini C, Magrini F, Bartorelli C: Left ventricular performance and related hemodynamic changes in Prinzmetal's variant angina pectoris. *Br Heart J* 1971;33:84–94.
40. Guazzi M, Polese A, Fiorentini C, Magrini F, Olivari MT, Bartorelli C: Left and right heart hemodynamics during spontaneous angina pectoris. Comparison between angina with ST segment depression and angina with ST segment elevation. *Br Heart J* 1975;37:401–413.
41. Guazzi M, Olivari MT, Polese A, Fiorentini C, Magrini F: Repetitive myocardial ischemia of Prinzmetal type without angina pectoris. *Am J Cardiol* 1976;37:923–927.
42. Maseri A, Severi S, De Nes M, L'Abbate A, Chierchia S, Marzilli M, Ballestra AM, Parodi O, Biagini A, Distante A: "Variant" angina: One aspect of a continuous spectrum of vasospastic myocardial ischemia. *Am J Cardiol* 1978;42:1019–1035.
43. Chierchia S, Brunelli C, Simonetti I, Lazzari M, Maseri A: Sequence of events in angina at rest: Primary reduction in coronary flow. *Circulation* 1980;61:759–768.
44. Maseri A, Chierchia S, Davies G, Glazier J: Mechanisms of ischemic cardiac pain and of silent myocardial ischemia. *Am J Med* 1985;79(34):7–11.
45. Nesto RW, Phillips RT: Asymptomatic myocardial ischemia in diabetic patients. *Am J Med* 1986;80(suppl 4c):40–47.
46. Blair RW, Weber RN, Foreman RD: Responses of thoracic spinothalamic neurones to intracardiac injections of bradykinin in the monkey. *Circ Res* 1982;51:83–94.
47. Mannheimer C, Carlsson CA, Vedin A, Wilhelmsson C: Transcutaneous electrical nerve stimulation (TENS) in angina pectoris. *Pain* 1986;26:291–300.
48. Murphy DF, Giles KE: Dorsal column stimulation for pain relief from intractable angina pectoris. *Pain* 1987;28:365–368.
49. Bishop VS, Malliani A, Thoren P: Cardiac mechanoreceptors, in Shepherd JT, Abboud FM, Geiger SR (eds): *Handbook of Physiology, Section 2 The Cardiovascular System,* Peripheral Circulation and Organ Blood Flow. Washington, DC, Am Physiol Soc, 1983, vol 3, pp 497–555.
50. Weidinger F, Hammerle A, Sochor H, Smelana R, Frass M, Glogar D: Role of Beta-endorphins in silent myocardial ischemia. *Am J Cardiol* 1986;58:428–430.
51. Wall PD: Future trends in pain research. *Phil Trans R Soc* (Lond) 1985;B308:393–401.
52. Wall PD, Woolf CJ: Muscle but not cutaneous C-afferent input produces prolonged increases in the excitatory responses of the flexon reflex in the cat. *J Physiol* 1984;356:428–430.
53. Woolf CJ, Wall PD: Relative effectiveness of C primary afferent fibers of different origin of the flexon reflex in the rat. *J Neurosci* 1986;6:1433–1442.
54. McMahon SR, Sykova F, Wall PD, Woolf CL, Gibson SJ: Neurogenic extravasation and substance P levels are low in muscle as compared to skin in the rat hindlimb. *Neurosci Lett* 1984;52:235–240.
55. Cook AJ, Woolf CJ, Wall PD, McMahon SR: Dynamic receptive field plasticity in rat spinal cord dorsal horn following C-primary afferent input. *Nature* 1987;325:151–153.
56. Barsky AJ: Palliation and symptomatic relief. *Arch Intern Med* 1986;146:905–909.
57. Biagini A, Emdin M, Michelazzi C, Testa R, Carpeggiani C, Mazzei MG, Andreotti F, L'Abbate A: The contribution of ventricular tachyarrhythmias to the genesis of cardiac

pain during transient myocardial ischemia in patients with variant angina. *Eur Heart J* 1988 (in press).
58. Procacci P, Zoppi M, Padeletti L, Maresca M: Myocardial infarction without pain. A study of the sensory functions of the upper limbs. *Pain* 1976;2:309–313.
59. Droste C, Greenlee MW, Roskamm H: A defective angina pectoris pain warning system: Experimental findings of ischemic and electrical pain test. *Pain* 1986;26:199–209.
60. Sigwart V, Grbie M, Payot M, Goy J, Essinger A, Fischer A: Ischemic events during coronary artery balloon obstruction, in Rutishauser W, Roskamm H (eds): *Silent Myocardial Ischemia*. Berlin, Springer-Verlag, 1984, pp 29–36.
61. Sylven C, Beerman B, Jonzon R, Brandt R: Angina pectoris like pain provoked by intravenous adenosine in healthy volunteers. *Br Med J* 1986;293:227–230.
62. Barnes PJ, Conradson TBG, Dixon CMS, Fuller RW, Maxwell DL: Effects of infused adenosine on cardiovascular and airway function in conscious man. *J Physiol* 1986;374:22P.
63. Malliani A: Homeostasis and instability: The hypothesis of tonic interaction in the cardiovascular regulation of negative and positive feedback mechanisms, in Lown B, Malliani A, Prosdocimi P (eds): *Neural Mechanisms and Cardiovascular Disease*. Fidia Research Series, Padova, Liviana Press, 1986, vol 5, pp 1–9.
64. Malliani A, Schwartz PJ, Zanchetti A: A sympathetic reflex elicited by experimental coronary occlusion. *Am J Physiol* 1969;217:703–709.
65. Malliani A, Pagani M, Lombardi F: Positive feedback reflexes, in Zanchetti A, Tarazi RC (eds): *Handbook of Hypertension, Pathophysiology of Hypertension Regulatory Mechanisms*. New York, Elsevier Science Publications, 1986, vol 8, pp. 69–81.
66. Hoberg F: Symptomatic versus asymptomatic ischemic episodes during Holter monitoring: patterns of high resolution trend recording of ST segment and heart rate. von Arnin TH, Maseri A (eds): *Silent Ischemia*. Darmstadt, FRG, Steinkopff-Verlag, 1987.
67. Littler WA, Honour J, Sleight P, Stott FD: Direct arterial pressure and electrocardiogram in unrestricted patients with angina pectoris. *Circulation* 1973;48:125–134.
68. Figueras J: Hemodynamic correlates of symptomatic and asymptomatic myocardial ischemia, in Singh BN (ed): *Silent Myocardial Ischemia and Angina,* New York, Pergamon Press, 1988.
69. Pagani M, Lombardi F, Guzzetti S, Rimoldi O, Furlan R, Pizzinelli P, Sandrone G, Malfatto G, Dell'Orto S, Piccaluga E, Turiel M, Baselli G, Cerutti S, Malliani A: Power spectral analysis of heart rate and arterial pressure variabilities as a marker of sympatho-vagal interaction in man and conscious dog. *Circ Res* 1986;59:178–193.

CHAPTER 5

Hemodynamic Correlates of Symptomatic and Asymptomatic Myocardial Ischemia

Jaime Figueras, MD

Reduced oxygen in the myocardial fiber results in an almost instant decrease in its contractile function,[1,2] because anaerobic metabolism is not sufficient to maintain the inotropic force even when the sources of adenosine triphosphate are not totally exhausted.[3] For the ischemic process to have an impact on the overall function of the heart, however, it is imperative that the compromised area be of certain magnitude.[4–6] Therefore, if less than 10 percent of the myocardium becomes ischemic, no detectable hemodynamic changes will likely occur.[6,7] Moreover, the size of the ischemic area also must reach a minimum to be possibly identified by the conventional methods of detecting ischemia. The degree of functional impairment is also affected by the site and intensity of ischemia. The hemodynamic changes produced by ischemia may further be influenced by extracardiac factors triggered by the ischemic myocardium[8,9] and by the effects of myocardial ischemia on the autonomic and central nervous systems. Thus, there is a complex interplay of factors that regulates the hemodynamic consequences of acute myocardial ischemia. In this chapter, an analysis of these factors is undertaken with particular emphasis on those occurring during ischemia at rest in patients with ischemic heart disease.

FUNCTIONAL AND HEMODYNAMIC CORRELATES OF MYOCARDIAL ISCHEMIA

Changes in Ventricular Function

Clinically, the hemodynamic changes associated with myocardial ischemia are comparable to those observed during experimental coronary occlusion. Thus, during exercise-induced ischemia in the catheterization laboratory[10–15] and during ambulatory monitoring of the pulmonary artery pressure,[16] increases in left ventricular filling pressure were detected before or at the onset of the ECG changes,[12,15] as in the case of changes in regional wall motion. With supine exercise, similar changes occur, but the ischemic threshold decreases[17,18] to the higher resting filling pressures that result from the larger end-diastolic volumes.[19,20] The fact that some investigators have found no decrease in threshold in this position,[21,22] may perhaps be explained by differences in patient population, the degree of recumbency, or both. When ischemia is produced by atrial pacing, regional and global function abnormalities are also elicited[23–25] with increases in left ventricular end-diastolic pressure, especially apparent at cessation of pacing,[23] that are ascribable to impaired ventricular relaxation[24,26,27] in view of no increases in end-diastolic volume.[24,28]

During spontaneous angina, increases in left ventricular filling pressures and decreases in stroke volume were also demonstrated (Table 5.1). The initial documentation of these hemodynamic changes was provided by Muller[29] and Johnson.[30] Roughgarden[31] was the first to describe the increase in pulmonary artery pressure associated with angina at rest.[32] Subsequent investigations confirmed these initial findings[33–42] (Figures 5.2 and 5.3). Decreases in cardiac output during spontaneous angina were initially reported by Rosland[43] in a single case and the decreases in stroke volume were first documented by Lecerof[34] in 3 patients, also in the catheterization laboratory as in the case of Rosland.[43]

Wall motion abnormalities during ischemia at rest also were demonstrated by radionuclide ventriculograms.[44] Most of this hemodynamic information was obtained from patients with advanced coronary artery disease, but also from a few with nonsignificant coronary stenosis in whom similar changes were found.[45]

Contrast ventriculography during spontaneous angina revealed abnormal early diastolic relaxation[46] and increases in end-systolic and end-diastolic volumes.[42] This impaired relaxation shifts the pressure-volume curve of the left ventricle upwards during ischemia.[27,47] The increases in left ventricular filling pressure during ischemia are more prominent in the presence of myocardial hypertrophy which reduces ventricular compliance[48,49] and during episodes associated with acute hypertension.[39,41] The latter not only increases afterload but may also further reduce ventricular distensibility by augmenting the contractile properties of the left ventricle due to the increased coronary perfusion pressure.[50]

The magnitude of the hemodynamic changes generally is modulated by the extent of the ischemic area, its intensity, and the status of the resting ventricular function and compliance. Thus, during spontaneous ischemia, a patient with severe triple-vessel disease and reduced resting ejection fraction and compliance, associated with a long history of effort angina and arterial hypertension, will tend to have much higher filling pressures and a smaller decrease in cardiac output than will a younger patient with single-vessel disease in whom severe transmural ischemia develops with no collaterals.

Careful continuous monitoring permits the correlation of hemodynamic and ECG changes.[33,36,37,41] These studies indicate that the onset of increases in left ventricular filling pressure precedes or at least coincides with the onset of the ECG changes, thus paralleling the experimental findings. Balloon angioplasty provides a model to study transient functional changes in the ventricle. Impairment in early relaxation can be detected 1 to 15 seconds after balloon occlusion, and by 50 seconds most ischemic segments become akinetic with late systolic outward displacement[51] with an increase in left ventricular end-diastolic pressure.[51,52] These mechanical changes clearly precede the ST-segment changes and have been documented angiographically and by two-dimensional echocardiography, not only during angioplasty,[53] but also during spontaneous angina or a positive ergonovine test.[54]

Table 5.1. Hemodynamic Changes During Angina at Rest

References	Author*	Year	n	CR	LVFP	RAP	CO	SV	SVR	BP†	HR†	Silent Ischemia
31	Roughgarden and Newman	1966	30	—	—	—	—	—	—	↑ 29%	↑ 30%	—
32	Roughgarden	1966	10	+	↑ (2)	—	—	—	—	↑ 26%	↑ 7%	—
33	Guazzi et al	1971	4	+	—	O	↓	—	—	↓	↑	+
34	Lecerof	1974	3	—	↑	—		↓	—	↑	↑	—
35	Cannom et al	1974	17	+	↑	—	—	—	—	↑	↑ 10%	—
36	Guazzi et al	1975	11	+	↑	↑	↓	↓	—	↑	Late ↑ O	+
37	Maseri et al	1975	5	+	↑	↑	—	—	—	↑	Late O	+
38	Gaasch et al	1975	4	—	↑	—	—	—	—	O	↑ O	—
39	Scheidt et al	1976	17	+	↑	—	—	—	—	↑	↑ 14%	—
40	Berndt et al	1977	7	+	↑	—	—	—	—	↑ O	↑	—
41	Figueras et al	1979	11	+	↑	↑	↓	↓	↑	↑	↑ O	+
42	Sharma et al	1980	14	—	↑	—	O	↓	—	O	↑	—
45	Maseri et al	1978	22	+	↑	—	—	—	—	↑	Late O	+
55	Chierchia et al	1980	6	+	↑	—	—	—	—	↑ ↓	↑	+

ABBREVIATIONS: BP = arterial blood pressure; CO = cardiac output; CR = continuous recording; HR = heart rate; LVFP = left ventricular filling pressure; RAP = right arterial pressure; SV = stroke volume; SVR = systemic vascular resistance; O = no change; — = not measured or assessed.

* The list of investigators cited is not exhaustive.

† The percentage indicates average change.

Changes in Blood Pressure

During spontaneous angina, as during exertional angina,[31] most authors, starting from the very early reports as carefully reviewed by Roughgarden,[31,32] reported increased blood pressure (Table 5.1). Initial intraarterial pressure monitoring indicated that such increases preceded the onset of pain.[32] It was later confirmed that these increases were progressive and striking,[36,39,41] particularly during pain (Figures 5.1 and 5.2) Continuous ECG and pressure recordings showed that the initial, and thus minor, changes in blood pressure very seldom precede the onset of ST-segment changes.[33,36,37,41,45] Moreover, when concomitant pulmonary artery pressure monitoring became available, the increases in blood pressure were found to accompany or follow the increases in pulmonary pressure, reflecting left ventricular dysfunction.[4,33,36,37] These trivial blood pressure changes at the very onset of ischemic ECG changes are consistent with little or no changes during short coronary artery occlusions with balloon angioplasty in patients with single-vessel disease involving either the left anterior descending or the right coronary artery.[52,56] Furthermore, in our experience and that of others,[57,58] there were also inconsequential changes in blood pressure or heart rate at the onset of the ST-segment changes during most positive responses to ergonovine, as observed in 18 consecutive patients with normal coronary arteries and in 25, also consecutive, with severe (>90%) coronary artery stenosis with either ST-segment elevation or depression during the test. Seemingly, Waters et al[58] documented an increase in blood pressure of only 10 mm Hg and no change in heart rate in a positive test with ST-segment elevation in 36 patients, 16 of whom had significant coronary artery stenosis. In agreement with previous investi-

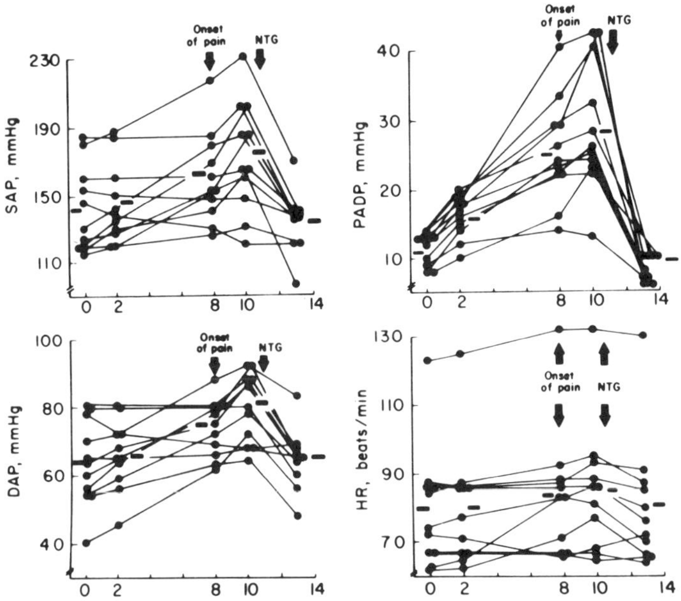

FIGURE 5.1. Sequential changes in systolic (SAP) and diastolic (DAP) arterial pressures, pulmonary artery diastolic pressure (PADP), and heart rate (HR) during spontaneous angina in 11 patients. Values are timed in regard to the onset of ECG changes from continuous recordings. The time of onset of pain, its peak, and the return to baseline are the average for all patients. Changes at the onset of ECG abnormalities are minimal except for pulmonary arterial diastolic pressure (PADP), which increases uniformly. After the onset of pain there is a further increase in blood pressure and PADP.

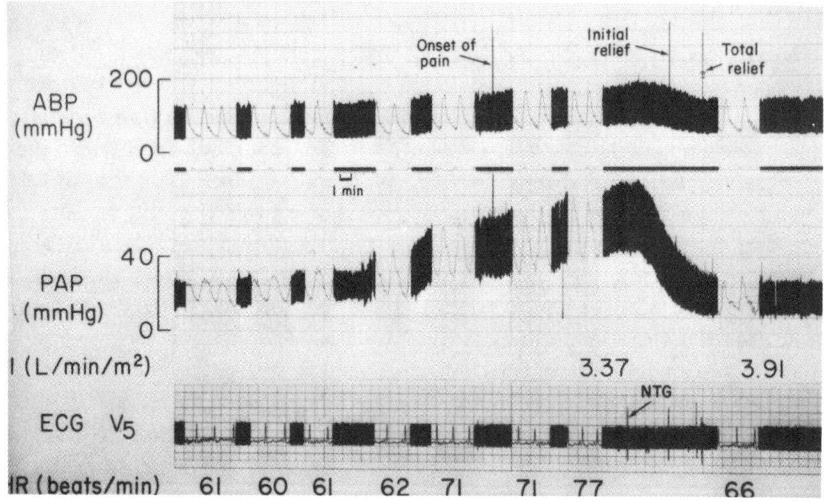

FIGURE 5.2. Continuous recording of arterial pressure (ABP), pulmonary artery pressure (PAP), and ECG during an episode of spontaneous angina. Cardiac index (CI) measurements before and after nitroglycerin are also indicated. Note that no increases in blood pressure or heart rate precede the onset of increases in pulmonary pressure which are accompanied by a decrease in cardiac index.

gators,[57–60] we encountered remarkable similarities between the ECG changes during spontaneous angina and those seen during ergonovine-induced myocardial ischemia. Thus, because the ECG changes that precede or coincide with the onset of pressure changes are already a "late" sign of ischemia, it is highly unlikely that they could be the cause of ischemia. Moreover, methoxamine-induced hypertension either did not produce ischemia even when pressures higher than those attained during angina had been achieved[61,62] or did in a few cases with an elevated resting left ventricular filling pressure[61] or at a much higher double product than during pacing-induced angina.[63] The hypertensive reaction may vary from crisis to crisis as observed during ambulatory blood pressure recordings.[64] It is attenuated by beta-blockers. Whether such increases in blood pressure are secondary to a reflex response to myocardial ischemia[65–67] or represent generalized vasoconstriction simultaneously affecting systemic and coronary circulations as documented in a clinical case[68] is uncertain. The latter is supported by the observation of Yasue et al[69] who found a simultaneous increase in blood pressure and the occurrence of a coronary spasm during administration of epinephrine to four patients. In contrast to hypertension, arterial hypotension is much less frequently seen during angina at rest, and it is generally associated with extensive coronary disease. More often, however, it is associated with intense transmural ischemia,[37] usually involving the inferior wall which is often accompanied by bradycardia due to stimulation of certain pressor receptors.[70–77] However, the increases in blood pressure during spontaneous angina are such that for all practical purposes, they can be considered an indirect sign of myocardial ischemia. For example, in our series of 75 consecutive patients with angiographically documented significant coronary artery disease with acute ECG changes during pain, 94 percent exhibited hypertension during most of their attacks, and in 16 patients without significant coronary stenosis, 73 percent also had increases in blood pressure during their painful ischemic episodes.

Changes in Heart Rate

The nature and pattern of changes in heart rate during spontaneous angina have been less controversial than are those in blood pressure. In most studies (Table 5.1), heart rate has been reported to increase by 10 to 20 percent, to remain unchanged, or to decrease. In observations during continuous ECG recordings, most of these changes occur after the onset of ischemia and especially after the onset of pain.[39,41,55] As with the changes in blood pressure, the overall changes in heart rate are similar during anterior or inferior ischemia. Nevertheless, there is a subset of patients who may develop bradycardia during severe transmural inferior ischemia which is generally associated with the presence of single-vessel disease, with or without significant coronary stenosis, and with virtually absent collaterals. The reported increases in heart rate during anterior ischemia, mostly referred to patients with nonsignificant coronary lesions,[72,73] in our experience are much less evident in those with significant stenosis who constitute the vast majority of patients with angina at rest.

It is therefore clear that these small changes in heart rate are unlikely to produce myocardial ischemia in most patients, especially when it is recognized that their resting heart rates range between 60 and 80 beats per minute[74] and that seldom do they exhibit an ischemic threshold during atrial pacing of less than 100 beats per minute.[40,62,74] In patients with fixed and severe coronary stenosis, the average heart rate during pain was 75 beats per minute, whereas the atrial pacing ischemic threshold among those with a positive test averaged 138 beats per minute.[74] Our experience now encompasses more than 130 similar patients with identical findings. However, Quyyumi et al[75] recently reported that in five patients, also with severe coronary disease, an increase in heart rate averaging 19 beats per minute preceded the onset of ST-segment depression during nocturnal angina, which reached a mean value of approximately 2.5 mm. To ascribe this intense ischemia to the small increases in heart rate appears somewhat unconvincing, at least relative to our pacing studies, some of which were also performed at night.[74] In no case, was there ST-segment depression of greater than 1.5 mm with pacing rates greater than 120 beats per minute. Thus, it is conceivable that additional factors contributed to the development of ischemia in at least some of the five patients studied by Quyyumi et al.[75]

It must be emphasized that even though we have noted a nocturnal decline in the pacing ischemic threshold[74] at least in our patients, it was still much higher than their heart rates observed during anginal episodes at night.[74] Papapietro et al[76] reported somewhat higher increases in heart rate during spontaneous angina, but some measurements were made immediately after pain and probably included some nitroglycerin effects. The relatively minor changes in heart rate during most episodes of angina at rest are similar to those seen during ischemia produced by a reduction in coronary blood flow during a positive ergonovine test[57–59] or during transient occlusion with balloon angioplasty.[52,56]

Electrocardiographic Changes: Elevation vs Depression of the ST Segment

Exercise-induced myocardial ischemia is associated with ST-segment depression due to the imbalance between oxygen supply and demand in the subendocardium. Recently, however, evidence in some patients has indicated the existence of a superimposed dynamic obstruction that may lead to transmural ischemia occurring spontaneously or during exercise.[72,78] During angina at rest, the ECG changes are somewhat differently distributed. Even though traditionally this form of angina has also been linked to electrical evidence of subendocardial ischemia, there is a growing awareness that as many or even more patients will experience transmural ischemia during their spontaneous episodes, expressed as ST-segment elevation but also as pseudonormalization of negative T waves.[77,79] This correlation has been validated by perfusion scintigraphy.[77,79] Some patients may present ventricular ectopic beats as the only electrical abnormality, whereas others may present inversion of the U wave.[80] The increasing use of the 12-lead electrocardiogram during spontaneous episodes of ischemia has increased the yield in diagnosing transmural ischemia.[81] Thus, the collective results of three large series[6,82,83] involving over 600 patients indicated that 40 to 50 percent had ST-segment elevation or positive T waves during pain. In general, patients with ST-segment depression tend to have a longer history of angina and more advanced coronary artery disease than do those with ST-segment elevation or normalization of negative T waves.[82–85] Hemodynamic changes during ischemia, however, are independent[41] of the type of the ECG changes (Figure 5.3). Thus, in contrast to initial reports[36] ST-segment elevation as in the case of ST-segment depression is much more frequently associated with hypertension than with hypotension.[31,61,86] Patients who develop hypotension with ST-segment elevation are very few and tend to exhibit severe coronary spasm over one-vessel disease, whereas most patients with ST-segment elevation during angina have severe stenosis of one or several vessels[87–89] and positive stress test results.[87] It has been well established that the leads involved in ST-segment elevation closely correspond to the area subtended by the stenosed coronary artery responsible for the ischemia during both exercise[90–93] and spontaneous angina.[94,95] They also correspond to the site of perfusion defects as detected by thallium-201 myocardial scintigraphy.[92,93] Angiographically, ST-segment elevation has been consistently correlated with total occlusion of the corresponding vessel, as during normalization of negative T waves[45,94] without significant collaterals. On the contrary, patients with ST-segment depression during

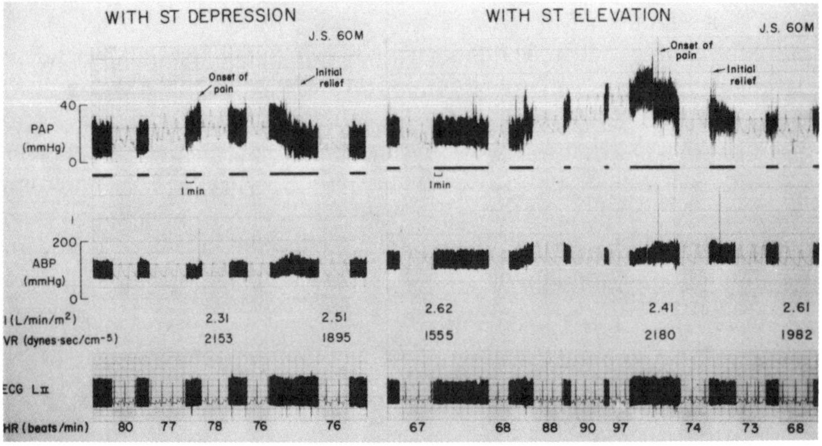

FIGURE 5.3. Continuous hemodynamic recordings during angina at rest associated with ST-segment depression (*left*) or ST-segment elevation (*right*). Changes are similar regardless of the direction of ST-segment shift. Decreases in cardiac index (CI) are accompanied by elevation of systemic vascular resistances in both cases. Changes, however, tend to be more prominent during ST-segment elevation. Abbreviations are given in Figure 5.2.

ischemia present diffuse narrrowing, incomplete occlusion,[94] or complete occlusion with a well-developed collateral circulation.[96,97] Also, they may present occlusion of smaller branches.[45,98] Accordingly, it was recently shown that among patients who present ST-segment depression during coronary balloon occlusion, collaterals are present or better developed than among those with ST-segment elevation.[99] Moreover, ST-segment elevation is highest in patients with totally absent collaterals.[52] In most episodes of angina at rest, ST-segment elevation is not preceded by ST-segment depression,[99] suggesting that as also occurs during positive ergonovine testing or during balloon occlusion,[99] the decrease in regional blood flow is precipitous. Very occasionally, there may be episodes of true myocardial ischemia associated with minimal or absent ECG changes, but with wall motion abnormalities[53,100] or elevated left ventricular end-diastolic pressure. However, most of these episodes without ST-T wave changes are unaccompanied by changes in blood pressure or other hemodynamic parameters[47] and do not respond to nitrites. In addition, most of these patients have normal or near normal coronary angiograms.

Observations During Myocardial Perfusion Studies

With the advent of myocardial scintigraphy it has been possible to substantiate a reduction of perfusion in the ischemic area during painful or painless episodes, whether they occur spontaneously,[77,79,101,102] during ergonovine administration,[45,101,103] or in exercise-induced ischemia.[92,102,103] As mentioned, in patients with ST-segment elevation or normalization of T waves during ischemia, there is good correlation between the ECG location of these changes and that of the area subserved by the stenotic artery.[77,79] Nevertheless, in those with ST-segment depression there is no such ECG-anatomic correlation.[79,102,104] The significance of these perfusion defects in patients with unstable angina, even in the absence of previous myocardial infarction, is often difficult to determine because resting perfusion defects may already be present in up to 40 percent of them[105,106] and may be attributable to delayed perfusion of the poststenotic area.[107] This flow reduction appears to be measurable with 133-xenon whenever the stenosis is severe enough (average 94%), which is frequently associated with local asynergy.[108]

Coronary Blood Flow Measurements

Several investigators have demonstrated that coronary blood flow increases insufficiently during exercise-induced ischemia induced by atrial pacing[109,110] in patients with significant coronary artery stenosis. In contrast, decreases in blood flow were shown duing spontaneous angina or ergonovine-induced ischemia[62,101,111] to be comparable to those observed during transient coronary occlusion produced by transluminal angioplasty.[56] Furthermore, coronary arteriography during spontaneous or even exercise-induced episodes of ischemia has identified a localized or a diffuse coronary spasm.[45,128,112] To date, most of the available observations during spontaneous angina in the catheterization laboratory point to the existence of a primary reduction in blood flow.[60,77,78,101] However, some of the methods used to measure coronary blood flow such as thermodilution may not be sensitive enough to detect relatively small changes. This might explain why MacDonald et al[113] failed to demonstrate changes in flow in a few patients with no apparent increases in myocardial oxygen consumption during angina at rest associated with ST-segment depression.

CLINICAL TYPES OF SPONTANEOUS ANGINA

In contrast to angina induced by active exercise, there are several forms of angina occurring at rest in which apparent provocative mechanisms are not readily identified. We recognize the following: nocturnal angina, postprandial angina, emotional angina, and postinfarction angina. Another variety is angina decubitus, but there is very little information about its incidence, mechanisms, and clinical-angiographic correlates. It will not be discussed herein.

Nocturnal Angina

The few existing reports on pressure[32,41] and cardiac output monitoring during ischemic episodes at night, while the patients are sleeping, demonstrate hemodynamic accompaniments that are identical to those at rest during the day time; however, the overall change is of a lesser magnitude.[41] It has been suggested that recumbency in these patients may favor ischemia by increasing left ventricular filling pressures and thus increasing wall tension at rest.[114] However, nocturnal angina usually occurs several hours after lying in bed, and it also occurs in patients who are bedridden in the hospital for several days.[41] In hospitalized patients with severe coronary artery disease and angina at rest, we found that pulmonary capillary wedge pressure remained unchanged at night during the pain-free intervals; moreover, as in normal subjects,[115,116] blood pressure and heart rate tended to fall.[41] Thus, we found no evidence of changes in resting hemodynamics that would decrease the ischemic threshold at night barring mild decreases in perfusion pressure that may be balanced by decreases in myocardial oxygen needs. More recently, however, we have found that in a significant number of patients, there is indeed a noticeable reduction in the ischemic threshold at night, as tested by atrial pacing.[74] These findings are in line with the higher nocturnal coronary vasoconstrictor sensitivity noted in some patients by ergonovine testing[79] or in selected patients by angiographic demonstration of exercise-induced coronary spasm in the early morning but not later in the day.[79] As a result, it is conceivable that the lower threshold seen at night during atrial pacing may be related to increased coronary tone,[74,117,118] whereas in those with advanced disease, timing is not as specific[123,118] even though it perhaps tended to develop earlier.[74] We have encountered similar findings as well as an early cluster of ischemic crises in the late evening-early night (Figure 5.4) when the patients are still alert.[74] Of interest, some patients experience angina just on awakening, be that in the morning or after an afternoon "nap," which reinforces the role of the autonomic nervous system in the origin of these ischemic attacks by possibly increasing coronary tone in these circumstances. Most patients are unable to recall any triggering element of their nocturnal angina, such as fear, nervousness, or bad dreams.[32,41] Some investigators have reported that in a few patients at least some episodes occur during light sleep associated with rapid eye movement,[119] but others have found no such relation.[120]

Postprandial Angina

This form of angina has long been considered a variety of effort-triggered angina,[121–123] although it has not been fully substantiated. On the contrary, we documented that there are no clearcut increases in the determinants of oxygen consumption during postprandial angina.[124] Typically, angina occurs during the meal or within the first

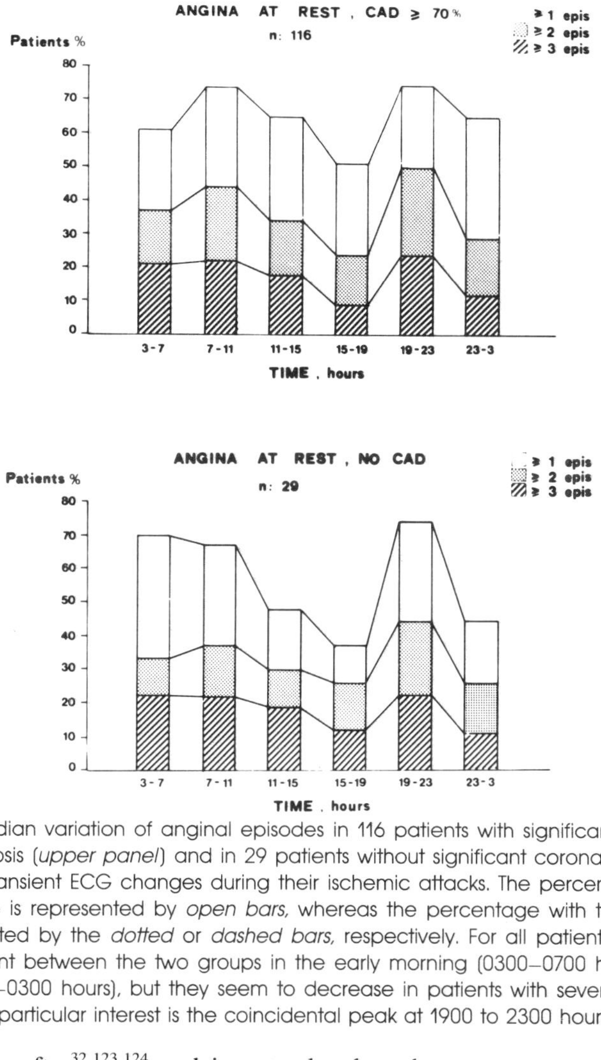

FIGURE 5.4. Circadian variation of anginal episodes in 116 patients with significant and fixed coronary artery stenosis (*upper panel*) and in 29 patients without significant coronary disease (*lower panel*), all with transient ECG changes during their ischemic attacks. The percentage of patients with one episode is represented by *open bars*, whereas the percentage with two or three episodes is represented by the *dotted* or *dashed bars*, respectively. For all patients, the trends are somewhat different between the two groups in the early morning (0300–0700 hours) and in the early night (2300–0300 hours), but they seem to decrease in patients with several episodes in a given interval. Of particular interest is the coincidental peak at 1900 to 2300 hours in both groups.

15 minutes thereafter[32,123,124] and is not related to the amount or type of food ingested;[32,124,125] this finding differs from the time-honored concept that postprandial angina linked to episodes occurring 1 or 2 hours later is (hypothetically) related to increases in circulating triglycerides.[126]

Food ingestion is known to be associated with increases in blood flow to the splanchnic area (diverting some flow from the periphery), increases in cardiac output, and decreases in systemic arterial resistance.[127–129] For instance, 30 minutes after a meal in normal volunteers, there is a modest increase in heart rate (10 beats/min) and cardiac output (0.6 l/min) and a decrease in systemic vascular resistance (4 mm Hg per minute per liter),[180] with no change in blood pressure. In addition, ejection fraction also increases postprandially by approximately 10 percent within the first 15 minutes and 20 percent at 30 minutes.[30] However, because the onset of ischemia is sometimes present within the first few bites of an apple or immediately after drinking a glass of milk, it is improbable that by this time, significant hemodynamic changes have preceded myocardial ischemia. In fact, through continuous hemodynamic recordings, no such changes have been noted before the onset of ischemia[124]

(Figures 5.5 and 5.6). Thus, contrary to the changes that occurred after a meal without angina, namely, an increase in cardiac output and a decrease in systemic vascular resistance with no change in ventricular filling pressure, postprandial angina was associated with the typical features of spontaneous ischemia: an increase in left ventricular filling pressure, a decrease in cardiac output, and an increase in blood pressure.[124] Overall, postprandial angina is associated with a higher heart rate than are spontaneous episodes unrelated to meals.[124] Even though the mechanism responsible for this form of angina remains unknown, it has been speculated that reflex increases in coronary tone may be elicited by the eating process.[130,131] As others,[121,124,132] we found that postprandial angina occurs in patients with particularly extensive coronary disease and almost never develops in patients with nonsignificant coronary disease. In the former group of patients the vasoconstrictor reflex is capable of producing a modest reduction in coronary flow, which becomes critical in patients with severely curtailed coronary reserve.

Angina Precipitated by Emotion

Emotional angina has also been considered a form of myocardial ischemia produced by increases in myocardial oxygen demands[121] secondary to increases in heart rate, blood pressure, and contractility, all due to increases in sympathetic activity. However, this hypothesis is not vindicated by controlled clinical observations. Thus, during the stress of right heart catheterization or insertion of an electrocatheter in pa-

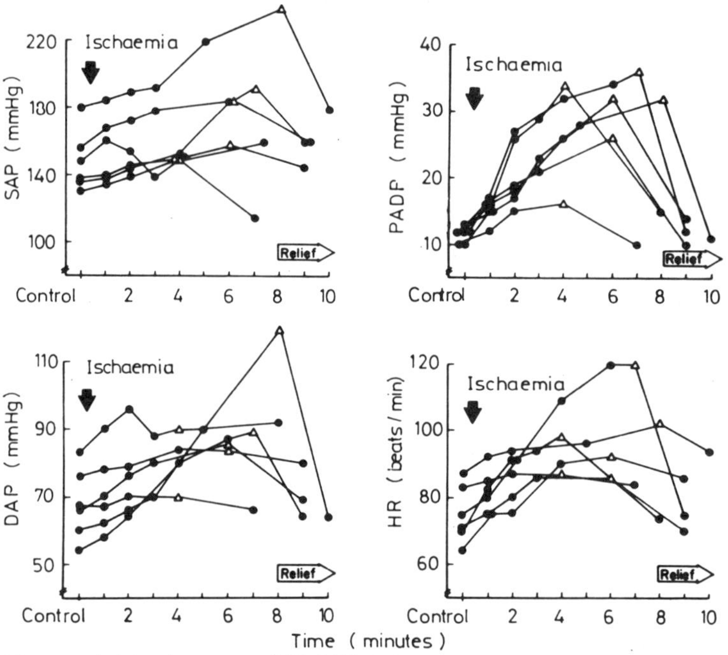

FIGURE 5.5. Changes in blood pressure (SAP, DAP), left ventricular filling pressure (PADP), and heart rate (HR) during postprandial angina in six patients. *Arrow* indicates the onset of ischemia as detected on the ECG, and the *open triangles* signify changes at the peak of pain. As during other episodes of angina at rest, hemodynamic changes are inconsequential at the onset of ischemia. During pain, changes, particularly those in left ventricular filling pressures, are remarkable. In this postprandial state, changes in heart rate tend to be greater than those during anginal attacks unrelated to meals. Abbreviations are given in Figure 5.1.

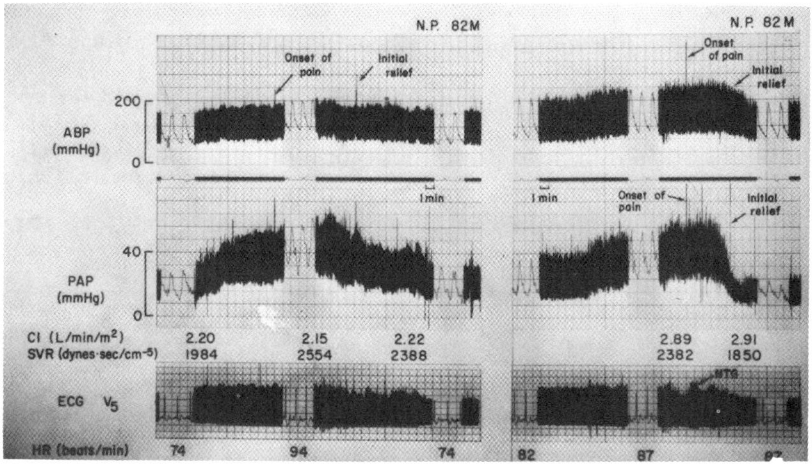

FIGURE 5.6. Hemodynamic changes during continuous pressure and ECG recordings during an episode of spontaneous angina (*right*) in the same patient. Changes are very similar except for the increases in heart rate which are greater during the postprandial episode. Abbreviations are given in Figure 5.2.

tients who present with a history of emotional angina, we consistently found that the double product at the onset of ischemia, during or immediately after the procedure, was only modest and clearly lower than that attained during angina induced by atrial pacing. Likewise, ST-segment depression developing during the stress of a quiz was associated with a lower double product than were equivalent ST-segment changes that developed during exercise.[133] We also noted that these patients demonstrate a high sensitivity to ergonovine, which produces the same ECG changes as those seen during emotionally evoked ischemia. Thus, these findings are consistent with the recently demonstrated coronary vasoconstriction during isometric exercise likely caused by increases in sympathetic tone and plasma catecholamine levels,[134] suggesting that emotional angina; at least in part, may also be related to coronary vasoconstriction in association with the increases in myocardial oxygen demands. In our experience, emotional angina is generally associated with severe coronary stenosis with multivessel involvement.

Postinfarction Angina

Some patients who have experienced acute transmural or nontransmural infarction develop spontaneous angina within the first few days of their hospital course.[135–141] These patients have a higher incidence of two- to three-vessel disease than do those without angina,[139,141] and the hemodynamic changes during the ischemic episodes are similar to all forms of acute myocardial ischemia and are generally associated with hypertension[137] (Figure 5.7). Spontaneous postinfarction angina also seems unrelated to increases in myocardial oxygen demands, because the double product is at most only slightly increased at the beginning of ischemia and is considered much lower during pain than during pacing-induced ischemia, which averages 140 beats per minute.[140] Moreover, some patients do not present ischemia during sustained pacing at 150 beats per minute.[140,141] Moreover, the ECG changes are localized in the same leads during pain as during the acute infarction[135–137] and are identical to those elicited during ergonovine-induced or spontaneous coronary spasm demon-

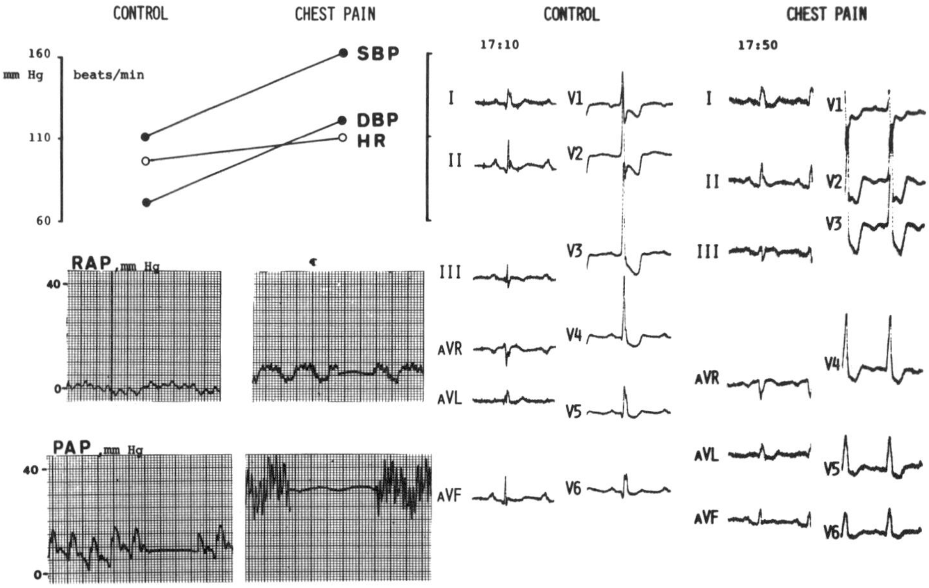

FIGURE 5.7. Changes in systolic (SBP) and diastolic (DBP) blood pressure, heart rate (HR), and right atrial (RAP) and pulmonary artery (PAP) pressures (*left panel*) during an episode of postinfarction angina associated with acute ECG changes (*right panel*). The observed increases in blood pressure and right and left ventricular filling pressure with a small change in heart rate are similar to those observed in other forms of rest angina.

strated angiographically.[142,143] Nevertheless, in some patients some episodes are protracted and poorly responsive to nitroglycerin, suggesting that transient coronary occlusion by platelet aggregates may also play an important role.[137]

SILENT ISCHEMIA

Although the precise incidence of silent ischemia remains controversial, its existence, whether exercise-induced or spontaneous, is now undeniable.[33,41,45,144–150] According to some investigators, more than 70 percent of the ischemic episodes are painless.[45,147,150] It may be difficult, however, to reconcile these figures with the low incidence of silent ischemia during ischemia produced by ergonovine[57,58] or by transient coronary occlusion during balloon angioplasty,[51,52,56] although it may be argued that these episodes are not particularly severe. Indeed, asymptomatic episodes tend to be shorter and less intense[118,151,152] and perhaps affect a smaller area of myocardium than that involved in painful ischemia.[146,153] The hemodynamic changes during painless episodes, probably first reported by Guazzi et al[33] in patients with angina at rest and later confirmed by others,[41,45,55] are identical to those associated with symptomatic attacks, but are of lesser magnitude and duration. In fact, during some episodes of silent ischemia in patients with severe coronary disease, no changes in end-systolic volume or in ejection fraction were detected by Iskandrian and Hakki.[154]

Changes in blood pressure and heart rate during painless ischemia follow the same patterns identified during painful episodes[33,36,41,55] (Figure 5.8). Similarly, they are also associated with the identical ECG changes[33,36,41,55] and occur in patients with significant coronary artery stenosis.[45] Furthermore, silent ischemia may also occur at any time during the day while having a circadian periodicity characteristic of that for heart rate and blood pressure.[155]

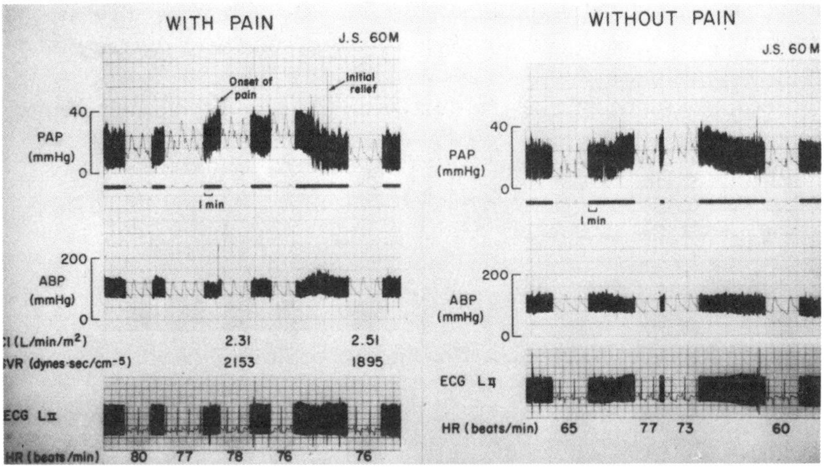

FIGURE 5.8. Hemodynamic changes during an episode of myocardial ischemia associated with pain and one without pain in the same patient. Upper panel shows recordings of pulmonary artery pressure (PA), middle panel arterial blood pressure (ABP) and lower panel the electrocardiogram (ECG). Both the symptomatic and asymptomatic episodes are not preceded by increase in heart rate or blood pressure and the overall changes are similar.

As in painful episodes, asymptomatic ischemia has been associated with angiographically demonstrated coronary spasm and a reduction in coronary blood flow as indirectly inferred from decreases in oxygen content in coronary sinus blood.[55,156] Also, perfusion defects in thallium-201 myocardial scintigrams were documented during painless exercise-induced ST-segment depression,[45,153,157] and changes in regional myocardial uptake of rubidium-82 using positron emission tomography have also been reported.[158]

SUMMARY AND CONCLUSIONS

During acute myocardial ischemia in man a distinct pattern of hemodynamic changes occurs which is similar to those observed in the experimental animal. The sequence of ECG and regional as well as global ventricular functional alterations indicates that mechanical changes are unquestionably the first to develop and are reflected in increases in ventricular filling pressures and reduced stroke volume. Clinically, these changes are associated with changes, mostly increases in blood pressure and heart rate, which are small and less consistent during spontaneous ischemia. Drug-induced hypertension has repeatedly failed to produce ischemia at levels of blood pressure achieved during angina at rest. Likewise, increases in heart rate by atrial pacing have also been unsuccessful in producing ischemia at the levels of double product attained during spontaneous attacks in most circumstances.

The patterns of hemodynamic changes are common to the different forms of angina at rest, namely, spontaneous, nocturnal, postprandial, emotional, and postinfarctional; they are also similar in exercise-induced angina although these increases in blood pressure may be modified by concomitant changes in catecholamine levels and systemic vascular resistance. Silent ischemia presents with the same hemodynamic accompaniments, but the overall changes are less striking and of shorter duration than those in symptomatic ischemia. In general, hemodynamic changes are independent of ECG changes. The site of ischemia in a few patients, particularly those with severe transmural inferior ischemia, may influence the pattern of hemodynamic changes. Finally, myocardial perfusion defects have been consistently detected during painful and painless episodes, and decreases in coronary blood flow have also been appreciated in both forms of transient ischemia. A study of the temporal sequence of hemodynamic and functional changes accompanying episodes of silent and symptomatic ischemia provides an insight into the underlying mechanisms and the nature of the imbalance of oxygen supply and demand in the myocardium. An understanding of the pathophysiologic mechanisms forms a rational basis for the therapy of myocardial ischemia.

REFERENCES

1. Tennant R, Wiggers CJ: The effect of coronary occlusion on myocardial contraction. *Am J Physiol* 1935;112:351–361.
2. Prinzmetal M, Schwartz LL, Corday E, Spritzler R, Bergman HC, Kruger HE: Studies on the coronary circulation. *VI Ann Intern Med* 1949;31:429–442.
3. Katz AM: Effects of interrupted coronary flow upon myocardial metabolism and contractility. *Prog Cardiovasc Dis* 1968;10:450–465.
4. Swan HJC, Forrester JS, Diamond G, Chatterjee K, Parmley WW: Hemodynamic spectrum of myocardial infarction and cardiogenic shock. A conceptual model. *Circulation* 1972;45:1097–1110.
5. Amsterdam EA: Function of the hypoxic myocardium. Experimental and clinical aspects *Am J Cardiol* 1973;32:461–471.
6. Kronenberg MW, Bron ML, Smith CW, Brorson L, Collins JC, Higgins SB, Vaughn WK, Rollo FD, Friesinger GC: Comparison of radionuclide and contrast ventriculography for detection and quantification of regions of myocardial ischemia in dogs. *J Clin Invest* 1981;67:1370–1381.
7. Rackley CE, Russell RO Jr, Mantle JA, Rogers WJ: Modern approach to the patients with acute myocardial infarction. *Curr Prob Cardiol* 1977;1:49–80.
8. Brown AM: Excitation of afferent cardiac sympathetic nerve fibers during myocardial ischemia. *J Physiol* 1967;190:35–45.
9. Malliani A, Schwartz PJ, Zanchetti A: A sympathetic reflex elicited by experimental coronary occlusion. *Am J Physiol* 1969;217:703–712.
10. Malmborg, RO: A clinical and hemodynamic analysis of factors limiting the cardiac performance in patients with coronary heart disease. *Acta Med Scand* 1965;177:426–438.
11. Parker JO, DiGiorgi S, West RO: A hemodynamic study of acute coronary insufficiency precipitated by exercise: with observations on the effect of nitroglycerin. *Am J Cardiol* 1966;17:470–483.
12. Weiner L, Dwyer EM, Cox JW: Left ventricular hemodynamics in exercise induced angina pectoris. *Circulation* 1968;38:240–249.
13. Lichtlen P: The hemodynamics of clinical ischemic heart disease. *Ann Clin Res* 1968;3:333–339.
14. Saltups A, McCallister BD, Hallermann FJ, Wallace RB, Smith RE, Frye RL: Left ventricular hemodynamics in patients with coronary artery disease and in normal subjects. Correlation with the extent of coronary artery lesions and the electrocardiogram. *Am J Med* 1971;50:8–19.
15. Upton MT, Rerych SK, Newman GE, Port S, Cobb FR, Jones RH: Detecting abnormalities in left ventricular function during exercise before angina and ST-segment depression. *Circulation* 1980;62:341–349.
16. Levy RD, Shapiro LM, Wright C, Mockus L, Fox K: Hemodynamic response to myocardial ischaemia during unrestricted activity, exercise testing, and atrial pacing assessed by ambulatory pulmonary artery pressure monitoring. *Br Heart J* 1986;56:12–18.
17. Thadani U, West RO, Mathew TM, Parker JO: Hemodynamics at rest and during sitting bicycle exercise in patients with coronary artery disease. *Am J Cardiol* 1977;39:776–783.
18. Currie PJ, Kelly MJ, Pitt A: Comparison of supine and erect bicycle exercise electro-

cardiography in coronary heart disease: Accentuation of exercise-induced ST depression by supine posture. *Am J Cardiol* 1983;52:1167–1173.
19. Holmgren A, Ovenfors CO: Heart volume at rest and during muscular work in the supine and the sitting position. *Acta Med Scand* 1960;167:267–274.
20. Poliner LR, Dehmer GJ, Lewis SE, Parkey RW, Blomqvist CG, Willerson JT: Left ventricular performance in normal subjects. *Circulation* 1980;62:528–534.
21. Freeman MR, Berman DS, Staniloff H, Elkayam U, Maddahi J, Swan HJC, Forrester JS: Comparison of upright and supine bicycle exercise in the detection and evaluation of extent of coronary artery disease by equilibrium radionuclide ventriculography. *Am Heart J* 1981;102:182–189.
22. Manyari DE, Kostuk WJ, Purves PP: Left and right ventricular function at rest and during bicycle exercise in the supine and sitting positions in normal subjects and in patients with coronary artery disease: Assessment by radionuclide ventriculography. *Am J Cardiol* 1983;51:36–42.
23. Parker JO, Ledwich JR, West RO, Case RB: Reversible cardiac failure during angina pectoris: Hemodynamic effects of atrial pacing in coronary artery disease. *Circulation* 1969;39:745–753.
24. Dwyer EM: Left ventricular pressure-volume alterations and regional disorders of contraction during myocardial ischemia induced by atrial pacing. *Circulation* 1970;42:111–119.
25. Pasternac A, Gorlin R, Sonnenblick EH: Abnormalities of ventricular motion induced by atrial pacing in coronary disease. *Circulation* 1972;45:1195–1205.
26. McLaurin LP, Rolett EL, Grossman W: Impaired left ventricular relaxation during pacing induced ischemia. *Am J Cardiol* 1973;32:51–59.
27. Mann T, Brodie BR, Grossman W, McLaurin LP: Effect of angina on the left ventricular diastolic pressure-volume relationship. *Circulation* 1977;55:761–766.
28. Barry WH, Brooker JZ, Alderman EL, Harrison DC: Changes in diastolic stiffness and tone of the left ventricle during angina pectoris. *Circulation* 1974;49:255–263.
29. Muller O, Rorvik K: Hemodynamic consequences of coronary heart disease with observations during anginal pain and on the effect of nitroglycerine. *Br Heart J* 1958;20:302–310.
30. Johnson JB, Fairley A, Carter C: Effects of sublingual nitroglycerin on pulmonary arterial pressure in patients with left ventricular failure. *Ann Intern Med* 1959;50:34–42.
31. Roughgarden JW, Newman EV: Circulatory changes during the pain of angina pectoris. *Am J Med* 1966;41:935–946.
32. Roughgarden JW: Circulatory changes associated with spontaneous angina pectoris. *Am J Med* 1966;41:947–961.
33. Guazzi M, Polese A, Fiorentini C, Magrini F, Bartorelli C: Left ventricular hemodynamic changes in Prinzmetal's variant angina pectoris. *Br Heart J* 1971;33:84–94.
34. Lecerof H: Central hemodynamics during spontaneous angina pectoris. *Br Heart J* 1974;36:1087–1091.
35. Cannom DS, Harrison DC, Schroeder JS: Hemodynamic observations in patients with unstable angina pectoris. *Am J Cardiol* 1974;33:17–22.
36. Guazzi M, Polese A, Fiorentini C, Magrini F, Olivari M, Bartorelli C: Left and right heart hemodynamics during spontaneous angina pectoris. Comparison between angina with ST segment depression and angina with ST segment elevation. *Br Heart J* 1975;37:401–413.
37. Maseri A, Mimmo R, Chierchia S, Marchesi C, Pesola A, L'Abbate A: Coronary artery spasm as a cause of acute myocardial ischemia in man. *Chest* 1975;68:625–633.
38. Gaasch WH, Adyanthaya AV, Pickering E, Quinones MA, Alexander JK: Prinzmetal's variant angina: Hemodynamic and angiographic observations during pain. *Am J Cardiol* 1975;35:683–690.
39. Scheidt S, Wolk M, Killip T: Unstable angina pectoris. Natural history, hemodynamics, uncertainties of treatment and the ethics of clinical study. *Am J Med* 1976;60:409–417.
40. Berndt TB, Fitzgerald J, Harrison DC, Schroeder JS: Hemodynamic changes at the onset of spontaneous versus pacing-induced angina. *Am J Cardiol* 1977;39:784–788.
41. Figueras J, Singh BN, Ganz W, Charuzi Y, Swan HJC: Mechanism of rest and nocturnal angina: Observations during continuous hemodynamic and electrocardiographic monitoring. *Circulation* 1979;59:955–968.

42. Sharma B, Hodges M, Asinger RW, Goodwin JF, Francis GS, Garner L: Left ventricular function during spontaneous angina pectoris: Effect of sublingual nitroglycerin. *Am J Cardiol* 1980;46:34–41.
43. Rosland GA: Hemodynamic observations during spontaneous angina pectoris. *Br Heart J* 1969;31:523–525.
44. Marzullo P, Parodi O, Schelbert HR, L'Abbate A: Regional myocardial dysfunction in patients with angina at rest and response to isosorbide dinitrate assessed by phase analysis of radionuclide ventriculogram. *J Am Coll Cardiol* 1984;3:1357–1366.
45. Maseri A, Severi S, DeNes M, L'Abbate A, Chierchia S, Marzilli M, Ballestra AM, Parodi O, Biagini A, Distante A: "Variant angina": One aspect of a continuous spectrum of vasospastic myocardial ischemia. *Am J Cardiol* 1978;42:1019–1035.
46. Sharma B, Behrens TW, Erlein TW, Hodges M, Asinger RW, Francis GS: Left ventricular diastolic properties and filling characteristics during spontaneous angina at rest. *Am J Cardiol* 1984;52:704–709.
47. Mann T, Goldberg S, Mudge GH Jr, Grossman W: Factors contributing to altered left ventricular diastolic properties during angina pectoris. *Circulation* 1979;55:14–20.
48. Spotnitz HM, Sonnenblick EM: Structural condition in the hypertrophied and failing heart. *Am J Cardiol* 1973;32:398–405.
49. Grossman W, McLaurin LP, Stefadouros MA: Left ventricular stiffness associated with chronic pressure and volume overloads. *Circ Res* 1974;35:793–800.
50. Ahn J, Apstein CS, Hood WB Jr: Contractile properties of the left ventricle: Direct effect of coronary artery perfusion pressure on diastolic wall stiffness and thickness (Abstract). *Clin Res* 1977;25:201A.
51. Serruys PW, Wijns W, Vanden Brand M, Meij S, Slager C, Schuurbiers JCH, Hugenholtz PG, Brower RW: Left ventricular performance, regional blood flow, wall motion, and lactate metabolism during transluminal angioplasty. *Circulation* 1984;70:25–36.
52. Cohen M, Rentrop P: Limitation of myocardial ischemia by collateral circulation during sudden controlled coronary artery occlusion in human subjects: A prospective study. *Circulation* 1986;74:469–476.
53. Hauser AM, Gangadharan V, Ramos RG, Gordon S, Timmis GC, Dudlets P: Sequence of mechanical, electrocardiographic and clinical effects of repeated coronary artery occlusion in human beings: Echocardiographic observations during coronary angioplasty. *J Am Coll Cardiol* 1985;5:193–197.
54. Distante A, Picano E, Moscarelli E, Palombo C, Benassi A, L'Abbate A: Echocardiographic versus hemodynamic monitoring during attacks of variant angina pectoris. *Am J Cardiol* 1985;55:1319–1322.
55. Chierchia S, Brunelli C, Simonetti I, Lazzari M, Maseri A: Sequence of events in angina at rest: Primary reduction in coronary flow. *Circulation* 1980;61:759–768.
56. Feldman RL, Conti CR, Pepine CJ: Regional coronary venous flow responses to transient coronary artery occlusion in human beings. *J Am Coll Cardiol* 1983;2:1–10.
57. Curry RC, Pepine CJ, Sabom MB, Feldman RL, Christie LG, Conti CR: Effects of ergonovine in patients with and without coronary artery disease. *Circulation* 1977;56–803–809.
58. Waters DD, Theroux P, Szalachcic S, Dauwe F, Crittin J, Bonan R, Mizgala HF: Ergonovine testing in a Coronary Care Unit. *Am J Cardiol* 1980;46:922–930.
59. Specchia G, Bramucci E, Angoli L, DeServi S, Mussini A, Marinoni GP, Ray M: Spontaneous and provoked coronary artery spasm: Are they the same? *Eur J Cardiol* 1978;8:581–588.
60. Feldman RL, Curry RC Jr, Pepine CJ, Mehta J, Conti CR: Regional coronary hemodynamic effect of ergonovine in patients with and without variant angina. *Circulation* 1980;62:149–159.
61. Figueras J, Cinca J: Acute arterial hypertension during spontaneous angina in patients with fixed coronary stenosis and exertional angina: An associated rather than a triggering phenomenon. *Circulation* 1981;64:60–68.
62. Figueras J, Cinca J, Guttierrez L, Segura R, Rius J: Prolonged angina pectoris and persistent negative T waves in the precordial leads: Response to atrial pacing and to methoxamine-induced hypertension. *Am J Cardiol* 1983;51:1599–1607.

63. Loeb HS, Saudye A, Croke RP, Talano JV, Klodnycky ML, Gunnar RM: Effects of pharmacologically-induced hypertension on myocardial ischemia and coronary hemodynamics in patients with fixed coronary obstruction. *Circulation* 1978;57:41–46.
64. Davies AB, Subramaniam VB, Cashman PMM, Raftery EB: Simultaneous recording of continuous arterial pressure, heart rate, and ST-segment in ambulatory patients with stable angina pectoris. *Br Heart J* 1983;50:85–91.
65. Staszewska-Barczak J: The reflex stimulation of catecholamine secretion during the acute stage of myocardial infarction in the dog. *Clin Sci* 1971;41:419–429.
66. Karlsberg RP, Penikoske PA, Cryer P, Corr PB, Roberts R: Rapid activation of the sympathetic nervous system following coronary artery occlusion: Relationship to infarct size, site and hemodynamic impact. *Cardiovasc Res* 1979;13:523–531.
67. Felder RB, Thames MD: The cardiogenic sympathetic reflex during coronary occlusion in anesthetized dogs. *Circ Res* 1981;48:685–692.
68. Gorlin R: Pathophysiology of cardiac pain. *Circulation* 1965;32:138–148.
69. Yasue H, Touyama M, Kato H, Tanaka S, Akiyama F: Prinzmetal's variant form of angina as a manifestation of alpha adrenergic receptor-mediated coronary spasm: Documentation by coronary arteriography. *Am Heart J* 1976;91:148–155.
70. Webb SA, Adgey AAJ, Pantridge JF: Autonomic disturbances at onset of acute myocardial infarction. *Br Med J* 1972;3:89–92.
71. Mark AL: The Bezold-Jarisch reflex revisited: Clinical implications of inhibitory reflexes originating in the heart. *J Am Coll Cardiol* 1983;1:90–102.
72. Perez-Gomez F, Martin de Dios R, Rey J, Aguado AG: Prinzmetal's angina reflex cardiovascular response during episode of pain. *Br Heart J* 1979;42:81–87.
73. Araki H, Anan T, Koiwaya Y, Nakagaki O, Takeshita A, Nakamura M: Reflex heart rate and blood pressure during ST-segment elevation in patients with variant angina. *Am Heart J* 1984;108:1273–1278.
74. Figueras J, Cinca J, Balda F, Moya A, Rius J: Resting angina with fixed coronary artery stenosis: Nocturnal decline in ischemic threshold. *Circulation* 1986;74:1248–1254.
75. Quyyumi AA, Mockus LJ, Wright CA, Fox KM: Mechanisms of nocturnal angina pectoris: Importance of increased myocardial oxygen demands in patients with severe coronary artery disease. *Lancet* 1984;2:1207–1209.
76. Papapietro SE, Niess GS, Paine TD, Mantle JA, Rackley CE, Russell RO Jr, Rogers WJ: Transient electrocardiographic changes in patients with unstable angina: Relation to coronary arterial anatomy. *Am J Cardiol* 1980;46:28–33.
77. Maseri A, Parodi O, Severi S, Pesola A: Transient transmural reduction of myocardial blood flow demonstrated by thallium-201 scintigraphy as a cause of variant angina. *Circulation* 1976;54:280–288.
78. Yasue H, Omote S, Takizawa A, Nagao H, Miwa K, Tanaka S: Circadian variation of exercise capacity in patients with Prinzmetal's variant angina: Role of exercise-induced coronary artery spasm. *Circulation* 1979;59:938–948.
79. Parodi O, Uthurralt N, Severi S, Bencivelli W, Michelassi C, L'Abbate A, Maseri A: Transient reduction of regional myocardial perfusion during angina at rest with ST-segment depression or normalization of negative T waves. *Circulation* 1981;63:1238–1247.
80. Miwa K, Murakami H, Kambara H, Kawai C: U wave inversion during attacks of variant angina. *Br Heart J* 1983;50:378–382.
81. McAlpin RN: Correlation of location of coronary arterial spasm with the lead distribution of ST-segment elevation during variant angina. *Am Heart J* 1980;99:55–64.
82. DeServi S, Ghio S, Ferraro M, Ardission D, Angoli L, Mussini A, Bramucci E, Salerno J, Vigano M, Montemartini C, Specchia G: Clinical and angiographic findings in angina at rest. *Am Heart J* 1986;111:6–11.
83. Marzilli M, Goldstein S, Trivelli M, Palumbo C, Maseri A: Some clinical considerations regarding the relation of coronary vasospasm to coronary atherosclerosis; A hypothetical pathogenesis. *Am J Cardiol* 1980;45:882–886.
84. Leclerq JF, LaValle JP, Mague C, Bouvrain Y: Correlation between angiographic and ECG signs location in unstable angina. *Eur J Cardiol* 1979;9:181–189.
85. Sclarovsky S, Davidson E, Strasberg B, Lewin RF, Arditti A, Wurtzael M, Agmon J: Unstable angina: The significance of ST-segment elevation or depression in patients

without evidence of increased myocardial oxygen demand. *Am Heart J* 1986;112:463–467.
86. Fischl SJ, Herman MV, Gorlin R: The intermediate coronary syndrome. Clinical angiographic and therapeutic aspects. *N Engl J Med* 1973;288:1193–1198.
87. MacAlpin R: Coronary spasm as a cause of angina. *N Engl J Med* 1973;288:788–789.
88. Higgins CB, Wexler L, Silverman JF, Schroeder JS: Clinical and arteriographic features of Prinzmetal's variant angina: Documentation of etiologic factors. *Am J Cardiol* 1976;37:831–839.
89. Bott-Silverman C, Heupler FA Jr, Yiannikas J: Variant angina: Comparison of patients with and without fixed severe coronary artery disease. *Am J Cardiol* 1984;54:1173–1175.
90. Fortuin NJ, Friesinger GC: Exercise-induced ST-segment elevation: Clinical, electrocardiographic and arteriographic studies in twelve patients. *Am J Med* 1970;49:459–466.
91. Longhurst JC, Kraus WL: Exercise-induced ST elevation in patients without myocardial infarction. *Circulation* 1976;60:616–629.
92. Dunn RF, Bailey IK, Uren R, Kelly DT: Exercise-induced ST-segment elevation: Correlation of thallium-201 myocardial perfusion scanning and coronary arteriography. *Circulation* 1980;61:989–995.
93. Waters DD, Chaitman BR, Bourassa MG, Tubau JF: Clinical and angiographic correlates of exercise-induced ST-segment elevation: Increased detection with multiple ECG leads. *Circulation* 1980;61:286–296.
94. Yasue H, Omote S, Takizawa A, Masao N, Hyon H, Nishida S, Horie M: Comparison of coronary arteriographic findings during angina pectoris associated with ST elevation or depression. *Am J Cardiol* 1981;47:539–546.
95. Fuchs RM, Achuff SC, Grunwald L, Yin FCP, Griffith LSC: Electrocardiographic localization in patients with one vessel disease. *Circulation* 1982;66:1168–1176.
96. DeServi S, Specchia G, Ardissino D, Falcone C, Mussini A, Angoli L, Bramucci E, Marinoni GP, Gavazzi A, Bobba P: Angiographic demonstration of different pathogenetic mechanisms in patients with spontaneous and exertional angina associated with ST-segment depression. *Am J Cardiol* 1980;45:1285–1291.
97. Tada M, Yamagishi M, Kodama K, Kuzuya T, Nanto S, Inoue M, Abe H: Transient collateral augmentation during coronary arterial spasm associated with ST-segment depression. *Circulation* 1983;67:693–698.
98. DeServi S, Specchia G, Angoli L: Coronary artery spasm of different degree as cause of angina at rest with ST-segment depression and elevation. *Br Heart J* 1979;42:110–112.
99. Macdonald RG, Hill JA, Feldman RL: ST-segment response to acute coronary occlusion: Coronary hemodynamic and angiographic determinants of direction of ST-segment shift. *Circulation* 1986;74:973–979.
100. Rovai D, Distante A, Moscarelli E, Morales M, Picano E, Palombo C, L'Abbate A: Transient myocardial ischemia with minimal electrocardiographic changes: An echocardiographic study in patients with Prinzmetal's angina. *Am Heart J* 1985;109:78–83.
101. Ricci DR, Orlick AE, Doherty PW, Cipriano PR, Harrison DC: Reduction of coronary blood flow during coronary artery spasm occurring spontaneously and after provocation by ergonovine maleate. *Circulation* 1978;57:392–395.
102. Uthurralt N, Davies GJ, Parodi O, Benivelli W, Maseri A: Comparative study of myocardial ischemia during angina at rest and on exertion using thallium-201 scintigraphy. *Am J Cardiol* 1981;48:410–417.
103. McLaughlin PR, Doherty PW, Martin RO, Goris ML, Harrison DC: Myocardial imaging in a patient with reproducible variant angina. *Am J Cardiol* 1977;39:126–129.
104. Fox RM, Hakki A, Iskandrian AS, Hackney J: Relation between electrocardiographic and scintigraphic location of myocardial ischemia during exercise in one-vessel coronary artery disease. *Am J Cardiol* 1984;53:1529–1531.
105. Wackers FJT, Lie KI, Liem KL, Sokole EM, Samson G, Vander Schoot JB, Durrer D: Thallium-201 scintigraphy in unstable angina pectoris. *Circulation* 1978;57:738–744.
106. Hakki A, Iskandrian A, Kane S, Amenta A: Thallium-201 myocardial scintigraphy and left ventricular function at rest in patients with rest angina pectoris. *Am Heart J* 1984;108:326–332.

107. Gewirtz H, Beller GA, Strauss HW, Dinsmore RE, Ziz LM, McKusick KA, Pohost GM: Transient defects of resting thallium scans in patients with coronary artery disease. *Circulation* 1979;59:707–713.
108. Nichols AB, Brown C, Han J, Nikoloff EL, Esser PD: Effect of coronary stenotic lesions on regional myocardial blood flow at rest. *Circulation* 1986;74:746–757.
109. Schmidt DH, Weiss MB, Casarella WJ, Fowler DL, Sciacca RR, Cannon PJ: Regional myocardial perfusion changes induced by atrial pacing in patients with coronary artery disease. *Circulation* 1976;53:807–819.
110. Maseri A, L'Abbate A, Pesola A, Michelassi C, Marzilli M, DeNes M: Regional myocardial perfusion during atrial pacing in patients with atherosclerotic coronary artery disease, at rest, and during angina pectoris induced by tachycardia. *Circulation* 1977;55:423–433.
111. Goldeberg S, Lam W, Mudge G, Green LH, Kushner F, Hirshfeld JW, Kastor JA: Coronary hemodynamic and myocardial metabolic alterations accompanying coronary spasm. *Am J Cardiol* 1979;43:481–487.
112. Dhurandar RW, Watt DL, Silver MD, Trimble AS, Adelman AG: Prinzmetal's variant form of angina with arteriographic evidence of coronary arterial spasm. *Am J Cardiol* 1972;30:902–905.
113. Macdonald RG, Feldman RL, Hill JA, Conti CR, Pepine CJ: Coronary hemodynamic response during spontaneous angina in patients with and patients without coronary artery spasm. *Am J Cardiol* 1985;56:41–46.
114. Levy RD, Cunningham D, Shapiro LM, Wright C, Mockus L, Fox K: Diurnal variation in left ventricular function: A study of patients with myocardial ischemia, syndrome X and or normal controls. *Br Heart J* 1987;57:148–153.
115. Messerli FH, Glade LB, Ventura HO, Dreslisnki GR, Suarez DH, MacPhee AA, Aristimuno GG, Cole FE, Frohlich ED: Diurnal variation of cardiac rhythm arterial pressure and urinary catecholamines in borderline and established hypertension. *Am Heart J* 1982;104:109–114.
116. Weber MA, Drayer JIM, Nakamura DK, Wyle FA: The circadian blood pressure pattern in ambulatory normal subjects. *Am J Cardiol* 1984;54:115–119.
117. Araki H, Koiwaya Y, Nakagaki O, Nakamura M: Diurnal distribution of ST-segment elevation and related arrhythmias in patients with variant angina: A study by ambulatory ECG monitoring. *Circulation* 1983;67:995–1000.
118. Mattiolo G, Cioni G, Andreoli C: Time sequence of anginal pain. *Clin Cardiol* 1986;9:165–169.
119. Quyyumi AA, Ethimou J, Quyyumi A, Mockus LJ, Spiro SG, Fox K: Nocturnal angina: Precipitating factors in patients with coronary artery disease and in those with variant angina. *Br Heart J* 1986;56:346–352.
120. Karacon I, Williams RY, Taylor WJ: Sleep characteristics of patients with angina pectoris. *Psychosomatics* 1969;10;280–289.
121. Friedberg CK: *Diseases of the Heart*, Philadelphia and London, WB Saunders, 1966, p 712.
122. Vatner SF, Franklin D, Van Citters RL: Coronary and visceral vasoactivity associated with eating and digesting in the conscious dog. *Am J Physiol* 1970;219:1380–1385.
123. Goldstein RE, Redwood DR, Rosing DR, Beiser GD, Epstein SE: Alterations in the circulatory response to exercise following a meal and their relationship to postprandial angina pectoris. *Circulation* 1971;44:90–100.
124. Figueras J, Singh BN, Ganz W, Swan HJC: Hemodynamic and electrocardiographic accompaniments of resting postprandial angina. *Br Heart J* 1979;43:402–409.
125. Klakeg CH, Pruitt RD; Burchell HB: A study of electrocardiogram recorded during exercise tests on subjects in the fasting state and after the ingestion of a heavy meal. *Am Heart J* 1955;49:614–625.
126. Kuo PT, Joyner CR Jr: Angina pectoris induced by fat ingestion in patients with coronary artery disease. Ballistocardiographic and electrocardiographic findings. *JAMA* 1955;158:1008–1013.
127. Abramson DI, Fierst SM: Peripheral vascular changes in man during digestion. *Am J Physiol* 1941;133:686–693.
128. Reininger EJ, Sapirstein LA: Effect of digestion on the distribution of blood flow in the rat. *Science* 1957;126:1176.

129. Fagan TC, Sawyer PR, Gourley LA, Lee JT, Gaffney TE: Postprandial alterations in hemodynamics and blood pressure in normal subjects. *Am J Cardiol* 1986;58:636–641.
130. Brown JM, White CJ, Sobol SM, Lull RaJ: Increased left ventricular ejection fraction after a meal: Potential source of error in performance of radionuclide angiography. *Am J Cardiol* 1983;51:1709–1711.
131. Gilbert NC, Fenn GK, Le Roy GV: The effect of distension of abdominal viscera on the coronary blood flow and on angina pectoris. *JAMA* 1940;115:1962–1967.
132. Morrison LM, Swalm WA: Role of gastrointestinal tract in production of cardiac symptoms. *JAMA* 1940;114:217–223.
133. Cohen LS, Elliott WC, Klein MD, Gorlin R: Coronary heart disease: Clinical cinearteriographic and metabolic correlations. *Am J Cardiol* 1966;17:153–168.
134. Brown BG, Lee AB, Bolson EL, Dodge HT: Reflex constriction of significant coronary stenosis as a mechanism contributing to ischemic left ventricular dysfunction during isometric exercise. *Circulation* 1984;70:18–24.
135. Schiffer F, Hartley LH, Schulman CL, Abelman WH: Evidence for emotionally induced coronary arterial spasm in patients with angina pectoris. *Br Heart J* 1980;44:62–66.
136. Stenson RE, Flamm MD Jr, Zaret BL, McGowan RL: Transient ST-segment elevation with postmyocardial infarction angina: Prognostic significance. *Am Heart J* 1975;89:449–454.
137. Marmor A, Sobel BE, Roberts R: Factors presaging early recurrent myocardial infarction ("extension"). *Am J Cardiol* 1981;48:603–610.
138. Figueras J, Cinca J, Valle V, Rius J: Prognostic implications of early spontaneous angina after acute transmural myocardial infarction. *Int J Cardiol* 1983;4:261–272.
139. Bosch X, Theroux P, Waters DD, Pelletier GB, Roy D: Early postinfarction ischemia: Clinical, angiographic, and prognostic significance. *Circulation* 1987;75:988–995.
140. Figueras J, Cinca J, Santana L, Rius J: Peri-infarction zone at risk during the first 5 days after an acute myocardial infarction: Electrocardiographic evidence. *Am J Cardiol* 1984;53:433–438.
141. Figueras J, Candell J, Cinca J, Segura R, Ortega D, Angel J, Rius J: Risk of myocardium adjacent to infarcted myocardium: Electrocardiographic, metabolic and scintigraphic evidence within the first week of acute myocardial infarction. *Am J Cardiol* 1986;57:1034–1040.
142. Koiwaya Y, Torii S, Takeshita A, Nakagaki O, Nakamura M: Postinfarction angina caused by coronary arterial spasm. *Circulation* 1982;65:275–280.
143. Moran TJ, French WJ, Abrams HF, Criley JM: Postmyocardial infarction angina and coronary spasm. *Am J Cardiol* 1982;50:197–202.
144. Gettes LS: Painless myocardial ischemia. *Chest* 1974;66:612–613.
145. Cohn PF: Severe asymptomatic coronary artery disease. A diagnostic, prognostic and therapeutic puzzle. *Am J Med* 1977;62:565–568.
146. Cole JP, Ellestad MH: Significance of chest pain during treadmill exercise: Correlation with coronary events. *Am J Cardiol* 1978;41:227–232.
147. Schang SJ Jr, Pepine CJ: Transient asymptomatic ST-segment depression during daily activity. *Am J Cardiol* 1977;39:396–402.
148. Stern S, Tzivoni D: Dynamic changes in the ST-T segment during sleep ischemic heart disease. *Am J Cardiol* 1973;32:17–20.
149. Cecchio AC, Dovellini EV, Marchi F, Pucc P, Santoro GM, Faccini PF: Silent myocardial ischemia during ambulatory electrocardiographic monitoring in patients with effort angina. *J Am Coll Cardiol* 1983;1:934–939.
150. Singh BN, Nademanee K, Figueras J, Josephson MA: Hemodynamic and electrocardiographic correlates of symptomatic and silent ischemia: Pathophysiologic and therapeutic implications. *Am J Cardiol* 1986;58:3B–10B.
151. Chierchia S, Lazzari M, Freedman B, Brunelli C, Maseri A: Impairment of myocardial perfusion and function during painless myocardial ischemia. *J Am Coll Cardiol* 1983;1:924–930.
152. Carboni GP, Lahiri A, Cashman PM, Raftery EB: Ambulatory heart rate and ST-segment depression during painful and silent myocardial ischemia in chronic stable angina. *Am J Cardiol* 1987;59:1029–1034.
153. Reisman S, Berman DS, Maddahi J, Swan HJC: Silent myocardial ischemia during

treadmill exercise: Thallium scintigraphic and angiographic correlates, (Abstract). *J Am Coll Cardiol* 1985;5:406.

154. Iskandrian AS, Hakki A: Left ventricular function in patients with coronary heart disease in the presence or absence of angina pectoris during exercise radionuclide ventriculography. *Am J Cardiol* 1984;53:1239–1243.
155. Rocco MB, Barry J, Campbell D, Nabel E, Cook EF, Goldman L, Selwyn AP: Circadian variation of transient myocardial ischemia in patients with coronary artery disease. *Circulation* 1987;75:395–400.
156. Biagini A, Mazzei MG, Carpeggani C, Testa R, Antonelli R, Michelassi C, L'Abbate A, Maseri A: Vasospastic ischemic mechanism of frequent asymptomatic transient ST-T changes during continuous electrocardiographic monitoring in selected unstable angina patients. *Am Heart J* 1982;103:13–20.
157. Bailey IK, Griffith LSC, Rouleau J, Strauss HW, Pitt B: Thallium-201 myocardial perfusion imaging at rest and during exercise. Comparative sensitivity to electrocardiography in coronary artery disease. *Circulation* 1977;55:79–87.
158. Deanfield JE, Shea M, Ribiero P, de Landsheere CM, Wilson RA, Horlock P, Selwyn AP: Transient ST-segment depression as a marker of myocardial ischemia during daily life. *Am J Cardiol* 1984;54:1195–1200.

CHAPTER 6

Circadian Rhythms and Ischemic Heart Disease with Particular Reference to Transient Myocardial Ischemia

Michael B. Rocco, MD and Andrew P. Selwyn, MD

Circadian rhythms are cyclic variations that form repetitive patterns over 24-hour periods. The presence of such patterns in biologic systems has been reported for centuries. However, only in the past two decades have a large variety of biologic rhythms and their potential association with cardiovascular disease processes been described. The temporal patterns of the clinical manifestations of coronary artery disease may be influenced by many of the normal biologic periodicities observed in humans (Table 6.1). Plasma cortisol is known to peak at the time of wakening.[1] Plasma catecholamine levels increase during early morning hours after rising.[2] This heightened sympathetic activity may influence cardiovascular function. Heart rate and systolic and diastolic blood pressures are known to increase in the early morning hours and peak in the mid-morning.[3] Indeed, when blood pressure is recorded in the time before and after rising, it can be shown that the major increase occurs abruptly at the time of rising.[4] Studies using noninvasively determined systolic time intervals report a morning increase in cardiac output and ventricular contractility.[5] Recent reports describe an increase in platelet aggregability[6,7] and a decrease in fibrinolytic activity[8,9] in the morning hours. Increases in hematocrit and blood viscosity have also been observed in the morning. These rhythmic phenomena, acting alone or in combination, may alter cardiovascular responses selectively at different times of the day and thus result in varying clinical expressions of cardiac syndromes. An appreciation of the circadian periodicity of cardiovascular disorders may provide insights into the mechanisms of such disorders and aid in the effective design of pharmacologic regimens for their control. The purpose of this chapter is to discuss aspects of this subject with particular reference to transient myocardial ischemia in subsets of patients with coronary artery disease.

DAILY RHYTHMS IN CARDIOVASCULAR DISEASE

Many epidemiologic and observational studies demonstrate the existence of distinct temporal patterns for the clinical manifestations of cardiovascular disease (Table 6.2).

Table 6.1. Cardiovascular Functions Subject to Circadian Periodicity and Factors That May Influence Them

I. Normal cardiovascular functions with circadian rhythms
   A. Blood pressure
   B. Heart rate
   C. Myocardial contractility
   D. ? coronary tone

II. Factors with circadian rhythms that may influence cardiovascular function
   A. Cortisol
   B. Catecholamines
   C. Platelet aggregability
   D. Fibrinolytic activity
   E. Blood viscosity
   F. Hematocrit

MYOCARDIAL INFARCTION

Numerous studies report a peak onset of pain from myocardial infarction occurring between 6 AM and 12 PM. In one of the earliest studies in a large population, Master[10] reported a peak onset of myocardial infarction at 10 AM. Other studies by Steven[11] and Muller et al[12] described a bimodal distribution with a major peak occurring between 9 and 10 AM and a secondary peak occurring in the evening. The study by Muller et al,[12] based on the data base of the Multicenter Investigation of the Limitation of Infarct Size, is the most recent report. It is of particular importance because it confirmed a morning peak in the incidence of myocardial infarction based not only on the assessment of symptoms, but also on the objective determination of the onset of myocardial infarction from extrapolation of carefully constructed creatinine kinase-MB curves (Figure 6.1).

SUDDEN DEATH

In a recent investigation of approximately 2,200 death certificates from the state of Massachusetts in 1983, the nearly 400 sudden cardiac deaths reported displayed a prominent circadian pattern with a primary peak occurring between 7 and 11 AM.[13] Many other studies similarly reported a peak in total mortality and cardiovascular related deaths in the morning hours.[14,15] There are certain limitations in defining the precise cause and timing of death in studies employing death certificate analysis, particularly with reference to unwitnessed deaths occurring throughout the night. However, a recent report from the Framingham Heart Study population in which more precise records for determining the time and cause of death were used reported a peak incidence of sudden cardiac death from 7 to 9 AM[16] (Figure 6.2). This was true even when assumptions about the time of unwitnessed deaths were made in a

Table 6.2. Cardiovascular Disorders Exhibiting Circadian Periodicity

Angina
Exercise induced ischemia
Ischemia during ambulatory monitoring
Myocardial infarction
Sudden cardiac death
Ventricular premature contractions

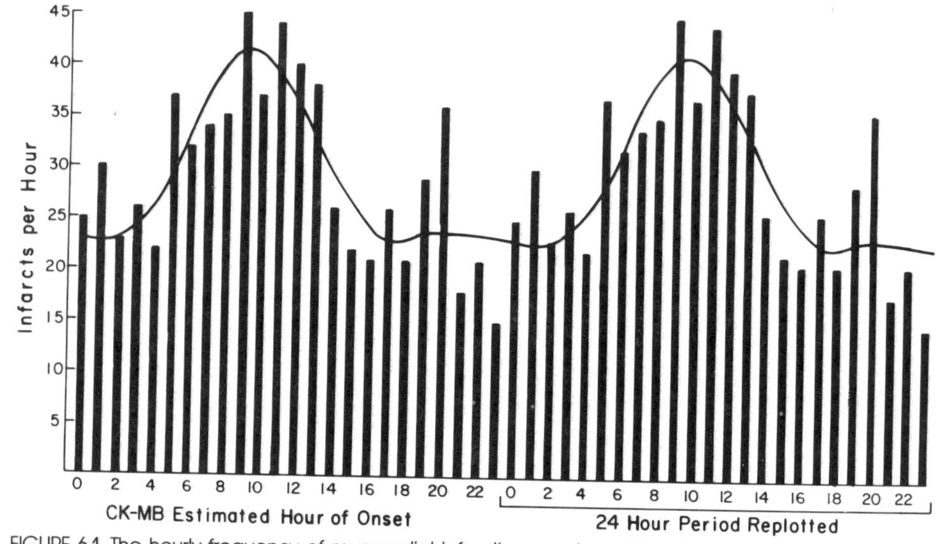

FIGURE 6.1. The hourly frequency of myocardial infarction onset as determined by the CK-MB method. There is a primary peak at 9 AM.[12] (Reproduced with the permission of the authors and the *New England Journal of Medicine.*)

manner likely to diminish the possibility of detecting an increased incidence in the morning. The authors further suggest that both sudden cardiac death secondary to myocardial ischemia or infarction and primary arrhythmic sudden cardiac death display this temporal pattern. Indeed, 24-hour ambulatory monitoring demonstrated an increased frequency of both atrial and ventricular arrhythmia between 6 and 9 AM.[17] However, at present the role of such arrhythmias in the pathogenesis of sudden arrhythmic deaths has not been elucidated.

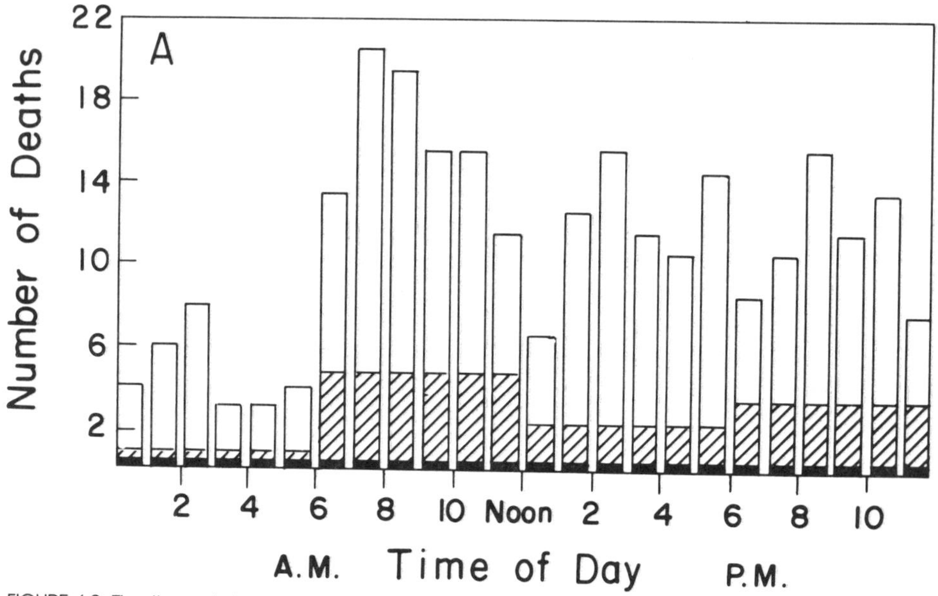

FIGURE 6.2. The time of day of 264 definite sudden cardiac deaths in the Framingham Heart Study.[16] The hourly risk of sudden cardiac death is approximately 70 percent higher from 7 to 9 AM than the average risk during the rest of the day. (Reproduced with the permission of the authors and the *American Journal of Cardiology.*)

TRANSIENT MYOCARDIAL ISCHEMIA DETECTED BY SYMPTOMS AND EXERCISE TESTING

Recent reports of the variable daily expression of angina and both symptomatic and asymptomatic ischemia detected by ECG analysis suggest a possible association between ischemia and the daily rhythm of infarction and sudden death. Physicians have long observed that episodes of angina at rest as well as exertional symptoms of anginal pectoris are more likely to be precipitated in the morning hours. Patients with Prinzmetal's angina are reported to have an increased frequency of attacks between 2 and 4 AM.[18] It was demonstrated that patients with coronary disease are more likely to develop ST-segment depression and angina at lower thresholds during exercise testing in the morning than in the afternoon. In a study from West Germany, Kenkels et al,[19] using a predetermined degree of ST-segment depression (0.15 mV) and the onset of angina to terminate an exercise test, observed that the worst exercise tolerance occurred at 8 AM when compared with similar tests performed at 11 AM, 2 PM, and 5 PM. Yasue et al[20] examined the responses of 13 patients with variant angina pectoris during exercise tests performed in the morning between 5 and 8 AM and the afternoon between 3 and 4 PM. Although all 13 patients developed attacks of angina during the morning tests, only 2 of the 13 patients experienced similar symptoms during the afternoon test even though the exercise workloads and total duration of exercise were greater in the afternoon.

TRANSIENT MYOCARDIAL ISCHEMIA DETECTED BY AMBULATORY MONITORING

More recently, continuous ambulatory monitoring of the electrocardiogram was used to detect and quantify episodes of symptomatic and asymptomatic ischemic ST-segment depression in patients with coronary artery diesase who are monitored during routine daily activities.[21–25] Rocco et al[24] examined the diurnal distribution of ischemic ST-segment depression in 32 patients with known coronary artery disease and chronic stable angina undergoing ambulatory monitoring (Figures 6.3 and 6.4A and B). A total of 251 distinct episodes of ST-segment depression were recorded, only 13 percent of which were associated with symptoms. A significantly greater number of episodes (39% of the total daily episodes) and total duration of ischemia in minutes (46% of the total ischemic time) occurred between 6 AM and 12 noon when compared with other times of the day. In fact, when the frequency distribution of episodes per hour was corrected for the variable time of waking, the early morning peak was even more striking, with approximately 20 percent of all ischemic episodes occurring during the first and second hours after rising. Although twice as many ischemic episodes occurred during the morning hours after rising compared to the evening hours before sleep, there were no significant differences in the characteristics of the episodes in terms of total duration, maximal ST-segment depression, heart rate at onset, associated physical activity level, or associated symptoms. The continuous 24-hour monitors allowed for determination of a threshold heart rate for the development of ischemic ST-segment depression in each patient. A comparison of morning and evening time periods demonstrated that patients were more likely to develop ischemic episodes when their heart rate exceeded the threshold range in the morning compared to the evening. This circadian variation in the frequency of and threshold for ischemic episodes in ambulatory patients with coronary artery disease

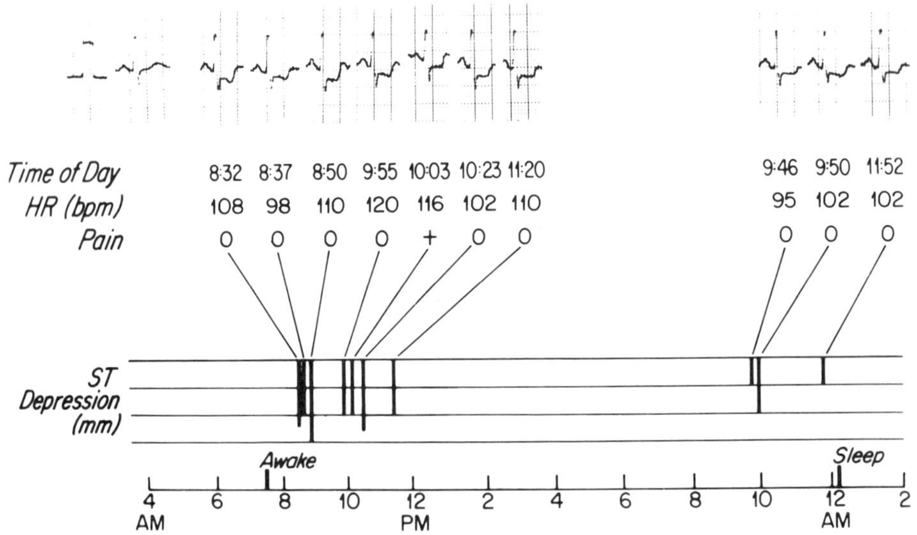

FIGURE 6.3. Typical 24-hour ambulatory monitoring results in a 65-year-old man.[24] Seven of 10 discrete episodes of ST-segment depression occurred during the first 3 to 4 hours after awakening. Only a single episode is associated with angina. (Reproduced with the permission of authors and the American Heart Association.)

is of particular interest and potential clinical importance, because this pattern parallels that reported for the onset of myocardial infarction and the occurrence of sudden cardiac death.

In a recent study, Nademanee et al[25] examined circadian periodicity in 68 patients with chronic stable angina and in 9 patients with Prinzmetal's angina. As in our own studies,[24] in patients with chronic stable angina, both silent and painful episodes had a peak occurrence in the morning and early afternoon hours (between 8 AM and 3 PM); the smallest number of episodes were between 1 and 5 AM (Figure 6.5). In contrast, in Prinzmental's angina, no clear periodicity in the distribution of ischemic events was seen; however, a greater number of symptomatic episodes at night was previously reported.[26] In addition, although a correlation between peak heart rate and the occurrence of ischemic episodes was reported in chronic stable angina, a similar correlation was not present in Prinzmetal's angina. The observed differences in the periodicity of ischemic episodes in chronic stable angina and Prinzmetal's angina may reflect differences in the mechanism of ischemia in these ischemic syndromes. Whether ischemic episodes exhibit a circadian periodicity in unstable angina is not known.

POSSIBLE MECHANISMS OF INCREASED MORNING ISCHEMIA IN CHRONIC STABLE ANGINA

Exogenous factors such as variations in physical activity level, emotional stimuli, or timing of the use of cigarettes or caffeine may interact to produce enhanced ischemic activity in the morning hours after awakening. However, it is likely that the previously cited endogenous rhythms in cardiovascular function at least contribute to, if not primarily explain, these phenomena. Morning increases in plasma catecholamine levels may contribute to the increased heart rate, blood pressure, and myocardial contractility described in the morning hours. The extrinsic stimuli associated with rising may further enhance sympathetic activity and its effect on these

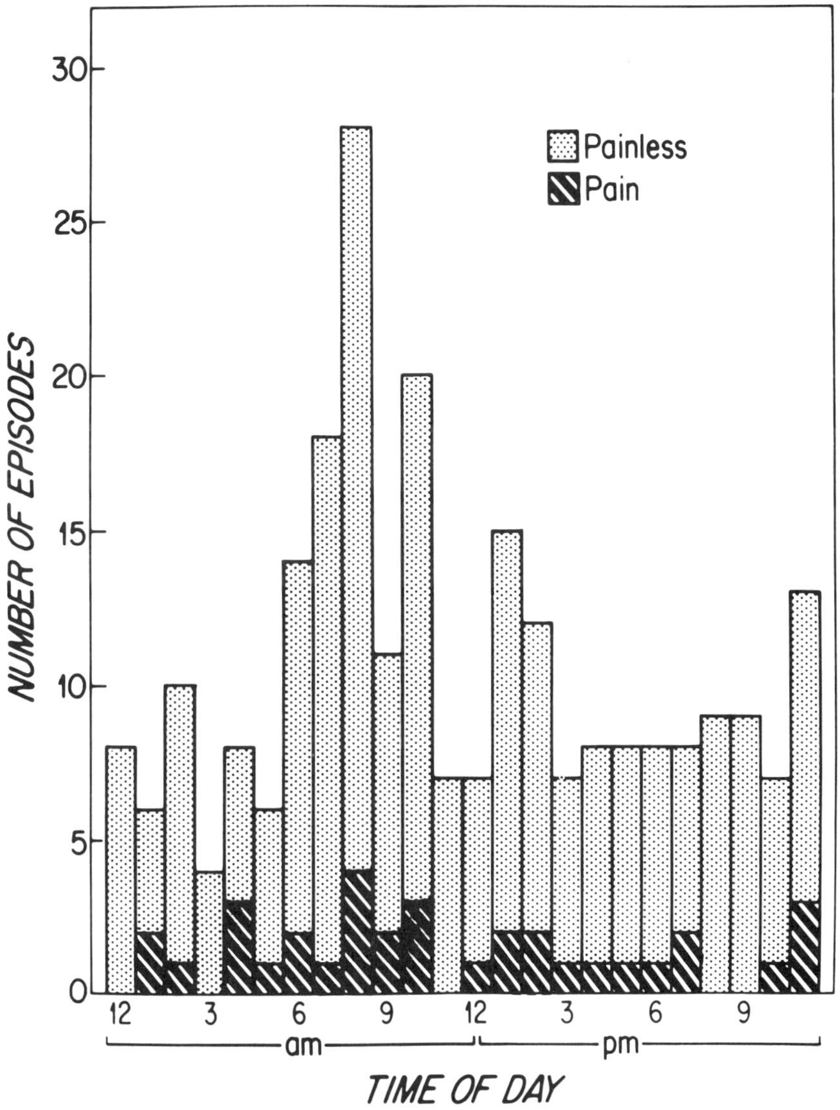

FIGURE 6.4A. The hourly frequency of episodes of ischemic ST-segment depression in 24 patients with coronary disease monitored off therapy is greatest at 8 AM.[24] (Reproduced with the permission of the authors and the American Heart Association.)

primary determinants of myocardial oxygen demand. This early morning increase in myocardial demand may precipitate myocardial ischemia in patients with significant coronary stenoses.

Diurnal changes in coronary artery tone and blood flow may also play a role in the development of ischemia in patients with coronary artery disease. Yasue et al[27] examined temporal differences in the size of large epicardial coronary arteries and their response to nitroglycerin in patients with variant angina. This angiographic study demonstrated that the dilating response of the coronary artery to nitroglycerin was greater in the morning than in the afternoon. The authors speculated that temporal differences in vasomotor tone of the epicardial coronary arteries may at least partially explain the clinical variability in symptoms and exercise response that they

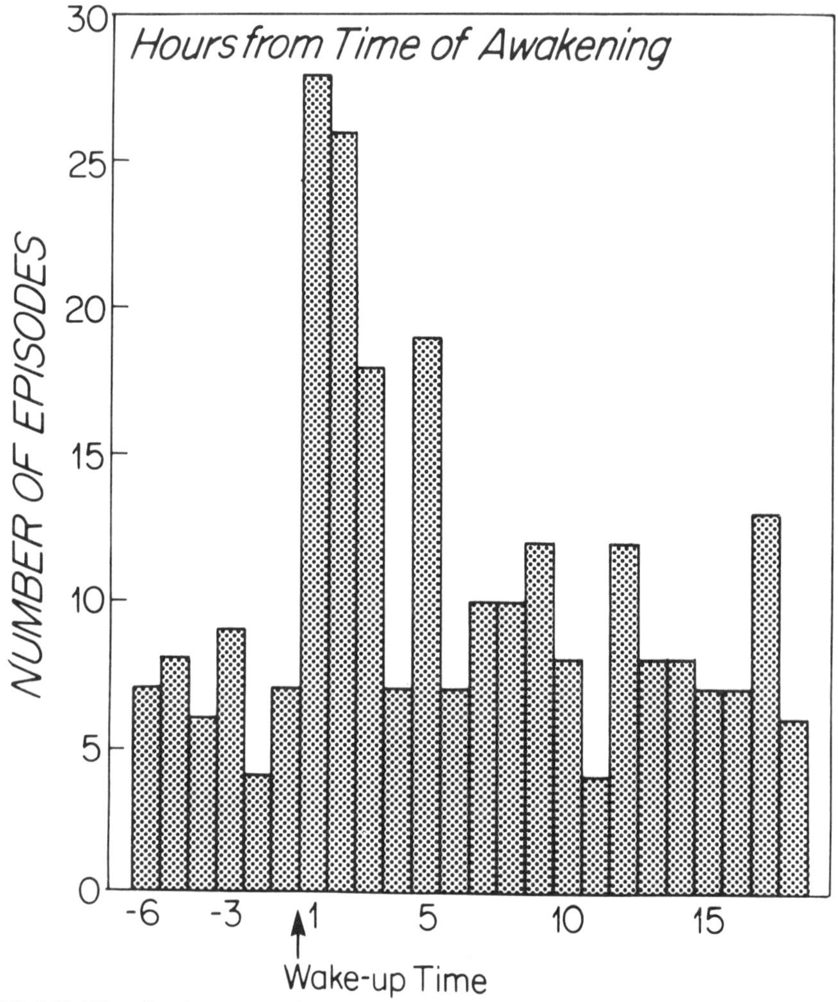

FIGURE 6.4B. When the frequency of episodes is displayed hourly from the time of awakening, the peak activity occurs in the first and second hour after rising.[24] (Reproduced with the permission of the authors and the American Heart Association.)

observed in similar patients. This increase in coronary tone may be due to altered levels of circulating catecholamines in the morning or possibly a heightened morning responsiveness of vascular receptors to vasoconstrictor stimuli. If circulating catecholamines and sympathetic activity are low during sleep, coronary vascular receptor sensitivity may increase during the night. On awakening, the substantial increase in circulating catecholamines may interact with vascular receptors with heightened sensitivity, resulting in increased tone over the subsequent hours. Continuing daytime increased sympathetic activity may make receptors less sensitive to stimuli, resulting in decreased coronary tone and a higher threshold for ischemia at other times of the day.

The role of platelet plugging and thrombosis in the pathogenesis of myocardial infarction has recently received much attention.[28] Recent reports indicate that the tendency of platelets to aggregate is increased in the morning and further suggest that this enhanced platelet aggregability is associated with morning rising and the

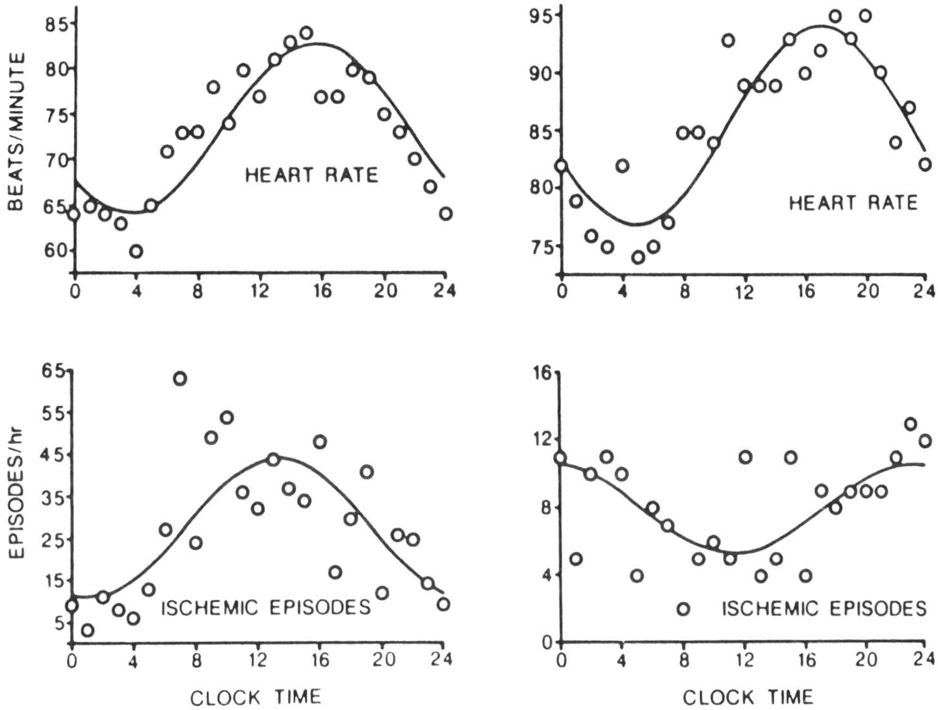

FIGURE 6.5. Circadian variation in heart rate changes and occurrence of ischemic episodes in patients with chronic stable angina (*left*) and Prinzmetal's angina (*right*) by cosinar analysis.[25] More important, there is a parallel correlation between peak heart rate and the occurrence of ischemic episodes in chronic stable angina. However, a similar correlation is not seen in Prinzmetal's angina. (Reproduced with the permission of the authors and the *American Journal of Cardiology*.)

assumption of an upright posture.[6,7] A trough in fibrinolytic activity[8,9] and increases in hematocrit and blood viscosity were also observed in the morning. These factors may result in a relatively hypercoagulable state at this time of day and therefore a greater tendency for thrombosis and interruption of coronary blood flow. In addition, the morning rise in arterial pressure may increase the likelihood of rupture of an atheromatous plaque. This acute change in arterial luminal geometry and a potentially thrombus-prone site may be an important step in the sequence of events leading to myocardial infarction and its complications. Furthermore, the increased activity of the sympathetic nervous system may contribute to the development of a primary arrhythmia and subsequent sudden death.

A relative imbalance in myocardial oxygen demand and coronary blood supply as the result of an interaction of these factors may be more prominent in the early morning hours than at other times of the day and thus result in a lower morning threshold for the development of myocardial ischemia and its complications (Figure 6.6). This imbalance and the resulting ischemia may be transient. However, the additional influences of pressure-induced deformations of atheromatous plaques and an increased tendency for thrombus formation may transform a stable into an unstable situation, resulting in infarction and possible sudden cardiac death. Certainly, further studies of the physiologic changes operative during this vulnerable morning period are needed to elucidate the isolated or aggregate role of these various factors in the clinical manifestations of cardiovacular disease.

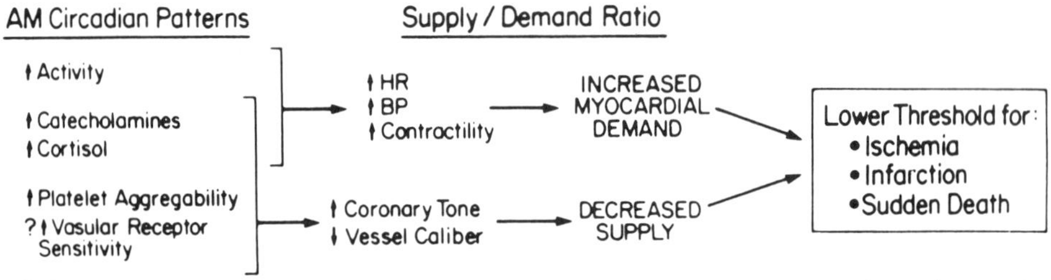

FIGURE 6.6. Hypothetical mechanisms causing morning increases in symptomatic and asymptomatic ischemic coronary events.

PHARMACOLOGIC EFFECTS ON CIRCARDIAN PERIODICITY IN MYOCARDIAL ISCHEMIA

Drug therapy has been shown to alter many of the observed circadian rhythms in cardiovascular disease. Metoprolol decreases nocturnal blood pressure and attenuates early morning blood pressure rise. Other drugs with beta-blocking activities such as atenolol reduce blood pressure during the day, but offer little effect during the rapid phase of blood pressure rise in the morning. The drug labetolol, which combines alpha-adrenergic blocking activity with beta-blocking activity, reduces the phase of rapid rise in the early morning.[29] In contrast, calcium-channel blockers may reduce heart rate and blood pressure without having an overall effect on circadian periodicity.[30]

The pharmacologic effects of these agents may influence the diurnal expression of ischemic activity in patients. Recent preliminary observations of Rocco et al,[31] employing 24-hour ambulatory monitoring of the ST segment during treatment with titrated doses of labetolol or propanolol, demonstrated that both drugs are effective in abolishing the normal morning increase in ischemic activity usually observed in patients with coronary artery disease. Similarly, a recent study by Imperi et al[32] indicated that metoprolol not only reduced the frequency and duration of silent myocardial ischemic episodes but also attenuated the circadian variation of such episodes documented by Holter recordings in patients with chronic stable angina. It is of note that the morning increase in the onset of myocardial infarction cited by Muller et al,[12] was not present in a subset of patients who were being treated with beta-blockers at the time of their presentation. These clinical observations may be explained by the role of beta-blockade in reducing the effects of catecholamines on the morning changes in vascular tone, platelet aggregability, and myocardial oxygen demand. This lack of a morning peak in infarction and the reduction in the recurrence rate of myocardial infarction with beta-blocker therapy[33] raise important questions about the relations between diurnal patterns of ischemic heart disease activity and prognosis in patients with coronary artery disease.

COMMENTS AND CONCLUSIONS

Twenty-four-hour rhythms in the normal and pathophysiologic function of the cardiovascular system are well described and may result from reproducible cyclic patterns in external environmental stimuli and endogenous biologic functions. Parallels of these rhythms with those of the clinical manifestations of coronary artery disease (including symptoms, exercise responses, reversible ischemia during ambulatory monitoring, onset of myocardial infarction, and sudden cardiac death) may provide valuable clues to the mechanisms that lead to myocardial infarction and sudden cardiac death.

Greater than one-half million individuals who are asymptomatic or mildly symptomatic with stable angina pectoris develop an acute myocardial infarction annually in the United States.[34] Over half the sudden deaths that occur each year in this country are due to significant coronary artery disease.[35] Observations from Holter monitoring suggest that ischemic ST-segment depressions precede the appearance of lethal arrhythmias in certain of these cases.[36] A better understanding of the factors that influence the changing patterns of ischemic disease activity over 24-hour periods may help to determine the mechanisms that transform a chronic stable condition into an acute catastrophic one. Therapeutic approaches may then be devised to better control myocardial ischemia and subsequently lead to a decrease in cardiac morbidity and mortality. It is possible, for example, that the frequently used medical regimens and dosing schedules of drugs may not provide patients with adequate pharmacologic protection during the time of day when they are at the greatest risk of developing ischemia: the first few hours soon after awakening. Conversely, that few episodes of ischemia in chronic stable angina occur between 12 midnight and 5 AM suggests that 24-hour "protection" from the consequences of ischemia may not be necessary in all cases. Whether specific drug therapies aimed at eliminating the morning increases in ischemic activity (by improving the relative morning mismatch in supply and demand) will have a beneficial effect on prognosis in patients with coronary artery disease remains to be tested. It is true that most of our present understanding of circadian rhythms in cardiovascular disease is based on observational studies and proposed associations. Nevertheless, these patterns suggest that ischemic heart disease activity is a dynamic and changing process that needs to be better understood in order to define new treatment strategies for myocardial ischemia designed to make further inroads into the morbidity and mortality figures of coronary artery disease.

REFERENCES

1. Weitzman ED, Fujushima D, Hogeire C, Roffwarg H, Gallagher TF, Hellman L: Twenty-four hour pattern of the episodic secretion of cortisol in normal subjects. *J Clin Endocrinol Metab* 1971;33:14–22.
2. Turton MB, Deegan T: Circadian variations of plasma catecholamine, cortisol and immunoreactive insulin concentrations in supine subjects. *Clin Chim Acta* 1974;55:389–397.
3. Millar-Craig MW, Bishop CN, Raftery EB: Circadian variation of blood pressure. *Lancet* 1978;1:795–797.
4. Floras JS, Jones JV, Johnston JA, Brooks DE, Hassan MO, Sleight P: Arousal and the circadian rhythm of blood pressure. *Clin Sci Mol Med* 1978;55:395–397s.
5. Wertheimer L, Hassen AZ, Delamn AJ. The 24-hour (circadian) rhythm of the cardiovascular disease. *Chronobiologia* 1982;9:195–201.
6. Tofler GH, Czeisler CA, Rutherford J, Williams GH, Muller JE. Increased platelet aggregability after arising from sleep (abstr.) *J Am Coll Cardiol* 1986;7(Suppl A):116A.
7. Brezinski DA, Sintomen S, Tofler GH, Schafer AI, Willich SN, Czeisler CE, Muller JE, Williams GH: Morning increases in platelet aggregability associated with assumption of the upright posture (Abstract). *Circulation* 1987;76:IV–366.
8. Rosing DR, Brakman P, Redwood DR, Goldstein RE, Beiser GD, Astrup T, Epstein SE: Blood fibrinolytic activity in man. Diurnal variation and the response to varying intensities of exercise. *Circ Res* 1970;27:171–184.
9. Petralito A, Magiafico RA, Gibino S, Cuffari MA, Miano MF, Fiore CE: Daily modifications of plasma fibrinogen, platelets, aggregation, Howell's time PTT, TT and an-

tithrombin III in normal subjects and in patients with vascular disease. *Chronobiologia* 1982;9:195–201.
10. Master AM: The role of effort and occupation (including physicians) in coronary occlusion. *JAMA* 1960;174:942–948.
11. Regional Office of Europe, World Health Organization. Myocardial infarction community registers: Results of a WHO international collaborative study coordinated by the regional office for Europe. *Public Health in Europe,* no. 5, Copenhagen, 1976;1–232.
12. Muller JE, Stone PH, Turi ZG, Rutherford JD, Czeisler CA, Parker C, Poole WK, Passamani E, Roberts R, Robertson T, Sobel BE, Willerson JT, Braunwald E, MILIS Study Group: Circadian variation in the frequency of onset of acute myocardial infarction. *N Engl J Med* 1985;313:1315–1322.
13. Muller JE, Ludmer PL, Willich SN, Tofler GH, Aylmer G, Klangos I, Stone PH: Circadian variation in the frequency of sudden cardiac death. *Circulation* 1987;75:131–138.
14. Smolensky M, Halberg F, Sargent F: Chronobiology of the life sequence, in Itoh S, Ogata K, Yoshimura H (eds): *Advances in Climatic Physiology.* New York, Springer-Verlag, 1972, pp 281–318.
15. Mitler MM, Hajdukovic RM, Hahn PM, Kripke DF: Circadian rhythm of death time: Cause of death versus recorded death time in New York City (Abstract). *Sleep Res* 1985;14:306.
16. Willich SN, Levy D, Rocco MB, Tofler GH, Stone PH, Muller JE: Circadian variation in the incidence of sudden cardiac death in the Framingham Heart Study Population. *Am J Cardiol* 1987;60:801–806.
17. Brisse B, Bender F, Gradause D, Gulker H. Schwippe G, Bramann H, Kuhs H: Circadian changes of heart rate and arrhythmias (Abstract). *Chronobiologia* 1979;6:81.
18. Karoiwa A: Symptomatology of variant angina. *Jpn Circ J* 1978;42:459–476.
19. Kenkels U, Blumchen G, Ebner F: Zur Problematick vone Belastungsprufungen in Abhangigkeit von der Tageszeit bei Patienten mit Koronarinsuffizienz. *Herz Kreisal* 1977;9:343–347.
20. Yasue H, Omote S, Takizawa A, Nagao M, Miwa K, Tanaka S: Circadian variation of exercise capacity in patients with Prinzmetal's variant angina; role of exercise-induced coronary arterial spasm. *Circulation* 1979;59:938–948.
21. Deanfield JE, Selwyn AP, Chierchia S, Maseri A, Ribeiro P, Krikler S, Morgan M: Myocardial ischaemia during daily life in patients with stable angina; its relation to symptoms and heart rate changes. *Lancet* 1983;2:753–758.
22. Schang SJ, Pepine CJ: Transient asymptomatic ST-segment depression during daily life activity. *Am J Cardiol* 1977;39:396.
23. Cecchi AC, Dovellini EV, Marchi F, Pucci P, Santoro GM, Fazzini DF: Silent myocardial ischemia during ambulatory electrocardiographic monitoring in patients with effort angina. *J Am Coll Cardiol* 1983;1:934.
24. Rocco MB, Barry J, Campbell S, Nabel E, Cook EF, Goldman L, Selwyn AP: Circadian variation of transient myocardial ischemia in patients with coronary artery disease. *Circulation* 1987;75:395–400.
25. Nademanee K, Intarachot V, Josephson MA, Singh BN: Circadian variation in occurrence of transient overt and silent myocardial ischemia in chronic stable angina and comparison with Prinzmetal angina in men. *Am J Cardiol* 1987;60:494–498.
26. Yasue H, Omate S, Takizawa A, Nagao M, Miwa K, Janaka S: Circadian variation of exercise capacity in patients with Prinzmetal angina: Role of exercise induced coronary arterial spasm. *Circulation* 1979;59:938–947.
27. Yasue H, Touyama M, Kato H, Tanaka S, Akiyama F: Prinzmetal's variant form of angina as a manifestation of alpha-adrenergic receptor-mediated coronary artery spasm: Documentation by coronary arteriography. *Am Heart J* 1976;91:148–155.
28. Davies MJ, Thomas AC: Thrombosis and acute coronary-artery lesions in sudden cardiac ischemic death. *N Engl J Med* 1984;310:137.
29. Raftery EB: The effects of beta-blockade therapy on diurnal variation of blood pressure. *Eur Heart J* 1983;4:61–64.
30. Subramanian VB: Clinical and research applications of ambulatory Holter ST-segment and heart rate monitoring. *Am J Cardiol* 1986;58:11B–20B.
31. Rocco MB, Nabel E, Mead K, Barry J, Selwyn AP: Effects of beta vs. alpha-beta blockade on transient myocardial ischemia (Abstract). *Circulation* 1987;76:IV–277.

32. Imperi GA, Lambert CR, Coy K, Lopez L, Pepine LJ: Effects of titrated beta-blockade (metoprolol) on silent myocardial ischemia in ambulatory patients with coronary artery disease. *Am J Cardiol* 1987;60:519–524.
33. The Norwegian Multicenter Study Group: Timolol-induced reduction of mortality and reinfarction in patients surviving acute myocardial infarction. *N Engl J Med* 1981;304:801–807.
34. Graves EJ: Summary: National hospital discharge survey. Rockville, Md: Sept. 18, 1984. National Center for Health Statistics (Advance data no. 101).
35. Liberthson RR, Nagel EL, Hirschman JC, Nussenfeld SR, Blackbourne BD, Davis JH: Pathophysiologic observations in prehospital ventricular fibrillation and sudden cardiac death. *Circulation* 1974;49:790–798.
36. Gradman AH, Bell PA, DeBusk RF: Sudden death during ambulatory monitoring. Clinical and electrocardiographic correlations. Report of a case. *Circulation* 1977;55:210–211.

PART B

Prevalence

CHAPTER 7

Prevalence and Significance of Asymptomatic Coronary Artery Disease

Peter F. Cohn, MD

Coronary artery disease represents a major public health problem in many parts of the world, and myocardial ischemia is one of the common expressions of this disease. Physicians have long been taught that chest pain or some other well-recognized anginal equivalent invariably accompanies myocardial ischemic episodes. However, in the last 5 to 10 years this tenet has seriously been challenged; a growing body of data recognizes that silent ischemia is a frequent manifestation of coronary artery disease.[1] Therefore, coronary artery disease can be not only severe and extensive, but also asymptomatic. Many of these asymptomatic lesions are still active, that is, capable of producing ischemia under certain circumstances. The resulting event, silent myocardial ischemia (also referred to as silent ischemia), is defined as objective evidence of myocardial ischemia (via direct or indirect measurements of left ventricular function, perfusion, metabolism, or electrical activity) without chest pain or other anginal equivalents. It can occur in a variety of settings, as described in the next section.

PREVALENCE

In 1981, we[2] proposed classifying patients with silent ischemia into three clinical types to help clarify the prevalence, detection, prognosis, and management of this syndrome. In our classification (Table 7.1), Type 1 includes persons with ischemia who are totally asymptomatic, never having experienced any signs or symptoms of cardiovascular disease. Type 2 includes persons who are asymptomatic after myocardial infarction but still demonstrate active (but painless) ischemia. Type 3 consists of patients with both angina and silent ischemia.

Estimates of the prevalence of these three types of silent ischemia have been made by extrapolating statistics from studies in the literature to the population at large. Because the number of studies is limited, these estimates must be viewed cautiously. Nevertheless, they do provide some idea of the scope of the problem. Figures for Type 1 patients are based on surveys of apparently healthy populations who undergo noninvasive screening with exercise testing followed by coronary arteriography.[3,4] From these studies, it appears that 2.5 to 10 percent of middle-aged men have asymptomatic but active coronary artery disease. If the lower figure is used as a conser-

Table 7.1. Clinical Classification of Patients with Silent Myocardial Ischemia

Type I.	Persons who are totally asymptomatic.
Type II.	Persons who are asymptomatic after myocardial infarction, but still demonstrate active ischemia.
Type III.	Persons with angina who are asymptomatic with some episodes of myocardial ischemia, but not others.

vative estimate, at least 1 to 2 million men in the United States between the ages of 35 and 60 years have Type 1 silent ischemia. It should be reemphasized that exercise ST-segment abnormalities *alone* are not sufficient for the diagnosis of coronary artery disease in the general population; these findings must be confirmed with other procedures, as will be discussed subsequently. Figures for postinfarction (Type 2) patients can be calculated from the results of low-level exercise tests performed after acute infarction. About 70 percent of postinfarction patients are suitable for such testing,[5] that is, their course has not been complicated by angina, severe heart failure, or high-grade ventricular arrhythmias. Theroux et al[6] studied 210 postinfarction patients; 64 had positive exercise responses, with 27 having angina and ST-segment depression and 37 having painless ST-segment depression. Thus, 18 percent of their total population—and 58 percent of the positive responders—had silent ischemia. In a study of 103 postinfarction patients in whom exercise testing could not be performed because of high-grade ventricular arrhythmias or severe ventricular dysfunction, Gottlieb et al[7] found that 39 patients had ST-segment depression, with 30 (29%) having at least one episode of painless ST-segment depression. In Type 3 patients, 24- to 96-hour ambulatory electrocardiographic (Holter) monitoring was performed in 423 patients with angina and angiographically documented coronary artery disease in five studies.[8–12] Painless ST-segment depression on the Holter monitor was present in 40 percent (168) of the 423 patients. In the four studies in which the number of episodes of ST-segment depression was noted, 1,862 of the total of 2,583 episodes were painless (72%). In two studies of unstable angina,[13,14] 66 of 119 patients (56%) continued to have silent ischemia on Holter monitoring even though their chest pain had abated on an intensive medical regimen. Positive exercise tests in patients with angina have a 42 percent chance of being silent.[15,16]

As indicated from these comments, estimating the prevalence of silent myocardial ischemia requires accurate methods of detection. At present, the detection of silent ischemia depends largely on the use of ambulatory ECG monitoring and exercise ECGs as well as related exercise radionuclide or echocardiographic procedures.

The exercise test is a useful screening procedure for detecting silent ischemia in asymptomatic postinfarction patients because the diagnosis of underlying coronary artery disease is almost certain. In the general population, however, the exercise test must be used with more caution and false-positive results are common. Exercise tests to detect silent coronary artery disease should be recommended only in selected individuals and not in the public at large. Appropriate individuals are those at high risk for developing coronary artery disease because of multiple risk factors (elevated cholesterol levels, hypertension, diabetes, and cigarette smoking) or a family history of premature coronary artery disease, or both. Diabetic populations seem especially suitable for screening because visceral neuropathy could contribute to the lack of pain from myocardial ischemia.[17] Unless an exercise test is strongly positive (>2 mm ST-segment depression in Stage I or II of the Bruce protocol), its results should be confirmed by a radionuclide procedure (such as thallium-201 perfusion imaging[18]) before a totally asymptomatic person is either labeled as having coronary artery disease or referred for coronary arteriography for anatomic definition.

The low-level exercise test in the postinfarction patient is still the most common way of detecting silent ischemia, but once detected, the frequency of ischemic episodes can be documented by Holter monitoring.[19] Holter monitoring can also be used when exercise testing is contraindicated.[7] For Type 2 individuals, the decision to define coronary anatomy with arteriography is less controversial, because it is based on more than just the presence of silent ischemia—infarction has occurred.

Type 3 patients can also be detected by exercise testing, but Holter recordings are more useful because they document out-of-hospital events. The Holter monitor has been used as an ischemic event recorder since the early 1970s, when Stern, Tzivoni, and colleagues[20] reported their experiences. Concern about frequency responses of the Holter devices as well as lack of standardization of different monitoring systems and their data analysis components raised serious questions about the reliability of their findings. This was unfortunate because many of the early observations made by these investigators concerning the frequency of painless ischemia during daily out-of-hospital activities have since been confirmed with more modern devices. The earlier problems have largely been overcome because of recent technologic advances combined with appropriate testing protocols to detect spurious ST-segment depression due to positional changes, hyperventilation, and the like. Crucial to the reliability of Holter ST-segment findings have been the validation studies of Deanfield et al,[9,21,22] in which simultaneous myocardial perfusion studies confirmed the ischemic nature of the ST-segment depression recorded during Holter monitoring. The studies of Deanfield et al showed a pattern of reduced rubidium-82 uptake that was often identical in both painful and painless episodes in the same patient. These studies clearly demonstrated that in a population with angina and known coronary artery disease (all patients had undergone coronary arteriography), the ST-segment abnormalities recorded on Holter monitoring were valid indicators of myocardial ischemia. About 75 percent of the out-of-hospital ischemic episodes were painless, a figure almost exactly that reported several years earlier by Schang and Pepine.[23] Most ischemic events occurred during nonexertion-related activities.

In addition to its use in documenting silent ischemia in anginal patients, the Holter monitor can do the same in asymptomatic populations. There is justified concern, however, about the meaning of ST-segment changes in patients without angina unless the coronary anatomy is defined and there is associated evidence of myocardial ischemia via thallium-scintigraphy, exercise radionuclide angiography, and the like. Three recently reported studies involving 34 patients[24–26] suggest that if an exercise test documents silent myocardial ischemia in an asymptomatic individual—and coronary arteriography confirms the diagnosis of coronary artery disease—then the Holter monitor can be used to record the frequency of out-of-hospital silent ischemia in these patients. In our study,[25] 10 patients had a total of 64 ischemic episodes (lasting 798 minutes) during 480 hours of monitoring. A striking finding in this study was the circadian variation of the ischemic events, with nearly half occurring between 6 AM and noon. This confirmed the earlier findings of Rocco et al[27] in 32 patients with angina. The temporal relation of these events and a similar peak incidence of myocardial infarction[28] may well have a common thread: increased platelet aggregability.[29] Current AM as well as FM devices for recording ischemic episodes are valid.[30] AM Holter devices are most reliable when correlated with standard exercise ECGs, using a method proposed recently by Tzivoni et al.[31] In this method, patients wear Holter devices during exercise protocols to test all components of the recording and analyzing system. The newest technology—real-time event recorders with the ability to provide ECG printouts of ischemic episodes—will allow long periods of monitoring, perhaps 5 to 7 days. However, the reliability of these devices should be carefully validated against conventional Holter systems.[32]

CLINICAL SIGNIFICANCE

Type 1 Silent Ischemia

Prognostic studies in asymptomatic persons are either epidemiologic or anatomic. Only the latter have arteriographic data, although both employ exercise tests. Anatomic studies provide arteriographic evidence that the ECG and perfusion abnormalities are associated with discrete coronary stenoses. Even though only the latter provide "hard" data in small numbers of persons, the epidemiologic studies are also important because of what can be inferred from the wealth of data inherent in large surveys. A study by Giagnoni and associates,[33] for example, demonstrated that asymptomatic healthy men with a positive exercise test, compared to negative responders, had a risk ratio for developing cardiac events of 5.55:1 over a 10-year follow-up period. The two groups were matched for age, sex, and the presence of coronary risk factors. Other recent surveys of this type with similar findings are the MRFIT study[34] and the Lipid Research Clinics Mortality Follow-Up Study.[35] In the latter, a positive exercise test was associated with a cumulative mortality of 11.9 percent over 8.1 years mean follow-up time versus 1.2 percent over 8.6 years for men with a negative test result. Most of these deaths were due to coronary artery disease.

Although the epidemiologic studies suggest that latent coronary artery disease accounts for the mortality trends, they cannot prove it unless autopsies are performed. During life, the gold standard for anatomic definition is still the coronary arteriogram. In this regard, the Norwegian study of Erikssen and Thaulow[3] has been particularly valuable in providing careful follow-up data in 50 men with Type 1 silent ischemia.

Although the number of patients in this study is small, the duration of follow-up is of particular interest. After 8 years,[3] 3 subjects died, 7 had myocardial infarction, 16 had angina pectoris, and 27 had more severe ECG abnormalities during the exercise stress test. Only 17 had remained unchanged clinically when compared with the baseline study.

At the end of 12.5 years,[36] 11 subjects had died, 8 of the remaining subjects developed acute myocardial infarction; 18 had angina pectoris and 24 of the remaining men alive demonstrated angiographic evidence of progression of coronary disease.

The mortality rate was 35 percent (yearly mortality 3%) in those subjects with three-vessel disease at baseline, 22 percent with two-vessel disease, and only 7 percent with single-vessel disease. The number of coronary events among the men with three-vessel disease is shown in Figure 7.1. It is evident that death occurred mainly after 10 years. It is of interest that only one subject died without having developed angina or myocardial infarction before death.

Sudden death has also been associated with Type 1 silent ischemia. Sharma et al[37] found many instances of exercise-induced silent ischemia in 15 patients (see

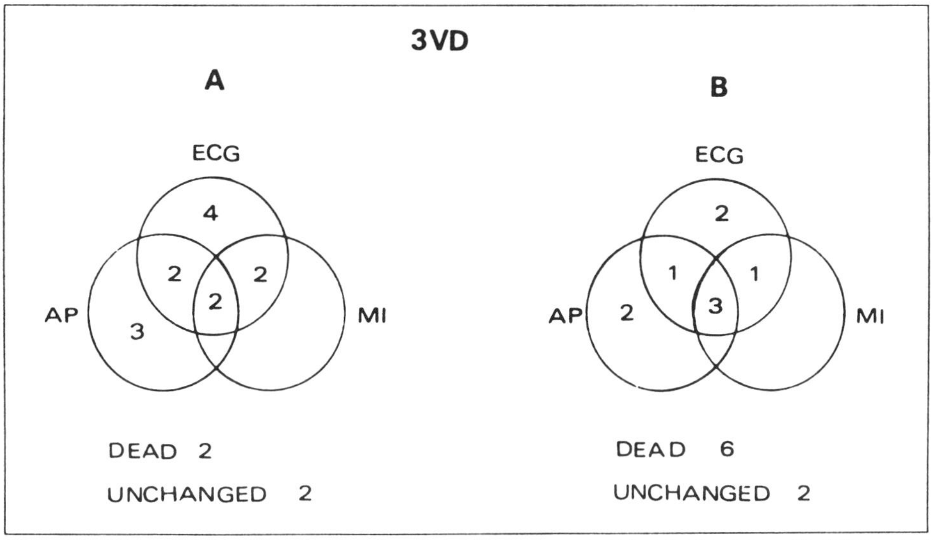

FIGURE 7.1. Venn diagram showing the number of coronary events among men with three-vessel disease (3VD) at the baseline examination. (*A*) findings at 8 years and (*B*) findings at 12.5 years of follow-up. AP = angina pectoris, MI = myocardial infarction, ECG = electrocardiographic abnormalities. (From Erikssen et al[36] with the permission of the authors and the publisher.)

Chapter 16) resuscitated from out-of-hospital sudden death; 9 of these patients had no prior history of heart disease. These data support other, indirect findings: about 50,000 of the 250,000 sudden death victims in this country per year have no prior history of heart disease, yet when autopsies are performed, these apparently healthy persons have evidence of advanced arteriosclerotic disease in their coronary arteries and scars in their myocardium[38] (see Chapter 16).

Type 2 Silent Ischemia

Compared to that in Type 1 patients, prognosis is worse in Type 2 patients, especially when left ventricular dysfunction is present. Again the most striking findings are in the three-vessel disease group. Three different long-term studies (albeit with different populations) have reported yearly mortality in the 5 to 6 percent range. These include the National Institutes of Health study,[39] the Duke-Harvard study,[40] and the Coronary Artery Surgery Study (CASS).[41,42] In one of the CASS studies, Weiner et al[42] showed that 7-year mortality in nonoperated postinfarction patients with silent ischemia was 24 percent, nearly identical to that of patients with angina (23%) and significantly higher than that of patients with negative exercise test results (12%, $p < 0.001$). In this study, patients in the three-vessel disease group had the highest mortality (43%, or about 6% per year). The NIH study further suggests that within the overall three-vessel disease group, there is a subgroup at even higher risk of cardiac death (8 to 9% per year) because of a combination of reduced exercise tolerance, severe ST-segment depression, and a marked decrease in the radionuclide-derived exercise ejection fraction.

Exercise tests performed 2 to 3 weeks after infarction showed an adverse short-term (1-year) prognosis associated with silent ischemia.[6] Holter monitoring in Type 2 patients who were not suitable for exercise testing also demonstrated that silent ischemia was a significant predictor of 1-year mortality.[7]

CONCLUSIONS

Silent ischemia can now be detected with reasonable certainty using stress testing, radionuclide procedures, and Holter monitoring. It is frequent in coronary patients, even asymptomatic ones. The Type 1 patients that are most worrisome, based on Erikssen's data, are those with three-vessel disease. To help make management recommendations, a strong case can be made for performing coronary arteriography in asymptomatic persons most likely to have advanced disease because of strongly positive exercise test results.

Type 2 patients are much more likely than Type 1 patients to come to the attention of the clinician. A positive exercise test alone (with or without pain) is often sufficient reason to recommend coronary arteriography, but in some instances radionuclide procedures or Holter monitoring may also be employed. The clinical importance of persistent myocardial iscehmia in the postinfarction patient cannot be overemphasized. Furthermore, with increasingly more of these patients being diagnosed, the "differences" between painful and painless myocardial ischemia in terms of prognosis and therapy are being blurred. This is as it should be. Ischemia is ischemia—pain is just one of its descriptors.

REFERENCES

1. Cohn PF: *Silent Myocardial Ischemia and Infarction*. New York, Marcel Dekker, 1986.
2. Cohn PF: Asymptomatic coronary artery disease. *Mod Concepts Cardiovasc Dis* 1981;50:55–60.
3. Erikssen J, Thaulow E: Follow-up of patients with asymptomatic myocardial ischemia, in Rutishauser W, Roskamm H, (eds): *Silent Myocardial Ischemia*. Berlin: Springer-Verlag, 1984, pp 156–164.
4. Langou RA, Huang EK, Kelley MJ, Cohen LS: Predictive accuracy of coronary artery calcification and abnormal exercise test for coronary artery disease in asymptomatic men. *Circulation* 1980;62:1196–1202.
5. Epstein SE, Palmeri ST, Patterson RE: Evaluation of patients after acute myocardial infarction. *N Engl J Med* 1982;307:1487–1492.
6. Theroux P, Waters DD, Halphen C, Debaisieux JC, Mizgala HF: Prognostic value of exercise testing soon after myocardial infarction. *N Engl J Med* 1979;301:341–346.
7. Gottlieb SH, Gerstenblith G, Achuff SC, Mellits ED, Gottlieb SO: Ischemic ST segment changes by ambulatory Holter predict one year mortality in high risk post-infarct patients (Abstract). *Circulation* 1986;74(Suppl II):58.
8. Cecci AC, Dovellini EV, Marchi F, Pucci P, Santoro GM, Fazzini PF: Silent myocardial ischemia during ambulatory electrocardiographic monitoring in patients with effort angina. *J Am Coll Cardiol* 1983;1:934–939.
9. Deanfield JE, Maseri A, Selwyn AP, et al: Myocardial ischemia during daily life in patients with stable angina: Its relation to symptoms and heart rate changes. *Lancet* 1983;2:753–758.
10. Quyyumi A, Wright CM, Mockus LJ, Fox KM: How important is a history of chest pain in determining the degree of ischaemia in patients with angina pectoris? *Br Heart J* 1985;54:22–26.
11. Tzivoni D, Gavish A, Benhorin J, Keren A, Stern S: Myocardial ischemia during daily activities and stress. *Am J Cardiol* 1986;58:47B–50B.
12. Carboni GP, Lahiri A, Cashman PMM, Raftery EB: Ambulatory heart rate and ST-segment depression during painful and silent myocardial ischemia in chronic stable angina pectoris. *Am J Cardiol* 1987;59:1029–1034.
13. Nademanee K, Intarachot V, Josephson MA, Rieders D, Mody FV, Singh BN: Prognostic significance of silent myocardial ischemia in patients with unstable angina. *J Am Coll Cardiol* 1987;19:1–9.

14. Gottlieb SO, Quyang P, Mellits ED, Gerstenblith G: Silent ischemia as a marker for early unfavorable outcomes in unstable angina. *N Engl J Med* 1986;314:1214–1216.
15. Lindsey H Jr, Cohn PF: "Silent" myocardial ischemia during and after exercise testing in patients with coronary artery disease. *Am Heart J* 1978;95:441–447.
16. Falcone C, deServi S, Poma E, Campana C, Scire A, Montemartini C, Specchia G: Clinical significance of exercise-induced silent myocardial ischemia in patients with coronary artery disease. *J Am Coll Cardiol* 1987;9:295–299.
17. Chipkin SR, Frid D, Albert JS, Baker SP, Dalen JE, Aronin N: Frequency of painless myocardial ischemia during exercise tolerance testing in patients with and without diabetes mellitus. *Am J Cardiol* 1987;59:61–65.
18. Guiney TE, Pohost GM, McKusick KA, Beller GA: Differentiation of false- from true-positive ECG responses to exercise stress by thallium-201 perfusion imaging. *Chest* 1981;23:4–10.
19. Cohn PF, Sodums MT, Lawson WE, Vlay SC, Brown EJ Jr: Frequent episodes of silent myocardial ischemia after apparently uncomplicated myocardial infarction. *J Am Coll Cardiol* 1986;8:982–985.
20. Stern S, Tzivoni D: Early detection of silent ischaemic heart disease by 24-hour electrocardiographic monitoring of active subjects. *Br Heart J* 1974;36:481–486.
21. Deanfield JE, Shea M, Kensett M, Horlock P, Wilson RA, deLandsheere CM, Selwyn AP: Silent myocardial ischaemia due to mental stress. *Lancet* 1984;2:1001–1005.
22. Deanfield JE, Shea MJ, Wilson RA, Horlock P, deLandsheere CM, Selwyn AP: Direct effects of smoking on the heart: Silent ischemic disturbances of coronary flow. *Am J Cardiol* 1986;57:1005–1009.
23. Schang J, Pepine CJ: Transient asymptomatic ST-segment depression during daily activity. *Am J Cardiol* 1977;39:396–402.
24. Campbell S, Barry J, Rebecca GS, Rocco MB, Nabel EG, Wayne RR, Selwyn AP: Active transient myocardial ischemia during life in asymptomatic patients with positive exercise tests and coronary artery disease. *Am J Cardiol* 1986;57:1010–1016.
25. Cohn PF, Lawson WE: Characteristics of silent myocardial ischemia occurring during out-of-hospital activities in asymptomatic coronary patients. *Am J Cardiol* 1987;59:746–749.
26. Coy KM, Imperi GA, Lambert CR, Pepine CJ: Silent myocardial ischemia during daily activities in asymptomatic men with positive exercise test responses. *Am J Cardiol* 1987;59:45–49.
27. Rocco MB, Barry J, Campbell S, Nabel E, Cook EF, Goldman L, Selwyn AP: Circadian variation of transient myocardial ischemia in patients with coronary artery disease. *Circulation* 1987;75:395–400.
28. Muller JE, Stone PH, Turi ZG, et al: Circadian variation in the frequency of onset of acute myocardial infarction. *N Engl J Med* 1985;313:1315–1322.
29. Tofler GH, Brezinski D, Schafer AI, Czeisler CA, Rutherford JD, Willich SN, Gleason RE, Williams GH, Muller JE: Concurrent morning increase in platelet aggregability and the risk of myocradial infarction and sudden cardiac death. *N Engl J Med* 1987;316:1514–1518.
30. Lambert CR, Imperi GA, Pepine CJ: Low-frequency requirements for recording ischemic ST-segment abnormalities in coronary artery disease. *Am J Cardiol* 1986;58:225–229.
31. Tzivoni D, Benhorin J, Gavish A, Stern S: Holter recording during treadmill testing in assessing myocardial ischemic changes. *Am J Cardiol* 1985;55:1200–1203.
32. Barry J, Campbell S, Nabel EG, Mead K, Selwyn AP: Ambulatory monitoring of the digitized electrocardiogram for detection and early warning of transient myocardial ischemia in angina pectoris. *Am J Cardiol* 1987;10:483–488.
33. Giagnoni E, Secchi MB, Wu SC, Morabito A, Oltrona L, Mancarella S, Volpin N, Flossa L, Bettazzi L, Arangio G, Sachero A, Folli G: Prognostic value of exercise EKG testing in asymptomatic normotensive subjects: A prospective matched study. *N Engl J Med* 1983;309:1085–1089.
34. Multiple Risk Factor Intervention Trial Research Group: Exercise electrocardiogram and coronary heart disease mortality in the Multiple Risk Factor Intervention Trial. *Am J Cardiol* 1985;55:16–24.
35. Gordon DJ, Elelund L-G, Karon JM, Probstfield JL, Rubenstein C, Sheffield LT, Weiss-

feld L: Predictive value of the exercise test for mortality in North American men: The Lipid Research Clinics Mortality Follow-Up Study. *Circulation* 1986;2:252–261.
36. Erikssen L, Cohn PF, Thaulow E, Mowinckel P: Silent myocardial ischemia in middle aged men: Long term clinical course, in Arnim TV, Maseri A (eds): *Silent Ischemia: Current Concepts and Management*. Darmstadt, Steinkopff, 1987, 45–51.
37. Sharma B, Asinger R, Francis GS, Hodges M, Wyeth RP: Demonstration of exercise-induced painless myocardial ischemia in survivors of out-of-hospital ventricular fibrillation. *Am J Cardiol* 1987;59:740–745.
38. Warnes CA, Roberts WC: Sudden coronary death: Relation of amount and distribution of coronary narrowing at necropsy to previous symptoms of myocardial ischemia, left ventricular scarring and heart weight. *Am J Cardiol* 1984;54:65–73.
39. Kent KM, Rosing DR, Ewels CJ, Lipson L, Bonow R, Epstein SE: Prognosis of asymptomatic or mildly symptomatic patients with coronary artery disease. *Am J Cardiol* 1982;49:1823–1831.
40. Cohn PF, Harris P, Barry WH, Rosati RA, Rosenbaum P, Waternaux C: Prognostic importance of anginal symptoms in angiographically defined coronary artery disease. *Am J Cardiol* 1981;47:233–237.
41. Passamani E, David KB, Gillespie MJ, Killip T, the CASS Principal Investigators and their Associates: A randomized trial of coronary artery bypass surgery: Survival of patients with a low ejection fraction. *N Engl J Med* 1985;312:1665–1671.
42. Weiner DA, Ryan TJ, McCabe CH, Luk S, Chaitman BR, Sheffield LT, Tristani F, Fisher LD: Significance of silent myocardial ischemia during exercise testing in patients with coronary artery disease. *Am J Cardiol* 1987;59:725–729.

CHAPTER 8

Silent Myocardial Ischemia During Daily Activities in Asymptomatic Patients with Positive Treadmill Tests

Carl J. Pepine, MD, Kevin Coy, MD,
and Charles Lambert, MD

Coronary artery disease in its asymptomatic form has generated considerable interest. Pathologic and arteriographic study of asymptomatic patients with coronary artery disease indicates that many patients have severe and extensive disease that is indistinguishable from that found in symptomatic patients.[1,2] These studies, however, cannot be used to determine whether the coronary artery disease is severe enough to cause transient myocardial ischemia. Until recently, these determinations were made in the exercise laboratory using stress testing designed to expose an imbalance between myocardial oxygen supply by diseased arteries and increasing demands of exercise. Although this approach yields useful information, it is incomplete in that it does not indicate whether these patients have transient ischemic episodes "in the field." Recently, numerous studies in patients with symptomatic coronary disease showed that most episodes of myocardial ischemia that occur during ordinary life are asymptomatic or silent.[3–5] Furthermore, most silent episodes in daily life are not associated with the high level of activity or tachycardia seen in these same patients during exercise testing. These findings support the view that in real-life situations exercise stress and extreme degrees of relatively "fixed" atherosclerotic coronary disease may not be required to cause transient ischemia. Instead, this new information suggests that during ordinary daily activities, other processes may transiently narrow coronary arteries, leading to alterations in flow of sufficient magnitude to cause ischemia. Thus, the traditional concept that totally asymptomatic patients thought to be in a relatively early stage of disease are free of ischemia may not be free of myocardial ischemia. Decreases in coronary artery diameter at sites of noncritical coronary stenosis could reduce regional blood flow in asymptomatic patients, resulting in silent ischemia and events. In addition, analysis of the sequence of changes preceding ischemia in patients in the asymptomatic phase may lead to identification of causes responsible for disturbances in coronary blood flow. They may act as trigger mechanisms for active ischemia in real life as well as mechanisms responsible for evolution of symptoms or events.

The purpose of this chapter is twofold: (1) to present data obtained in our laboratory from a previously published study[6] dealing with detection of ischemia out of the hospital in asymptomatic patients with positive stress tests, and (2) to examine the available data dealing with myocardial ischemia detected during daily life in such patients.[7,8]

STUDIES IN OUR LABORATORY

Patient Selection

Patients were selected from those referred for exercise ECG stress tests performed at our hospitals over a period of 13 months. A modified Bruce protocol was used with a Quinton treadmill, and 12-lead electrocardiograms were recorded using Marquette recorders. From approximately 1,500 patients exercised, 56 were asymptomatic and had ≥2.0-mm ST-segment depression without symptoms suggesting angina during the test. Thirty-nine of these patients were excluded from further study because of left ventricular hypertrophy, conduction abnormalities, baseline ST-T-wave abnormalities, labile ST-T waves, medications known to influence the ST segment (eg, digoxin and antiarrhythmics), and preexcitation. The remaining 17 men constituted the study subjects. Although none had angina, several were known to have coronary artery disease (ie, previous silent or unrecognized myocardial infarctions and abnormal coronary angiograms).

Seventeen patients (mean age 62, range 42 to 77 years) without symptoms who had ischemic responses *S* (>1.0-mm horizontal or downsloping ST-segment depression), persisting for 80 ms past the J point during exercise testing, were studied. All patients then underwent ambulatory ECG monitoring for 72 hours using an Oxford Medilog II FM recorder and kept a detailed daily diary recording activities and symptoms. An episode of ischemia was defined as a period when at least 1 mm of horizontal or downsloping ST-segment depression occurred, was present 60 ms after the J point, and persisted for more than 60 seconds.[3] At least 60 seconds of return of the ST segment to baseline was required before another episode was counted. Each patient underwent coronary angiography using standard techniques. A ≥50 percent diameter reduction in a major epicardial branch was considered evidence of severe coronary artery disease. The extent of coronary artery disease was classified according to the number of arteries containing severe stenosis.

RESULTS

Patient Characteristics

All patients reported in their diaries that they were performing ordinary daily activities without angina or other cardiac-related symptoms. All but one, a 70-year-old man, had at least one coronary risk factor such as elevated serum cholesterol, diabetes, tobacco use, or systemic hypertension. Most had multiple risk factors. Two patients had Q waves ≥0.04 seconds in duration on their baseline electrocardiograms that were thought to reflect past silent myocardial infarctions.

Exercise Test Responses

Exercise Test Findings:

Exercise stress test responses are summarized according to peak stage achieved, blood pressure at the onset of ischemic-type ST-segment depression, maximum ST-segment depression at peak stage, and heart rate at the onset of ST-segment depression

(Table 8.1). All patients had the onset of ST-segment depression at a peak heart rate of 135 beats per minute or less with the exception of one whose rhythm was atrial fibrillation. Each had a greater than 10 mm Hg increase in systolic blood pressure at peak exercise and at least 2 mm of ST-segment depression during exercise. Exercise was terminated when either the patient became fatigued or ≥2 mm of ST-segment depression was observed.

Coronary Angiographic Findings:

Twelve of the seventeen patients had severe coronary artery disease. The remaining five patients had either normal coronary arteries or only very minor irregularities. The angiographic results are given in Table 8.1.

Ambulatory Electrocardiographic Monitor Findings:

During monitoring periods, no patients recorded symptoms in their diaries. One patient (number 12) withdrew from the study at the end of the first day of monitoring. He had no ST-segment shifts during the hours monitored and was excluded from further consideration because of the limited ambulatory ECG monitoring period; however, he was subsequently found to have coronary artery disease. All of the remaining 16 patients completed three separate 24-hour ambulatory ECG monitoring periods as planned, which yielded a total of 1,154 hours of high quality recordings ranging from 64 to 72 hours per patient. Five patients had no episodes of ischemia during ambulatory ECG monitoring out of the hospital.

Episodes of ischemia were identified in the remaining 11 patients whose findings are summarized in Table 8.2. The total number of ischemic episodes was 69. There were 6.3 ± 7.5 (mean ± SD) episodes per patient. The total ischemic time was 1,240 minutes with a mean of 113 ± 171 minutes per patient (range 3 to 608 minutes).

Heart rates at the onset of 75 percent (52 of 69) of the ischemic episodes recorded during daily activity were lower than heart rates recorded at the onset of the same magnitude of ST-segment depression occurring during exercise testing. Episodes of silent ischemia occurred during ordinary daily activities and were very similar to those associated with silent ischemia in patients with angina pectoris previously reported from this and other laboratories.[3] The magnitude of ischemic ST-segment shifts recorded during daily activity ranged from 1 to 10 mm. In seven patients the magnitude of ST-segment depression was the same or greater during daily activity compared with that recorded at peak exercise.

Patients who were found to have multivessel coronary disease had many more silent ischemic episodes than did those with only one-vessel disease (Figure 8.2). The duration of ambulatory monitoring apparently was related to the ability to detect an ischemic episode during daily life. Of the 11 patients with severe coronary disease, 6 had an ischemic episode detected within 24 hours of the start of ambulatory monitoring. Two additional patients had an episode detected after 40 hours of ambulatory monitoring, and three other patients required 72 hours of ambulatory monitoring before an episode of ischemia was detected (Figure 8.1). This need for extended ambulatory monitoring is further emphasized by analyzing individual patient variability in silent myocardial ischemia. All but 3 of the 11 patients had at least one 24-hour period of monitoring during which no ischemic episodes were recorded. Twenty-four hours of ambulatory monitoring identified only 6 of the 11 patients with silent ischemia, whereas 72 hours of ambulatory monitoring identified all 11 patients.

Table 8.1. Summary of Patient Characteristics, Exercise Treadmill Test (ETT), and Coronary Angiography*

					ETT				Coronary Angiography		
Patient	Age (yr)	ECG	CAD Risk Factors	Previous MI†	Stage	BP at Onset ST†	Max ST† (mm)	HR at Onset ST†	LAD	LCx	RCA
1	69	NL	T	0	III	110/70	3	110	0	20%	80%
2	64	L. Ax	FH, T	0	II	172/84	2	122	<20%	100%	100%
3	57	IMI	T	+	II	180/90	2	130	90%	100%	100%
4	65	AMI	T	+	1/2	156/76	2	120	30%	0	100%
5	54	NL	T	0	I	150/80	2	128	70%	70%	100%
6	77	L. Ax.	T	0	I	174/76	2	100	90%	80%	100%
7	65	NL	T	0	1/2	135/80	2	105	100%	80%	<20%
8	42	NL	HTN	0	1/2	170/95	3	100	90%	100%	100%
9	70	NL	0	+	I	140/85	4	88	100%	0	20%
10	57	NL	DM, Chol	0	II	194/75	2	124	95%	80%	0
11	66	L. Ax.	HTN, T	0	1/2	140/80	4	110	80%	95%	100%
12‡	58	NL	FH, Chol	0	I	180/90	3	130	75%	100%	90%
13	61	NL	DM, FH, T	0	1/2	160/90	2	135	0	0	30%
14	70	AF	T	0	1/2	120/60	2	176	0	40%	40%
15	67	NL	HTN	0	III	170/60	2	133	<20%	0	40%
16	61	NL	T	+	III	166/68	2	124	<20%	0	0
17	58	NL	HTN, FH, DM, T	0	I	150/85	2	135	0	<20%	30%
										0	0

ABBREVIATIONS: AF = atrial fibrillation; AMI = anterior MI; Chol = elevated serum cholesterol; DM = diabetes mellitus; FH = family history; HTN = hypertension; IMI = inferior MI; LAD = left anterior descending; L. Ax. = left axis deviation; LCX = left circumflex; NL = normal; RCA = right coronary artery; T = tobacco.

*From Coy et al.[6] Reproduced with permission of the *American Journal of Cardiology*.

† + = present; 0 = not present.

‡ = withdrew from study after 24 hours.

Table 8.2. Ambulatory Electrocardiographic Monitoring Results in the Eleven Patients with Severe Coronary Artery Disease*

Patient	No. of SMI Episodes	Duration of Episodes (min)	Total Ischemic Time (min)	HR at Onset of SMI	Maximum Magnitude of ST-Segment Depression (mm)	Duration of High Quality Recording (hr)	HR at Onset of ST† at ETT
1	1	6	6	85	1	72	110
2	8	5–33	153	96–120	3	72	122
3	1	35	35	80	1	69	130
4	4	3–20	47	87–105	2	72	120
5	1	3	3	115	1	69	130
6	5	10–75	171	70–100	4	66	100
7	1	10	10	108	2	64	105
8	1	5	5	100	2	72	100
9	32(1)	1–137	608	50–105	10	72	88
10	1	39	39	89	1	72	124
11	14(2)	3–40	163	68–115	4	70	110
Total	69	1–137†	1,240	50–120†	1–10†	770	88–130†
Mean ± SD	6.3 ± 9.5		113 ± 177				

* From Coy et al.[6]

† Range: (1) onset of 16 episodes was at HR > 88/min; (2) onset of 1 episode was at HR > 110/min.

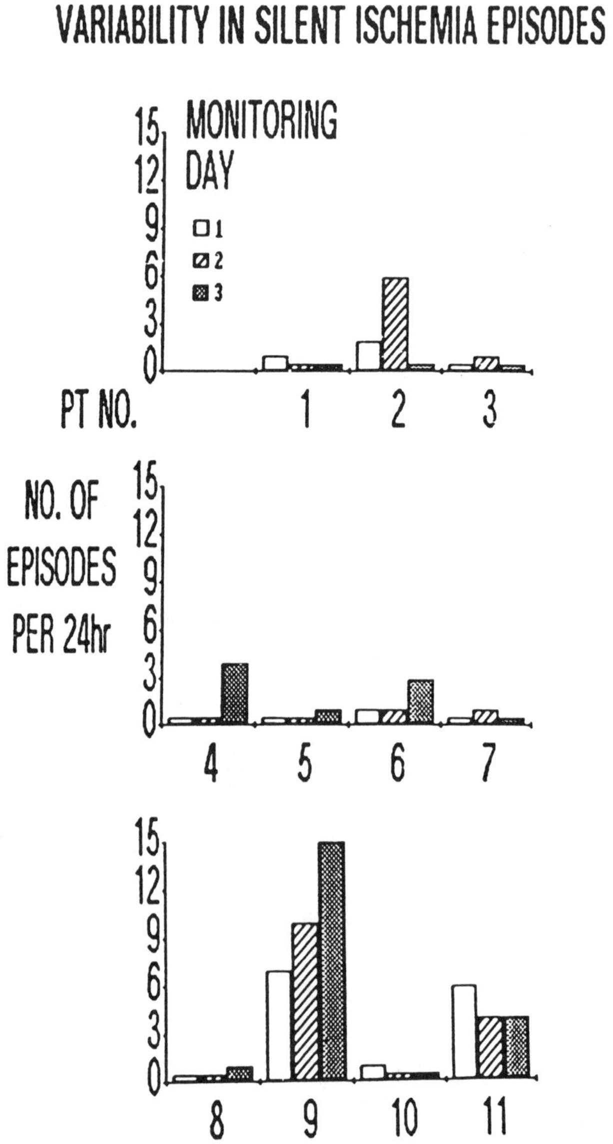

FIGURE 8.1. Summary of silent ischemic episodes in each of 11 patients during 3 consecutive days of monitoring. Note the wide day-to-day variability in many patients for each day of monitoring.

Analysis of daily variation in silent ischemia showed a trend for total ischemic time to increase after waking, as noted by us and others.[7–9] Although there was no statistically significant clustering of ischemia in any quarter of the day, lack of clustering was attributed to a single patient (number 9) who had nearly 200 minutes of silent ischemia occurring in the 1200 to 1800 and 1800 to 2400-hour quarters.

WORK BY OTHERS

Results of studies on silent ischemia during ambulant living reported by others are summarized along with our results in Table 8.3 and Figures 8.3 and 8.4. These 26 patients represent the worldwide experience in asymptomatic patients with coronary

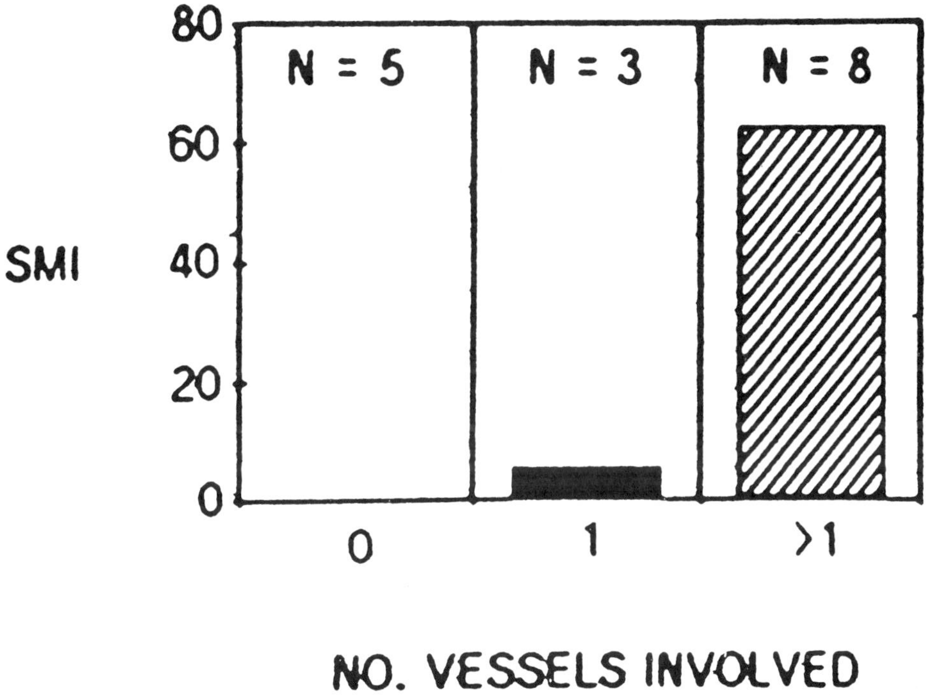

FIGURE 8.2. Total episodes of silent myocardial ischemia (SMI) per 72 hours and the extent of coronary artery disease in 11 asymptomatic subjects with positive exercise tests. N = number of patients.

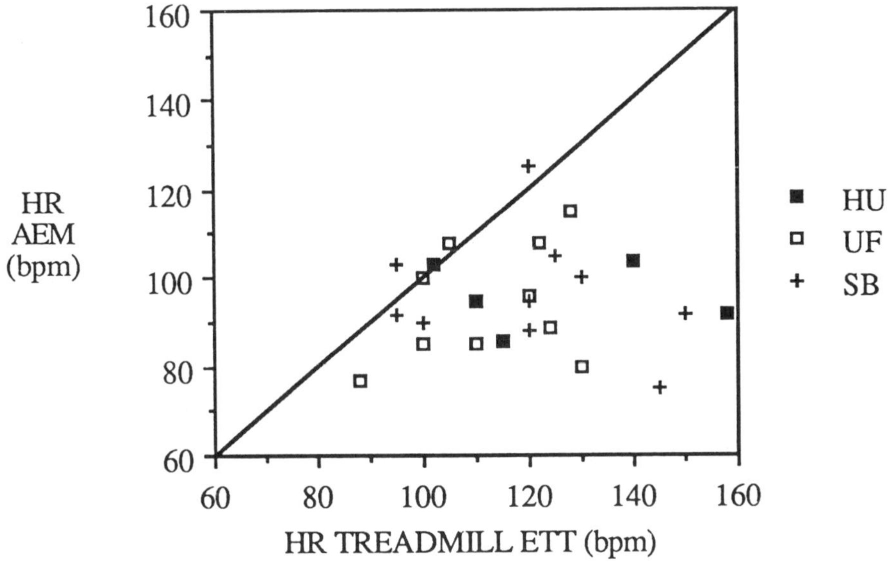

FIGURE 8.3. Relation between heart rate (HR) at onset of ischemia during treadmill exercise test (ETT, *horizontal axis*) and ambulant living (AEM, *vertical axis*). Heart rate during ischemia with ambulant living recorded by AEM was averaged for each patient from episodes occurring in each of the 26 asymptomatic men reported. HU = Campbell et al; UF = Coy et al; SB = Cohn et al. The line of identity is shown and the HR is uniformly high during exercise.

Table 8.3. Reported Asymptomatic Patients with Coronary Artery Disease (CAD) with Positive Exercise Treadmill Test and Silent Ischemia

Author (yr)/ No. Patients	Age (yr)	Old MI	MV CAD	AEM (hr)	SMI	Max AEM Ischemia No.	Time (min)	ST (mm)
Campbell[7], 1986								
5 men	51	4	5	48–96	2–13	13	622	5.0
Coy[6], 1987								
11 men	62	4	8	72	1–32	32	608	10.0
Cohn[8], 1987								
10 men	57	3	7	48	1–17	17	239	4.5
Totals								
26 men	57	11	20	48–96	1–32	32	622	10.0
(5%)	(42)	(74)						

ABBREVIATIONS: AEM = ambulatory electrocardiographic monitoring; MI = myocardial infarction; MV = multivessel; SMI = silent myocardial ischemia.

artery disease who were studied by ambulatory ECG monitoring. Campbell and coworkers[7] were the first to describe silent myocardial ischemia during daily activities detected by ambulatory monitoring in patients with painless, positive exercise tests. Four of the seven were taking no antiischemic medication when studied. These workers found five patients (age range 34 to 68) who had ≥1 mm of ST-segment depression lasting ≥30 seconds after 48 to 96 hours of monitoring per patient. Four of these five patients had at least one previous myocardial infarction, and all five had multivessel coronary artery disease. Most (68%) episodes were 10 minutes or less in duration and ranged from 1 to 253 minutes. Most (70%) had maximal ST-segment depression ranging from 1 to 2 mm, although one patient had approximately 5 mm of ST-segment depression. A small increase in heart rate preceded 65 percent of the episodes. However, 35 percent of the episodes were associated with no change or even a decline in heart rate before the onset of ischemia. Most episodes occurred at rest or during relatively light physical activity. Approximately 8 percent occurred

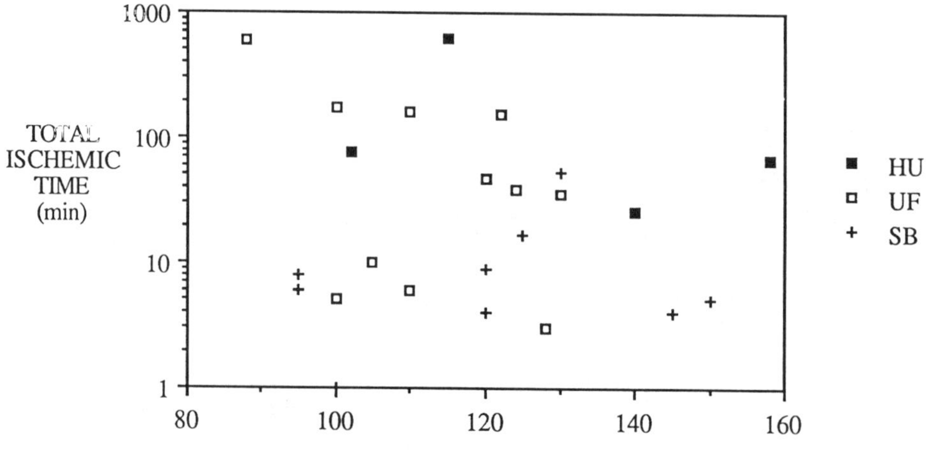

FIGURE 8.4. Relation between heart rate (HR) at onset of ischemia during treadmill exercise (ETT, *horizontal axis*) and the total ischemic time during ambulant living (AEM) for each of 26 asymptomatic patients. There is no apparent relation.

during sleep, and only 38 percent during exercise. Seventy-eight percent of the episodes were recorded during periods when the subjects reported that their mental activity was usual, and 14 percent during mental stress. A distinct diurnal variation was found in these five patients, with 57 percent of the episodes of ischemia occurring between 0600 and 1200 hours.

More recently, Cohn and Lawson[8] described results of studies in 10 asymptomatic patients with coronary disease who were monitored during daily activities while they were not receiving cardiac drugs. The age range of these patients was 41 to 74 years and three had a prior myocardial infarction. Multivessel coronary artery disease was present in seven of the patients whose ambulatory monitoring periods averaged 48 hours per patient. All 10 patients had silent myocardial ischemia during ambulatory monitoring, ranging from 1 to 17 episodes per monitoring period. The duration of silent ischemia was 798 (range 1 to 80) minutes over the monitoring period, and the magnitude of ST-segment depression ranged from 1 to 4.5 mm. Heart rate at the onset of these episodes ranged from 65 to 150 (mean 98) beats per minute and was less than that seen during treadmill exercise (mean 120) in the same patients. Striking circadian variation was noted, as 47 percent of the episodes occurred between 0600 and 1200 hours.

CLINICAL IMPLICATIONS

These findings suggest that silent myocardial ischemia during daily life is relatively common in patients with asymptomatic positive exercise tests who have coronary artery disease. In one study silent ischemia was found in five of seven patients, but only 48-hour monitoring periods were used in two patients in whom silent ischemia was not detected by ambulatory ECG monitoring. In our study it was found in 11 of 16 patients who completed all monitoring periods, but the five negative patients were not found to have coronary artery disease. In the Cohn study, silent ischemia was found by ambulatory ECG monitoring during daily life in 10 of 10 consecutive patients. These data, although limited to only 28 patients, suggest that silent ischemia occurs frequently in asymptomatic patients with positive treadmill exercise tests who have coronary artery disease. It should be noted that in most of these patients severe multivessel coronary artery disease was present. Silent ischemia in these asymptomatic patients seems to have the same characteristics as silent ischemia occurring during daily life in symptomatic patients.[3–5]

The course of asymptomatic patients with silent ischemia during daily life is unknown. However, there is ample evidence to indicate that asymptomatic, high risk patients with abnormal exercise ECG responses have a higher mortality from coronary artery disease than do patients with similar risk factors and normal exercise electrocardiographs.[10] Whether the presence of silent ischemia during daily life adds additional prognostic information over that imparted by other risk factors and the abnormal exercise response remains to be determined. However, silent ischemia detected by ambulatory ECG monitoring has been a positive factor strongly related to prognosis in many studies of symptomatic patients.[11–13]

The optimal duration of ambulatory ECG monitoring required to provide a reasonable specificity and sensitivity for the detection of silent ischemia during daily life is unknown. The literature on symptomatic patients undergoing ambulatory ECG monitoring for silent ischemia reveals monitoring periods that range from 12 to 72 hours. Seventy-two hours of ambulatory ECG monitoring were required to detect

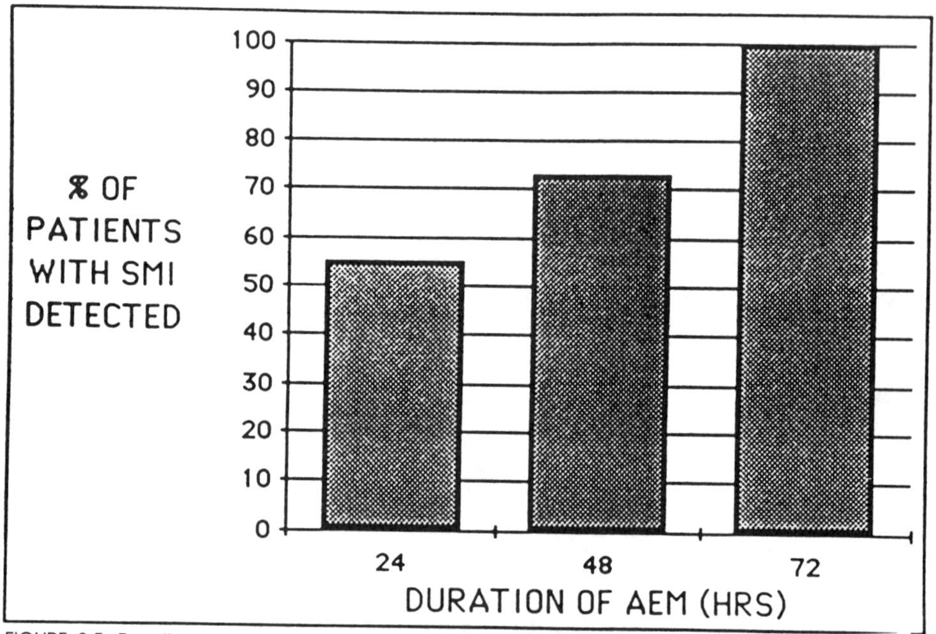

FIGURE 8.5. Duration of ambulatory ECG monitoring (AEM) required to identify silent myocardial ischemia (SMI) in 11 patients with severe coronary artery disease.[6] (Reproduced with permission of the *American Journal of Cardiology*.)

silent ischemia in some patients in our study (Figure 8.5), probably because silent ischemia occurred relatively infrequently in some individuals and also is known to be widely variable. The latter, however, simply reflects the numerous processes that have the ability to convert relatively quiescent coronary artery disease into active myocardial ischemia. These stressor processes are only now being recognized. Ambulatory monitoring in this asymptomatic group of patients may be of considerable use in the identification of those patients at risk for ischemic events. In such evaluations, however, the usefulness of ambulatory ECG monitoring will be lessened considerably if shorter monitoring periods are used. For this, the newer, longer use ambulatory ECG monitoring provided by digital recorders may offer a considerable advantage.

In summary, silent myocardial ischemia appears to be relatively common during active daily life in asymptomatic patients with positive exercise test responses and coronary artery disease. Information on the prevalence of this finding in the general population and what additional prognostic information ischemia provides during active life are anxiously awaited from studies in progress. In addition, the ability of certain therapeutic manipulations to alter silent ischemia in this group is of considerable interest.

REFERENCES

1. Warners CA, Roberts WC: Morphologic findings in sudden coronary death: A comparison of those with/those without previous symptoms of myocardial ischemia, in Pepine CJ (ed): *Cardiology Clinics: Silent Myocardial Ischemia*. Philadelphia, WB Saunders, 1986, vol 4, pp 607–615.
2. Lindsey HE, Cohn PF: "Silent" myocardial ischemia during and after exercise testing in patients with coronary artery disease. *Am Heart J* 1978;95:441–447.

3. Schang SJ, Pepine CJ: Transient asymptomatic ST segment depression during daily activity. *Am J Cardiol* 1977;39:396–402.
4. Deanfield JE, Selwyn AP, Chierchia S, Maseri A, Ribeiro P, Krikler S, Morgan M: Myocardial ischemia during daily life in patients with stable angina: Its relation to symptoms and heart rate changes. *Lancet* 1983;1:753–758.
5. Cecchi AC, Dovellini EV, Marchi F, Pucci P, Santoro GM, Fazzini PF: Silent myocardial ischemia during ambulatory electrocardiographic monitoring in patients with effort angina. *J Am Coll Cardiol* 1983;1:934–939.
6. Coy KM, Imperi GA, Lambert CR, Pepine CJ: Silent myocardial ischemia during daily activities in asymptomatic men with positive exercise test responses. *Am J Cardiol* 1987;59:45–49.
7. Campbell S, Barry J, Rebecca GS, Rocco MB, Nabel EG, Wayne RR, Selwyn AP: Active transient myocardial ischemia during daily life in asymptomatic patients with positive exercise tests and coronary artery disease. *Am J Cardiol* 1986;57:1010–1016.
8. Cohn PF, Lawson WE: Characteristics of silent myocardial ischemia during out-of-the-hospital activities in asymptomatic angiographically documented coronary artery disease. *Am J Cardiol* 1987;59:746–749.
9. Imperi GA, Lambert CR, Coy K, Lopez L, Pepine CJ: Effects of titrated beta blockade (metoprolol) on silent myocardial ischemia in ambulatory patients with coronary artery disease. *Am J Cardiol* 1987;60:519–524.
10. Multiple Risk Factor Intervention Trial Research Group. Exercise electrocardiogram and coronary heart disease mortality in the Multiple Risk Factor Intervention Trial. *Am J Cardiol* 1985;55:16–24.
11. Johnson SM, Mauritson DR, Winniford MD, Willerson JT, Firth BG, Cary JR, Hillis LD: Continuous electrocardiographic monitoring in patients with unstable angina pectoris: Identification of high-risk subgroup with severe coronary disease, variant angina, and/or impaired early prognosis. *Am Heart J* 1982;103:4–12.
12. Gottlieb SO, Weisfeldt ML, Ouyang P, Mellits ED, Gerstenblith G: Silent ischemia as a marker for early unfavorable outcomes in patients with unstable angina. *N Engl J Med* 1986;314:1214–1219.
13. Nademanee K, Intarachot V, Josephson M, Rieders D, Mody FV, Singh B: Prognostic significance of silent myocardial ischemia in patients with unstable angina. *J Am Coll Cardiol* 1987;10:1–9.

CHAPTER 9

Characteristics of Silent and Symptomatic Ischemia in Chronic Stable Angina

Comparison with Unstable and Vasospastic Angina

John E. Deanfield, MD

It is increasingly appreciated that transient myocardial ischemia is a major cause of myocardial scarring, infarction, and sudden death. Therefore, the character and causes of ischemia must be understood as it occurs in different subsets of patients with coronary artery disease.[1–3] Angina pectoris is the most frequent symptom accompanying transient regional myocardial ischemia. Indeed, its frequency, character, and trigger mechanisms have been for years the conventional means of determining the risk of adverse coronary events and assessing responses to treatment.

It is clear, however, from studies in and out of hospital, that angina pectoris underestimates the true incidence of myocardial ischemia, with many episodes being completely asymptomatic.[4,5] In hospital studies, thallium-201 scintigraphy,[6] ST-segment changes, increases in left ventricular end-diastolic pressure,[7] and increases in myocardial oxygen extraction[8] have all been reported without symptoms. Recent interest in this "silent ischemic activity" has been awakened by studies using ambulatory ECG monitoring which enables objective observations to be made in patients during their normal daily activities. These studies reveal a picture of disease activity that differs from that inculcated by traditional teaching. The newer information may necessitate a reevaluation of the overall clinical approach to the diagnosis, follow-up, and treatment of ischemic heart disease. This chapter examines the clinical characteristics of silent and symptomatic episodes of myocardial ischemia in different patient populations with coronary artery disease and the impact that assessment of total ischemic activity (symptomatic and silent) may have on the understanding of pathophysiology and patient management.

USE OF ST-SEGMENT CHANGE TO STUDY MYOCARDIAL ISCHEMIA

Ambulatory monitoring of ST-segment changes provides a unique method for obtaining objective information from patients over long periods of time during normal daily life rather than during the narrow "window" of the patient's brief visits to the hospital. Its value obviously depends on the reliability of the ST-segment deviation as a marker of ischemia and, in addition, on whether the character of the ST-segment change can be used to describe the character of the underlying myocardial ischemia. Initially, doubts about transient ST-segment changes, detected out of the hospital, arose because of the technical deficiencies of monitoring devices used in early studies and concern about the specificity of ST-segment change in the population.[9,10] The adoption of frequency-modulated monitors, improvement in amplitude modulated systems, and the recent introduction of digital recorders have significantly overcome the technical problems. These newer systems have allowed the detection as well as the quantitation of frequency and duration of ischemia with a high degree of reliability.

OBSERVATIONS IN NORMAL SUBJECTS AND IN PATIENTS WITH CHRONIC STABLE ANGINA

Our own observations in normal volunteers have revealed a very low incidence of significant ST-segment depression.[11] During 24-hours of monitoring, only 2 of 100 subjects, both aged more than 40 and both with risk factors for coronary disease, showed ST-segment depression that met study criteria and that have now been accepted for the detection of ischemia in patients. In patients with known coronary artery disease, the validity of the ST-segment deviation as a marker of ischemia, both with and without accompanying angina, has been extensively studied using rubidium-82 and positron emission tomography. The regional myocardial uptake of cations such as rubidium-82 provides a measure of myocardial blood flow that can be used to follow ischemic changes in individual patients in a number of physiologic circumstances.[12–14] In one study, regional disturbances of perfusion were found in 63 of 65 episodes of painful ST-segment depression (97%) and 30 of 30 (100%) painless episodes of ST-segment depression recorded in 30 patients with chronic stable angina[15] (Figure 9.1). In each case, the abnormal region of myocardium was always the same during painful and painless ischemia. Our studies using ambulatory monitoring of the electrocardiogram in patients with chronic stable angina and coronary disease demonstrated surprisingly prolonged episodes of ischemic ST-segment depression.[16] The median duration of episodes was approximately 20 minutes. Does this prolonged ST-segment depression indicate prolonged underlying myocardial ischemia? Studies using positron tomography suggest that prolonged abnormalities of regional myocardial uptake of rubidium-82 and myocardial perfusion are common after a number of triggers of ischemia. Indeed, clinical observations of pain and even ST-segment change frequently underestimate the duration of the ischemic disturbances in the ventricular myocardium.

A typical study showing the relation of angina, ST-segment depression, and reduced cation regional myocardial uptake after exercise-induced ischemia in a patient with chronic stable angina is shown in Figure 9.2. In 40 similar patients, the affected segment of myocardium was still significantly abnormal after 6 to 8 minutes in 46 of 52 tests, after 12 to 14 minutes in 32 tests, after 17 to 20 minutes in 15 tests, and after 23 minutes in 6 tests.[17] Similar studies in patients recovering after ischemic events also showed that the depth of ST-segment depression is a reasonable means of following the severity of ischemic disturbances in the myocardium. These investigations increase confidence in the use of ST-segment change to follow not just the incidence but also the character of ischemia outside the hospital.

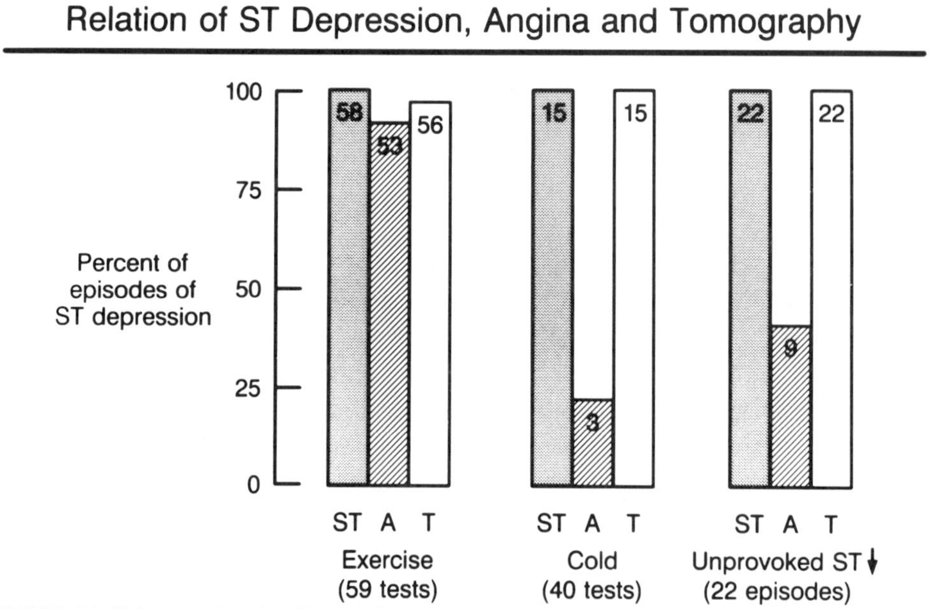

FIGURE 9.1. Histogram showing the relation between angina, ST-segment depression, and tomographic evidence of regional myocardial perfusion in 30 patients with chronic stable angina studied by positron tomography with rubidium-82.

PAINFUL AND PAINLESS ST-SEGMENT CHANGES

Our observation during 446 days of monitoring 30 patients with chronic stable angina and positive exercise tests over 18 months revealed 1,934 episodes of transient ST-segment depression (≥0.1 mV) with only 417 (24%) accompanied by angina pectoris.[16] This ratio of painful to painless episodes confirms the findings of other studies in chronic stable angina[4,5,18] and is similar to observations in unstable angina,[19,20] in variant angina,[8,18] and after myocardial infarction (Chapter 14). For example, in the study reported by Nademanee et al[20] who analyzed Holter recordings from 41 patients with unstable angina, there were 781 episodes of ischemia: 392 (50%) with ST-segment depression, 242 (31%) with ST-segment elevation, and the remainder with other ECG abnormalities. Only 154 (20%) of the 781 episodes were associated with angina. In a subsequent study[18] in which the characteristics of ischemia in chronic stable angina and in Prinzmetal's angina were examined, 90 percent of the episodes in either condition were silent. Eighty percent of the ischemic episodes of variant angina showed ST-segment elevation in patients with angiographically normal coronary arteries; in chronic stable angina all episodes demonstrated ST-segment depression. It was of interest that in this study, the ischemic episodes in patients with Prinzmetal's angina were short (mean 3 ± 2 minutes), but they occurred more frequently (mean 21 ± 18 per 24 hours). In contrast, the mean deviation of ischemic episodes in chronic stable angina was significantly longer (18 ± 23 minutes; $p < 0.01$), but the overall frequency of the attacks was significantly less (6 ± 4 per 24 hours; $p < 0.01$) than that in patients with variant angina.

Why should some episodes of ischemia be painful and others silent? The question has been extensively researched, but the mechanisms responsible for cardiac ischemic pain are complex and poorly understood (see Chapter 4). Certainly, the duration and severity of the ischemic insult do not appear to be sufficient to explain

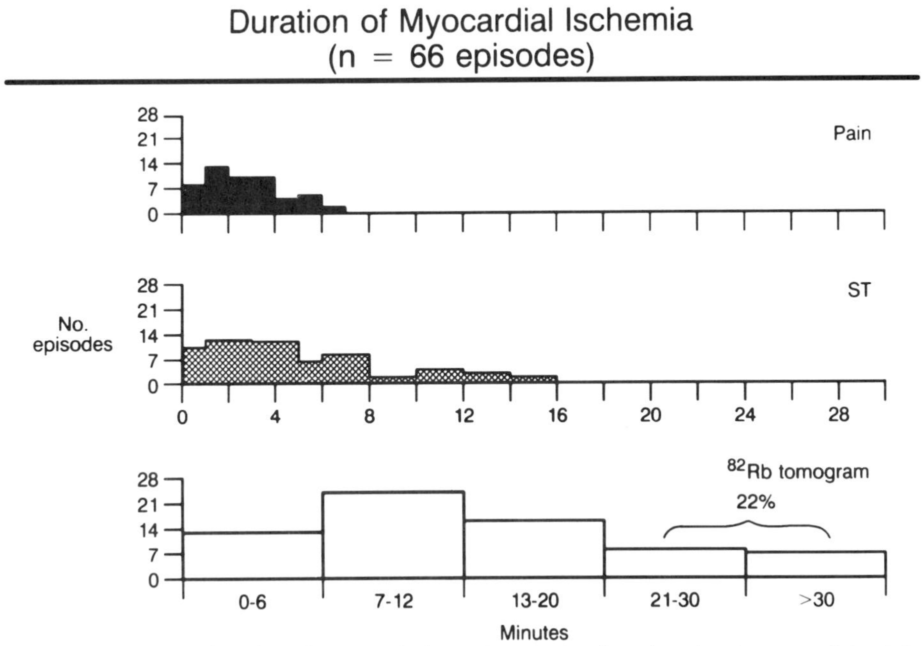

FIGURE 9.2. Relation of angina, ST-segment depression, and reduced regional myocardial uptake of rubidium-82(^{82}RB) during exercise-induced ischemia in a patient with chronic stable angina. Tomographic abnormalities persisted for much longer than either symptoms or ST-segment changes.

the presence or absence of symptoms. In our patients with chronic stable angina, symptomatic episodes lasted on the average slightly longer than asymptomatic episodes, and a higher proportion of episodes of severe ST-segment depression were accompanied by angina. However, there was considerable overlap between painful and painless episodes between and within patients. Similar findings were reported for patients with rest angina studied in the coronary care unit, with again no ECG features to reliably predict the presence of cardiac pain.[8]

PATHOPHYSIOLOGY OF SYMPTOMATIC AND SILENT MYOCARDIAL ISCHEMIA

Until recently myocardial ischemia was thought to occur when critical fixed coronary stenoses limit appropriate increases in coronary blood flow during periods of increased demand (see Chapter 2). It is now clear, however, that this traditional concept is not sufficient to explain recent clinical and experimental observations that suggest an active role for factors affecting coronary blood supply as well as myocardial oxygen demand in the genesis of ischemia.[21]

The first clinical situation in which this became apparent was variant angina.[22] Although rare, this syndrome demonstrated the ability of epicardial coronary arteries to alter their vasomotor tone and thus affect coronary blood flow. Studies by Chierchia and colleagues[23] in patients with rest angina showed that the first detectable abnormality during the ischemic event was an absolute fall in regional coronary blood flow, as indicated by a decrease in coronary sinus oxygen saturation which was then followed by ventricular dysfunction and in some cases ECG abnormalities and cardiac pain. Numerous investigations have consistently demonstrated "spasm" of epicardial coronary arteries in such circumstances.

In chronic stable angina, ECG monitoring outside the hospital also implicates transient changes in coronary blood flow in many circumstances. The majority of ischemic episodes during normal daily activities, both in our studies and those described by others, were not preceded by a significant increase in heart rate of the type that occurs during physical exercise.[16,24,25] Furthermore, episodes of ST-segment depression occurred at heart rates well below those that could be achieved during the rest of the day without ST-segment depression as well as below levels found at the onset of ST-segment depression during exercise testing in the hospital. Levels of heart rate and changes in heart rate preceding painful and painless ST-segment depression were indistinguishable (Figure 9.3). Further indirect evidence that the presence or absence of pain does not indicate differing pathophysiology comes from the circadian distribution of ischemic events throughout the day. We reported a peak in ischemic activity in patients with chronic stable angina between 6 and 9 AM, which is similar for painful and painless episodes.[26] This finding has been confirmed in a number of studies (see Chapter 6) that have revealed a more pronounced circadian variability when a correction for time of waking was introduced.[27] A number of factors potentially able to affect supply and demand may be responsible for these observations and require study.

To examine more directly the pathophysiologic character of painful and silent myocardial ischemia in patients with coronary disease, a study was designed to examine the disturbances of coronary supply and myocardial oxygen demand using positron emission tomography and rubidium-82 during provoked and "spontaneous" ischemic events.[28] Both exercise-induced and unprovoked ischemia with and without pain were accompanied by an absolute decrease in the regional myocardial uptake

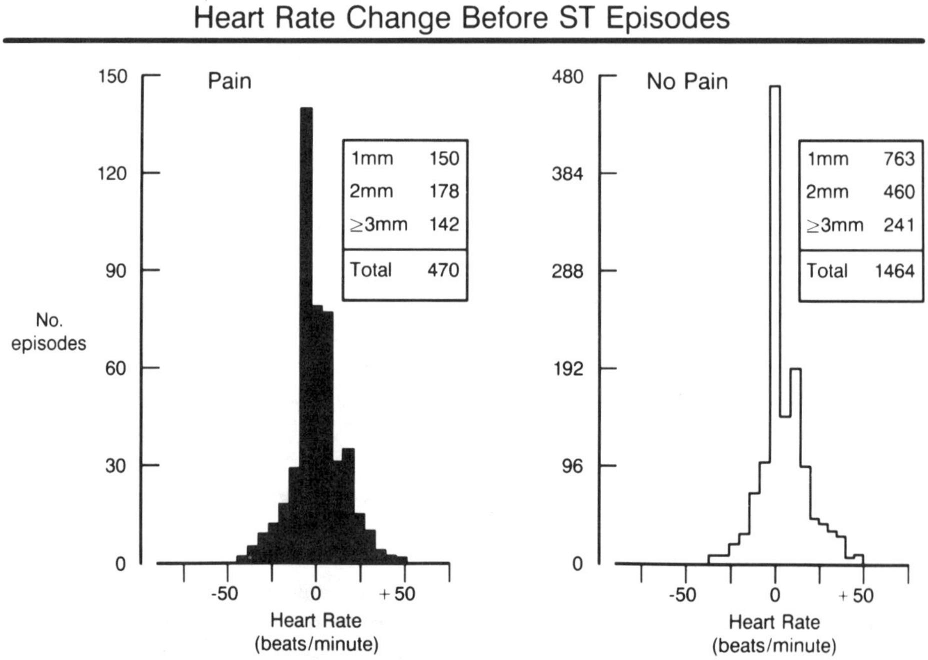

FIGURE 9.3. Histogram showing heart rate change during the minute preceding ST-segment depression in 1,928 episodes of ST-segment depression with and without angina recorded in 30 patients with chronic stable angina. There was no difference between painful and painless episodes. In 75 percent, the heart rate increased by less than 10 beats per minute during the preceding minute.

of rubidium-82 in the affected segment of the myocardium, suggesting a decrease in regional myocardial perfusion. The occurrence of angina and ST-segment depression was not related to the severity of decreased myocardial perfusion to this ischemic segment. These decreases in perfusion were indistinguishable during painful and painless ischemic episodes when comparisons where depression tended to occur when failure of supply was also accompanied by a significant increase in myocardial oxygen demand (and in response by greater increase in perfusion to remote myocardium). These findings add further powerful support for the inclusion of silent ischemic episodes as well as those accompanied by angina when activity of disease and therapeutic strategies are being assessed, because the potentially damaging disturbances of regional coronary blood flow are no different in silent and painful episodes with angina.

MECHANISMS FOR DISTURBED REGIONAL MYOCARDIAL PERFUSION

It is becoming increasingly clear that events in the epicardial coronary arteries, capable of affecting coronary blood supply, play an important role in most ischemic episodes. However, underlying mechanisms are likely to be different in different patient subgroups. For example, physiologic variation in epicardial coronary tone may profoundly affect coronary diameter and thus coronary perfusion when the lumen is already significantly narrowed by an atherosclerotic plaque. Conversely, focal inappropriate vasoconstriction or coronary "spasm" found in patients with variant angina is not simply an increase in physiologic constriction, but is probably due to local coronary artery hyperreactivity responding to a variety of different trigger stimuli.[29] This syndrome is uncommon, and there is good evidence that the basis of vasomotor disturbances seen in the much more common condition of chronic stable angina is very different (see Chapter 2). In a recent study, episodes of ST-segment changes during normal daily activities were compared in patients with variant angina and those with chronic stable angina.[18] The ECG changes were different (ST-segment elevation predominated in variant angina and was entirely absent in chronic stable angina); there was a clear circadian distribution of ischemia in chronic stable angina but a less distinctive one in Prinzmetal's angina. This subject is dealt with at length in Chapter 6.

Recent elegant work by Ludmer, Ganz, Nabel, Gordon, and Selwyn in Boston has expanded on experimental work to indicate that the integrity and function of the vascular endothelium play a crucial role in determining the vasomotor properties of epicardial coronary arteries in patients with atherosclerosis. Failure of the endothelial dependent relaxant factor (EDRF) to release accounts for the paradoxic vasoconstrictor response of human atherosclerotic epicardial coronary arteries to acetylcholine.[30] This was shown to parallel the vessel's vasomotor responses to more usual physiologic stimuli such as exercise and exposure to cold.[31,32]

PRACTICAL IMPLICATIONS

It is now clear that transient myocardial ischemia frequently occurs without angina pectoris in a wide variety of clinical settings including chronic stable angina and variant angina as well as following myocardial infarction. All evidence indicates that the character and severity of disturbed perfusion in painful and painless ischemia are identical, and therefore both may have to be considered when evaluating patients in terms of risk stratification for therapy. This view is supported by prospective studies in patients that indicate that the presence of silent ischemia identifies patient subgroups at high risk for adverse coronary events including myocardial infarction and sudden death. When silent events are considered together with angina in studies during patients' normal daily lives, a more comprehensive picture of disease activity can be obtained. Ischemia is frequent, prolonged, and variable, and the pathophysiologic basis appears to be different from traditional concepts involving both variable oxygen supply and demand. These findings are important in the investigation of underlying mechanisms responsible for ischemia in different clinical subgroups. Treatment strategies may increasingly need to consider asymptomatic ischemic activity as well as pain in an attempt to prevent myocardial damage and improve prognosis.

REFERENCES

1. Cohn PF, Braunwald E: Chronic ischemic heart disease, in Braunwald E (ed): *Heart Disease, a Textbook of Cardiovascular Medicine*. Philadelphia. WB Saunders, 1984, pp 1334–1344.
2. Sobel BE, Braunwald E: Coronary blood flow and myocardial ischemia, in Braunwald E (ed): *Heart Disease, a Textbook of Cardiovascular Medicine*. Philadelphia, WB Saunders, 1984, pp 1235–1241.
3. Weiner DA, Ryan TJ, McCabe CH, Chaitman BR, Sheffield LT, Ferguson JC, Fisher LF, Tristani F: Prognostic importance of a clinical profile and exercise test in medically treated patients with coronary artery disease. *J Am Coll Cardiol* 1984;3:772–780.
4. Stern S, Tzivoni D: Early detection of silent ischaemic heart disease by 24-hour electrocardiographic monitoring of active subjects. *Br Heart J* 1974;36:481–486.
5. Schang SJ Jr, Pepine CJ: Transient asymptomatic ST-segment depression during daily activity. *Am J Cardiol* 1977;39:396–402.
6. Maseri A, Parodi O, Severi S, Pesola A: Transient transluminal reduction of myocardial blood flow, demonstrated by thallium-201 scintigraphy, as a cause of variant angina. *Circulation* 1976;54:280–288.
7. Maseri A, Mimmo R, Chierchia S et al: Coronary artery spasm as a cause of acute myocardial ischemia in man. *Chest* 1975;68:625–633.
8. Chierchia S, Lazzari M, Freedman B, Brunelli C, Maseri A: Impairment of myocardial perfusion and function during painless myocardial ischemia. *J Am Coll Cardiol* 1983;1:924–930.
9. Bragg-Remschel DA, Anderson CM, Winkle RA: Frequency-response characteristics of ambulatory ECG monitoring systems and their implications for ST-segment analysis. *Amer Heart J* 1982;103:20–31.
10. Armstrong WF, Jordan JW, Morris SN, McHenry PL: Prevalence and magnitude of ST-segment and T-wave abnormalities in normal men during continuous ambulatory electrocardiography. *Amer J Cardiol* 1982;49:1638–1642.
11. Deanfield JE, Ribiero P, Oakley K, Krikler S, Selwyn AP: Analysis of ST-segment changes in normal subjects: Implications for ambulatory monitoring in angina pectoris. *Am J Cardiol* 1984;54:1321–1325.
12. Selwyn AP, Allan RM, L'Abbate A et al: Relation between regional myocardial uptake of rubidium-82 and perfusion: Absolute reduction of cation uptake in ischemia. *Am J Cardiol* 1982;50:112–121.
13. Zaret BL: Myocardial imaging with radioactive potassium and its analogues, in Holman BH, Sonnenblick EH, Lesch M (eds): *Principles of Cardiovascular Nuclear Medicine*. New York, Grune & Stratton, 1978, pp 49–53.
14. Prokop EK, Strauss WW, Shaw J: Comparison of regional myocardial perfusion determined by ionic potassium-42 and that determined by microspheres. *Circulation* 1979;50:978–984.

15. Deanfield JE, Shea M, Ribiero P et al: Transient ST-segment depression as a marker of myocardial ischemia during daily life. *Am J Cardiol* 1984;54:1195–1200.
16. Deanfield JE, Maseri A, Selwyn AP et al: Myocardial ischemia during daily life in patients with stable angina: Its relation to symptoms and heart rate changes. *Lancet* 1983;II:753–758.
17. Selwyn AP, Shea MJ, Deanfield JE, Wilson RA de Landsheere CM, Jonathan A, Horlock P, Jones T: Prolonged disturbances of ventricular myocardium following ischemic events in patients with coronary disease. *Circulation,* in press, 1988.
18. Nademanee K, Intarachot V, Josephson MA, Singh BN: Circadian variation in occurrence of transient overt and silent myocardial ischemia in chronic stable angina and comparison with Prinzmetal angina in men. *Am J Cardiol* 1987;60:494–498.
19. Johnson SM, Mauritson DR, Winniford MD et al: Continuous electrocardiographic monitoring in patients with unstable angina pectoris. Identification of high-risk subgroups with severe coronary disease, variant angina and/or impaired early prognosis. *Am Heart J* 1982;103:4–12.
20. Nademanee K, Intarachot V, Josephson MA, Singh BN: Characteristics and clinical significance of silent myocardial ischemia in unstable angina. *Am J Cardiol* 1986;58:26B.
21. Maseri A: The changing face of angina pectoris: Practical implications. *Lancet* 1983;1:746–749.
22. Prinzmetal M, Kennamer R, Merliss R et al: Angina pectoris; a variant form of angina pectoris. *Am J Med* 1959;27:375–88.
23. Chierchia S, Brunelli C, Simonetti I et al: Sequence of events in angina at rest; primary reduction in coronary flow. *Circulation* 1980;61:759–768.
24. Chierchia S, Gallino A, Smith G et al: Role of heart rate in pathophysiology of chronic stable angina. *Lancet* 1984;1:1353–1357.
25. Singh BN, Nademanee K, Figueras J, Josephson MA: Hemodynamic and electrocardiographic correlates of symptomatic and silent myocardial ischemia: Pathophysiologic and therapeutic implications. *Am J Cardiol* 1986;58:3B.
26. Deanfield JE, Shea MJ, Selwyn AP: Clinical evaluation of transient myocardial ischemia during daily life. *Am J Med* 1985;(suppl 3A):18–24.
27. Rocco MB, Barry J, Campbell S, Nabel E, Cook F, Goldman L, Selwyn AP: Circadian variation of transient myocardial ischemia in patients with coronary artery disease. *Circulation* 1987;75:395–400.
28. Selwyn AP, Deanfield JE, Shea MJ, Wilson R, de Landsheere CM, O'Brien J, Jones T: Differences in pathophysiology between painful and silent transient myocardial ischemia in coronary artery disease. *Circulation* in press, 1988.
29. Maseri A, Chierchia S: Coronary artery spasm: Demonstration, definition, diagnosis and consequences. *Prog Cardiovasc Dis* 1982;XXV:169–191.
30. Ludmer PL, Selwyn AP, Shook TL, Wayne RR, Mudge GJ, Alexander RW, Ganz P: Paradoxical vasconstriction induced by acetylcholine in atherosclerotic coronary arteries. *N Engl J Med* 1986;315:1046–1051.
31. Nabel EG, Ganz P, Gordon JB, Wayne RW, Selwyn AP: Atherosclerosis determines the response of coronary arteries to cold pressor stimulation (abstract). *J Am Coll Cardiol* 1987;9:68A.
32. Gordon JB, Ganz P, Nabel EG, Selwyn AP: Endothelial function influences the coronary vasomotor response to exercise. *Circulation* 1987;76(suppl IV):238.

CHAPTER 10

Silent Ischemia and Noradrenergic Tone in Ambulatory Hypertensives with Left Ventricular Hypertrophy and Stable Angina

Vincent DeQuattro, MD, Debora De-Ping Lee, MD, Shinobu Kimura, MD, Vinh Ngo, MD, Timothy Cox, Thuy Quang Pham, MD, and Kathryn Rigonan, MD

With the Technical Assistance of
Peter Wong, RDMS, RCPT, RRT

Hypertension is a major risk factor for coronary atherosclerosis and thereby the leading cause of death in the United States of America.[1] Ventricular ectopy[2] and reduced coronary reserve,[3] which are sequelae of hypertensive heart disease, appear to participate in the fatal event. Transient episodes of myocardial ischemia, most of which occur silently, are a source of morbidity and mortality in normotensive patients with coronary artery disease and might adversely affect prognosis in hypertensive patients.[4,5] The sympathetic nervous system may be involved in the pathogenesis of several features of the hypertensive cardiovascular diatheses: blood pressure elevation,[6] left ventricular hypertrophy,[7] and dynamic alterations in coronary artery vasomotor tone.[8]

In this study the role of noradrenergic tone in the genesis of silent myocardial ischemia was assessed in normotensive and hypertensive patients with stable angina. We measured left ventricular mass and silent myocardial ischemia, simultaneously with plasma norepinephrine, epinephrine, and normetanephrine, coincident with the tone alert of a real-time ECG monitor and obtained by a portable withdrawal pump, while the patients lived their normal daily lives. Furthermore, the effects of metoprolol, a cardioselective beta-blocker, on blood pressure, heart rate, silent ischemia, and sympathetic activity were studied.

METHODS

Patients

Ten normotensive and 20 hypertensive patients (both male and female) with stable angina (at least two or three anginal episodes per week) participated in this study. All these patients had evidence of exercise-induced myocardial ischemia during a placebo run-in period. They gave written informed consent, and the protocol was approved by the Institutional Research Review Committee. Hypertensive patients who were treated with hydrochlorothiazide in doses up to 100 mg per day were included in this study, but when their average blood pressure exceeded 160/104 mm Hg on three separate occasions, they were excluded. Patients with unstable angina, congestive heart failure, uncontrolled arrhythmias, and previous myocardial infarction were also excluded in this study.

Protocol

All antianginal drugs were stopped at the start of the study, but sublingual nitroglycerin was given for pain. After 3 weeks of placebo run-in period (Phase I), the patients were randomized to a double-blind cross-over trial: 3 weeks each with placebo and metoprolol 100 mg twice daily (Phases II and III) (Table 10.1). During Phase I, the patients underwent complete medical history, physical examination, routine laboratory tests, electrocardiography, echocardiography, and exercise stress test. At the end of Phases II and III, on two consecutive days, 48-hour Holter monitoring and 48-hour real-time electrocardiographic monitoring with Q-MED Monitor One (Q-MED) or Compas (Cardiac Care Units) were performed simultaneously. During this period, the patients were instructed to continue their daily routine and record a diary of their activities and behavior using a form developed by David Krantz, Ph.D., and Alan Rozanski, M.D. (Figure 10.1). On one of these days, the 24-hour ambulatory blood pressure was also monitored every 20 minutes using Spacelabs Model 5200. During silent ischemic episodes, when the tone was initiated by Q-MED or Compas and the patient had no chest pain, the patient also measured blood pressure by activating the monitoring device. On another day of this period, venous blood samples for plasma norepinephrine, epinephrine, and normetanephrine were taken at 30 minutes while supine and 60 minutes while standing. During the first silent ischemic event, two additional blood samples were obtained by the ambulatory blood

Table 10.1. Protocol and Procedures for Metoprolol Silent Ischemic Trial

PROTOCOL
Phase I: 3 weeks of placebo run-in
Medical history and physical examination
Routine laboratory test including ECG
Exercise tolerance test
Echocardiogram
Phase II and III: 3 weeks of double-blind cross-over; placebo or metoprolol 100 mg twice daily
Plasma catecholamines (supine, standing, and event)
Psychologic Testing
Instrumentation
Radionuclide studies
PROCEDURES
Instrumentation
48-hour Holter monitor
48-hour real-time ECG monitor (Q-MED/Compas)
24-hour ambulatory blood pressure
Cormed blood withdrawal pump for event blood samples
Psychologic Assessments
Jenkins Activity
Type A/B, anger in/out, hostility, anxiety, depression
Structured Interview—Type A/B
Radionuclide studies (MUGA)
Wall motion—during exercise, stroop color word test, serial 7's subtraction, and public speaking

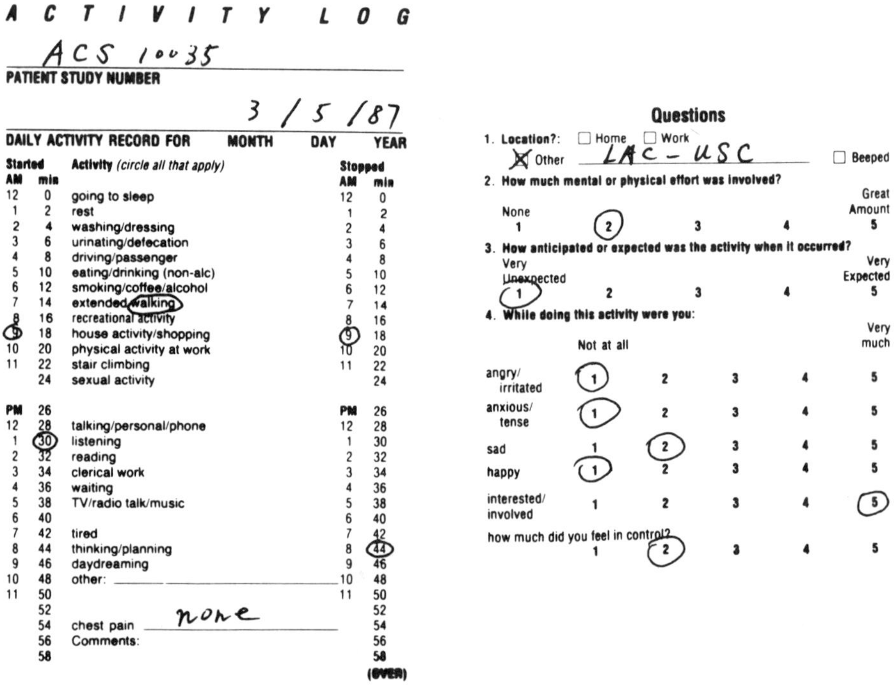
A C T I V I T Y L O G

ACS 10035
PATIENT STUDY NUMBER

3 / 5 / 87
DAILY ACTIVITY RECORD FOR MONTH DAY YEAR

Started AM	min	Activity (circle all that apply)	Stopped AM	min
12	0	going to sleep	12	0
1	2	rest	1	2
2	4	washing/dressing	2	4
3	6	urinating/defecation	3	6
4	8	driving/passenger	4	8
5	10	eating/drinking (non-alc)	5	10
6	12	smoking/coffee/alcohol	6	12
7	14	extended walking	7	14
8	16	recreational activity	8	16
9	18	house activity/shopping	9	18
10	20	physical activity at work	10	20
11	22	stair climbing	11	22
	24	sexual activity		24
PM	26		PM	26
12	28	talking/personal/phone	12	28
1	30	listening	1	30
2	32	reading	2	32
3	34	clerical work	3	34
4	36	waiting	4	36
5	38	TV/radio talk/music	5	38
6	40		6	40
7	42	tired	7	42
8	44	thinking/planning	8	44
9	46	daydreaming	9	46
10	48	other:	10	48
11	50		11	50
	52			52
	54	chest pain none		54
	56	Comments:		56
	58			58

(OVER)

Questions

1. Location?: ☐ Home ☐ Work ☒ Other LAC – USC ☐ Beeped
2. How much mental or physical effort was involved? None 1 (2) 3 4 5 Great Amount
3. How anticipated or expected was the activity when it occurred? Very Unexpected (1) 2 3 4 5 Very Expected
4. While doing this activity were you: Not at all ... Very much

angry/irritated	(1)	2	3	4	5
anxious/tense	(1)	2	3	4	5
sad	1	(2)	3	4	5
happy	(1)	2	3	4	5
interested/involved	1	2	3	4	(5)
how much did you feel in control?	1	(2)	3	4	5

Patient started walking at 9:30 a.m. Patient finished at 9:45 a.m. Patient was at the LAC/USC Medical Center. Behavioral questions self-explanatory.

FIGURE 10.1. Self-Report "Activity Log."

withdrawal pump (Cormed ML6). Also during Phases II and III, gated wall motion studies with gated equilibrium radionuclide technetium were performed and behavior patterns were assessed by the Jenkins activity survey[9] and structured interview.[10] Scales of anger,[11] hostility,[12] anxiety,[13] and depression[14] were also assessed by routine methods.

Echocardiogram

Two-dimensional and M-mode echocardiograms with Doppler were performed with the patients in the partial left lateral decubitus position, using an ATL ultramark IV. The following left ventricular measurements (mean of three cardiac cycles) were made according to the recommendations of the American Society of Echocardiography:[15] end-diastolic measurements of left ventricular internal dimension (LVID), interventricular septal thickness (IVS), and posterior wall thickness (PWT). Left ventricular mass was calculated by the following formula: LV mass $= 0.8 \times [1.04 \times (\text{LVID} + \text{LVS} + \text{PWT})3 - (\text{LVID})3] + 0.6$ g.[16] Measurements of left ventricular mass were divided by body surface area to obtain left ventricular mass index.

Exercise Stress Test

All patients underwent maximal or symptom-limited treadmill exercise stress test, following the standard Bruce protocol. A 12-lead electrocardiogram was performed and blood pressure recorded during the control period, at 1-minute intervals during exercise, and during recovery for 10 minutes. The exercise test was considered positive when the ST-segment depression (80 ms after the J point) greater than 1.0 mm in normotensive subjects and greater than 2.0 mm in hypertensive patients occurred and persisted for three consecutive beats.

Holter Monitoring

Bipolar leads were attached with the exploring electrodes usually at standard leads V_2 and V_5. Tracing was obtained by portable ECG recording (Del Mar Avionics, electrocardiocorder model 453). Tapes were analyzed with an interactive computer-based high-speed scanning system with features of audiovisual superimposed ECG presentation, arrhythmiagraphy display of R-R intervals, continuous ST-segment display, and an operator programming arrhythmia analyzer (Del Mar Avionics, Innovator model 760). Ischemic episodes were defined as transient downsloping or horizontal ST-segment depression (80 ms after the J point) of 1.0 mm or greater from baseline, lasting longer than 1 minute.

Real-Time Electrocardiographic Monitoring (Q-MED Monitor One and Compas)

Q-MED electrodes were attached in a lead CS5 configuration, with the negative reference over the sternum and positive electrode in the lead V_5 position. The earth electrode was attached over the right lower anterior ribs. For Compas, augmented unipolar leads were placed in the lead II, V_5, and aVF positions. The electrodes for Q-MED/Compas and Holter were placed as closely together as possible. The Q-MED and Compas algorithms exclude ectopic beats and noise and identify isoelectric, J, and J + 60-ms points in the beats classified as normal. Downsloping or horizontal ST-segment depression of at least 1 mm lasting more than 40 seconds represents the threshold for detection of an ischemic event. A tone was initiated by the Q-MED or Compas when the ST-segment amplitude was above this threshold for longer than 40 seconds.

Ambulatory Blood Withdrawal Pump

A thrombo-resistant butterfly needle with a nonthrombogenic tube was inserted into a forearm vein. After blood samples for plasma norepinephrine, epinephrine, and normetanephrine determinations were taken at 30-minute supine and 60-minute standing positions, the catheter was filled with heparinized saline solution and attached to a portable blood withdrawal pump (Cormed ML6), which was set to withdraw blood continuously at a rate of 1.0 ml/min into heparinized tubes. These procedures were performed during Holter and real-time ECG monitoring. The patients were asked to continue their normal daily lives. When the first tone was initiated by Q-MED/Compas and not accompanied by chest pain, two consecutive blood samples were withdrawn during the first 10 minutes and the subsequent 10 minutes. Plasma norepinephrine, epinephrine, and normetanephrine were measured by HPLC methods.[17] The sample ECG traces at that time were also inspected to confirm ischemic ST-segment changes.

Radionuclide Ventriculography

Patients were injected with 25 mCi of technetium-99m-labeled red blood cells. Imaging was performed using an all-purpose collimator and quarter-inch sodium iodine crystal. Imaging was performed during exercise and three separate mental tasks: stroop color word task, serial 7's subtraction from the number 4000, and a public speaking task in front of two observers for five minutes.[18]

Statistic Analysis

Computer analyses were performed at Los Angeles County/USC Medical Computer Center with Clinfo computer program. The data were presented as the mean ± standard error (SE). The results were analyzed using Students' *t* test for paired comparison: placebo versus metroprolol and supine versus event catecholamines. Duration and frequency of silent ischemic events were analyzed by Wilcoxon's signed rank test. Linear regression was used to test relations among blood pressure, catecholamines, silent ischemic events, ectopic beats, and left ventricular mass index. A p value of less than 0.05 was considered significant.

RESULTS

The first 17 patients, aged 59 ± 2 years (5 normotensive and 12 hypertensive subjects), with stable angina were analyzed and presented here.

Myocardial Ischemic Event

Before metoprolol treatment, 179 asymptomatic and 18 symptomatic episodes of >1.0-mm ST-segment depression were recorded in 13 of 17 patients (76%) during ECG monitoring. In these 13 patients, metoprolol decreased the frequency and duration of ST-segment depression episodes: from 8.7 ± 3 to 2.9 ± 2.4 (per 24 hours), $p < 0.1$, and from 101 ± 75 to 63 ± 62 (min/24 hours), $p < 0.01$, respectively. The silent ischemia did not appear to be closely related to increased physical activity. In one patient the silent ischemia occurred while lying down, although plasma norepinephrine and epinephrine were about two times higher than supine levels (Figure 10.2). In another patient, silent ischemia occurred during light physical activity (washing and dressing) with increased plasma normetanephrine (32%) and without change in plasma norepinephrine (Figure 10.3).

Ambulatory Blood Pressure and Heart Rate

Metoprolol decreased average systolic and diastolic blood pressure and heart rate from 138 ± 4/86 ± 3 to 127 ± 4/78 ± 2 mm Hg, $p < 0.01$, and from 80 ± 3 to 64 ± 2 beats/min., $p < 0.001$, respectively: The average diurnal and nocturnal blood pressures were derived from 0700 to 2100 hours and from 2100 to 0700 hours, respectively. The diurnal blood pressure was significantly higher than the nocturnal blood pressure during both placebo and metoprolol administration; 144 ± 4/89 ± 3 vs 135 ± 5/84 ± 3 mm Hg, $p < 0.05$, and 133 ± 4/82 ± 2 vs 125 ± 5/77 ± 2 mm Hg, $p < 0.01$, respectively. Generally, a pressor surge starts before awakening and continues until approximately noon. Maximum systolic blood pressure during

PATIENT JRM 10002 (HTN)
PLACEBO: Q-MED MONITOR TRACING

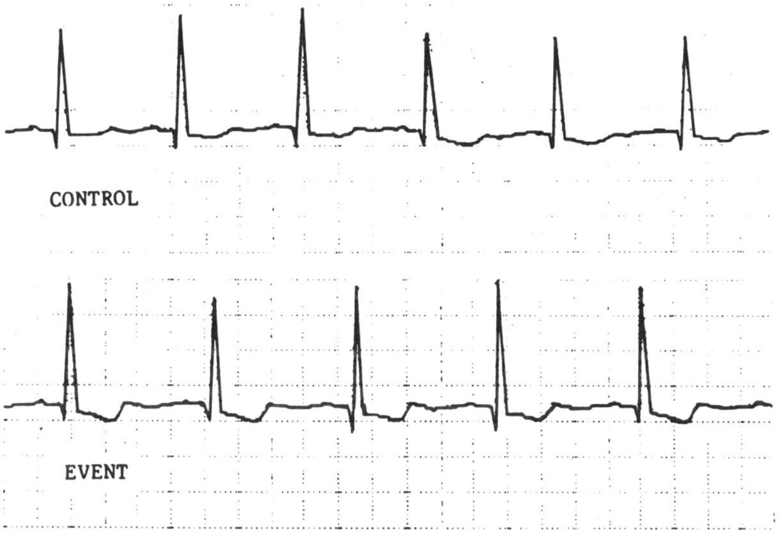

PATIENT WAS LYING DOWN.

CATECHOLAMINE	NE	E	NMN
SUPINE	572	15	226
EVENT	925	27	239

	BLOOD PRESSURE	HR
SUPINE	133/82 mmHg	73
STANDING	145/80 mmHg	72

NO HOLTER MONITOR DOCUMENTATION FOR THIS EVENT.

FIGURE 10.2. Q-med monitor tracing, control and event with simultaneous plasma catecholamines.

this period was significantly higher during placebo than during metoprolol administration: 173 ± 6 vs 159 ± 8 mm Hg, $p < 0.05$, but the percentage increments of maximum systolic blood pressure from nocturnal systolic blood pressure were similar: 29 ± 4% at placebo and 27 ± 5% at metoprolol administration, suggesting metoprolol did not blunt the pressor surge.

Blood pressure during the silent ischemic episode (150 ± 12/90 ± 7 mm Hg) was not different from the daytime blood pressure, but event heart rate exceeded that of the daytime pulse rate (96 ± 5 vs 81 ± 3, $p < 0.05$).

Plasma Catecholamines

Metoprolol did not change plasma norepinephrine, epinephrine, and normetanephrine either supine or standing. However, plasma norepinephrine and epinephrine were significantly increased on standing during both placebo and metoprolol administration, but the increment of normetanephrine on standing was not significant at placebo (Table 10.2). In 9 of 17 patients, 11 blood samples were taken with a Cormed withdrawal pump during silent ischemic episodes; 8 samples were taken during placebo and 3 during metoprolol. In these patients, the event plasma norepinephrine and

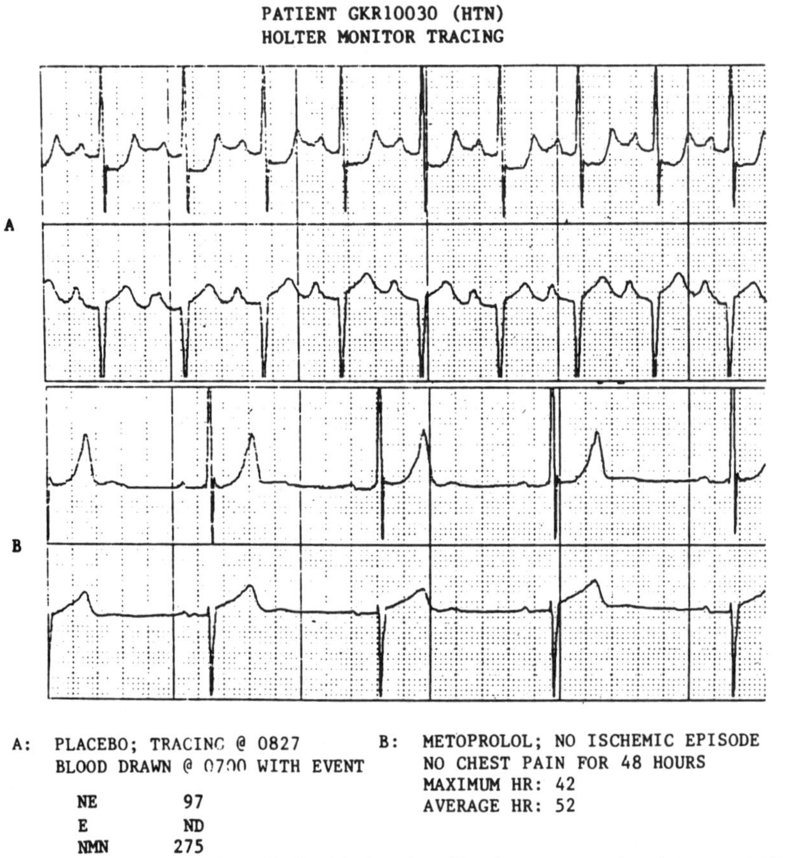

FIGURE 10.3. Holter monitor during (*A*) silent ischemia with plasma norepinephrine and (*B*) during no ischemia.

epinephrine levels, and the values 10 minutes after the event were significantly higher than the resting supine levels. However, the plasma normetanephrine level was unchanged (Table 10.3). Furthermore, in five patients, six event blood samples were taken during subdued physical behaviors (lying down or resting). Even in these patients, the plasma norepinephrine level at the event and 10 minutes after it was still significantly higher than those taken supine (Table 10.4).

Electrocardiography and Left Ventricular Mass

The electrocardiograms in 12 of our first 17 patients were normal, although left ventricular hypertrophy was detected by echocardiography in 4 of these 12. Five of the patients had abnormal ECGs; one had left ventricular hypertrophy on voltage criteria (LVMI = 117), one had T-wave inversion at rest (LVMI = 105), one had flat T waves (LVMI = 148), one had loss of R wave in precordial leads (LVMI = 111), and one had low voltage (LVMI = 105). Twelve of the first 17 patients (not the same 12 just mentioned) had perfusion abnormality on either MUGA or thallium or had significant coronary atherosclerosis on angiography. There was no anatomic or radionuclide evidence of ischemia in the remaining five patients. Holter monitoring for 96 hours was negative in one of the five patients and positive in four of five patients. Of these four, two had left ventricular hypertrophy determined by ECG

Table 10.2. Plasma Catecholamines, Supine and Standing, During Placebo and Metoprolol Therapy

	Placebo (n = 17)		Metoprolol (n = 17)	
Catecholamines	Supine	Standing	Supine	Standing
Norepinephrine (ng/l)	273 ± 29	513 ± 65*	258 ± 28	525 ± 53*
Epinephrine (ng/l)	22 ± 3	34 ± 4†	26 ± 2	44 ± 9‡
Normetanephrine (ng/l)	233 ± 18	263 ± 17	251 ± 28	305 ± 27†

Values are mean ± SE.

*p < 0.001 †p < 0.05 ‡p < 0.01 compared to supine.

or echocardiography. Left ventricular mass index was significantly increased in hypertensive subjects compared with normotensive subjects (130 ± 9 vs 105 ± 3 g/m^2, $p < 0.05$). Left ventricular mass index was significantly correlated with average ambulatory systolic blood pressure ($r = 0.57$, $p < 0.05$, n = 17) with placebo but not metoprolol administration (Figure 10.4). No significant correlation was found between left ventricular mass index and average ambulatory diastolic blood pressure, or plasma cathecholamines, ischemic episode (frequency or duration), or total ventricular ectopy either with placebo or metoprolol.

Behavioral and Radionuclide Study

We have yet to analyze behavioral and radionuclide assessments as related to blood pressure, plasma catecholamines, ischemic events, and left ventricular mass. However, silent ischemic events occurred in several patients during mental stress or sleeping without any physical activity.

DISCUSSION

Although 62 to 80 percent of patients with proven ischemic heart disease have "silent ischemia" as recorded on Holter monitoring,[19,20] 13 to 39 percent with normal coronary angiograms also have recorded ischemic events; of these, many are likely to be false. Because repolarization abnormalities occur frequently in patients with left ventricular hypertrophy, the false-positive rate may be higher in hypertensive subjects. Seventy-two percent of our patients had evidence of coronary ischemia on direct or indirect evaluation other than on Holter monitoring or ECG. Seventy-six percent of our patients with chronic stable angina had Holter evidence of silent ischemia. Furthermore, studies of these patients by positron emission tomography might have revealed perfusion abnormalities not detected by MUGA, thallium, or angio-

Table 10.3. Plasma Catecholamines During Supine Rest and Events

Catecholamines	Supine (n = 11)	Event (n = 11)	After Event (n = 11)
Norepinephrine (ng/l)	258 ± 41	508 ± 122*	410 ± 74*
Epinephrine (ng/l)	28 ± 4	40 ± 4†	45 ± 7†
Normetanephrine (ng/l)	234 ± 30	438 ± 123	263 ± 63

Values are mean ± SE.

*p < 0.01 †p < 0.05 compared to supine.

Table 10.4. Plasma Catecholamines During Subdued Behavior at Time of Silent Ischemic Events Compared with Supine Rest

Catecholamines	Supine (n = 6)	Event (n = 6)	After Event (n = 6)
Norepinephrine (ng/l)	292 ± 60	453 ± 99*	468 ± 104*
Epinephrine (ng/l)	28 ± 4	38 ± 5	47 ± 11
Normetanephrine (ng/l)	214 ± 28	210 ± 13	194 ± 11

Values are mean ± SE.

*$p < 0.05$ compared to supine.

graphy.[21] Conversely, they could represent the coronary flow reserve abnormality of left ventricular hypertrophy[22] rather than technical aberrations.

The coronary vasculature receives rich sympathetic innervation. Norepinephrine, the predominant neurotransmitter, causes profound vasoconstriction of the epicardial coronary vessels.[23] However, the relations of peripheral noradrenergic and adrenergic tone to the clinical syndromes of myocardial ischemia and infarction are controversial. Several studies in humans and laboratory animals concluded that sympathoadrenal involvement in myocardial ischemia was not significant; in humans with ischemia, both norepinephrine release[24] and plasma norepinephrine during ethanol-provoked ischemia[25] were unchanged from baseline. After experimental coronary artery occlusion, there was no change in coronary sinus norepinephrine content in the isolated perfused rat heart,[26] there was a reduction in coronary sinus norepinephrine in the intact dog,[27] and no change was noted in the norepinephrine content of coronary sinus or peripheral veins of the dog.[28] Furthermore, there was no increment in coronary sinus norepinephrine content in the dog even after experimental myocardial infarction.[29]

Plasma norepinephrine, however, increased in some patients with vasospastic angina preceding the anginal episode.[8] In another study of patients with coronary artery disease, those with multiple-vessel involvement had higher peripheral plasma norepinephrine content than did patients with single-vessel disease.[30] Both arterial and coronary sinus content of norepinephrine increased in some patients with ischemia

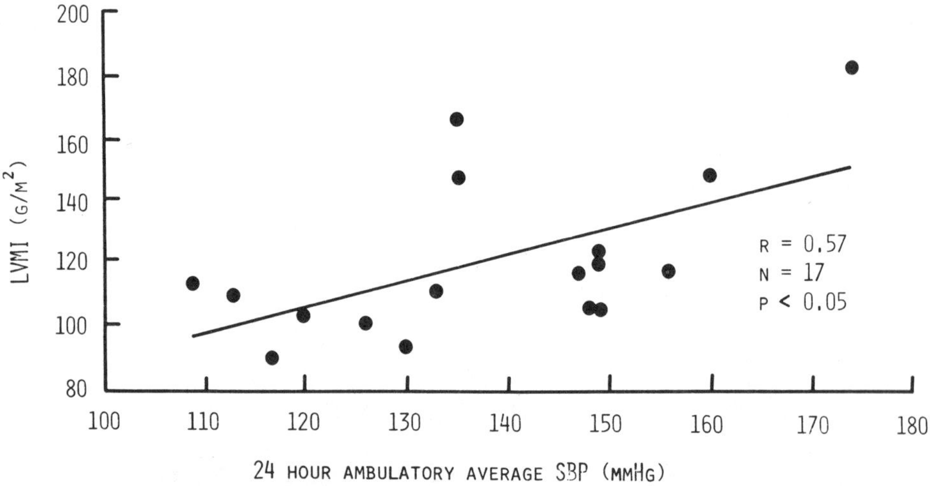

FIGURE 10.4. Correlation of average ambulatory systolic blood pressure with left ventricular mass index.

after the onset of spontaneous spasm.[31] Plasma norepinephrine and epinephrine increased during provoked effort angina in patients with coronary artery disease.[32] Furthermore, unlike the aforementioned findings, coronary ischemia in cats and in the isolated rat heart increased norepinephrine content after vagotomy[33] and norepinephrine release,[34] respectively.

The increased cardiovascular morbidity and mortality occurring in certain persons and in patients during life stress[35] may be related to intrinsic or behaviorally induced sympathetic and cardiovascular reactivity.[36,37] The evidence for adrenergic involvement during acute myocardial infarction derives from studies in humans; morbidity and mortality may be predicted by high levels of both norepinephrine and epinephrine[38,39] which may be ameliorated by propranolol therapy.[40] Other studies in humans describe the reduced alpha-2 receptors[41] and the elevated blood sugar level[40] as related to elevated plasma norepinephrine and epinephrine, which may follow acute myocardial infarction.

Evidence of a sympathoadrenal role in coronary vasomotion is found in both human and animal pharmacologic interventions. During coronary ischemia, propranolol blunts the chronotropic effects of endogenously released norepinephrine in dogs.[42] Nifedipine, while raising arterial and plasma norepinephrine levels before and during pacing angina, still improves coronary flow and delays the onset of ischemia.[43] The alpha agonist, clonidine, decreases both blood pressure and norepinephrine[44] and ST-segment elevation in humans.[45] The alpha antagonist, trimazosin, reduces coronary vascular tone with cold pressor stimulation, and still other evidence with yohimbine implicates the alpha-2 receptor in coronary vasospasm.[46] A serotonin antagonist reduced coronary sinus norepinephrine content and prevented arrhythmias in dogs after coronary ischemia.[47] Lidocaine also reduced the effects of coronary ischemia on norepinephrine release and arrhythmias.[48] Studies of patients with cerebral ischemia revealed a high prevalence of elevated plasma norepinephrine levels which appeared causally related to myocardial necrosis and ischemia.[39]

There is a paucity of evidence relating clinical, biochemical, and pharmacologic features of sympathoadrenal hyperactivity to syndromes of coronary ischemia in normotensive subjects, and there may even be less evidence for an adrenergic role in hypertension. However, there have been findings of disordered noradrenergic tone in the pathogenesis of primary hypertension and, independently, left ventricular hypertrophy. Over the last three decades, in studies of wide-ranging populations of patients in California,[6,49,50] Michigan,[51,52] and Ireland,[53,54] we found evidence of raised noradrenergic tone in urine, plasma, spinal fluid, and tissue in younger patients with mild hypertension and in some patients with systolic hypertension alone.[55] Despite extensive reviews that corroborated these findings,[56] the absence of evidence reported by some workers has served to muddy the waters.[57]

Although septal hypertrophy, as manifested by a prominent "Q-wave" in the lateral precordial leads, has long been related to a hyperactive, hyperadrenergic, and hyperdynamic heart, it is only in the last few years that left ventricular hypertrophy has been associated with quantitative measures of noradrenergic tone, specifically plasma norepinephrine.[58,59] Sympatholytic therapy has been more effective in decreasing blood pressure and causing hypertrophy to regress[22] than have equally potent doses of vasodilators that cause a reflex surcharge of noradrenaline. One of the missing links in understanding the relation of noradrenergic tone to the ischemic syndromes is the effect of sympathoadrenal activity on the genesis of coronary atherosclerosis. There are both direct and indirect mechanisms whereby the noradrenergic system can stimulate atherogenesis, because sympathoadrenal arousal mobilizes fat from tissue stores[60] as well as elevating blood pressure.

Thus, it is plausible to relate heightened noradrenergic tone to the anatomic and biochemical substrates of coronary ischemia, including raised afterload, left ventricular hypertrophy, reduced coronary reserve, increased myocardial oxygen requirements, and coronary atherosclerosis. The preliminary findings of this report suggest that in some patients with evidence of effort-related ischemia, heightened noradrenergic tone related to mental stress contributes to dynamic vasoconstriction in atherosclerotic coronary vessels and that the resultant inadequate flow produced ischemia. Other explanations for the elevated plasma norepinephrine level would include local and peripheral norepinephrine release as a consequence of ischemia. Evidence of this latter possibility seems far less than that of the former. Most studies in animals do not show changes in peripheral or coronary sinus plasma norepinephrine after experimental coronary occlusion. It is possible that the beep tone of the monitor device engendered sympathoadrenal alarm responses with the onset of ischemia. However, outwardly at least, most patients registered little concern with the intermittent sounding of the tone. The burden of carrying the equipment may have contributed to autonomic arousal in these patients, although plasma norepinephrine while supine and on standing was normal. Thus, the data suggest that silent ischemia in patients during subdued physical activity may have been preceded by sympathoadrenal arousal, contributing to altered vasomotor tone and ischemia. Pulse rates, but not blood pressure, were raised during the ischemic events. Thus, in addition to coronary flow changes, there apparently were increments in myocardial oxygen demand. Although we view plasma norepinephrine and epinephrine as the most reliable biochemical markers of sympathetic nerve tone, the stability of normetanephrine in vitro confers extra value, because immediate centrifugation and refrigeration of the sample were not always possible.[61] In a few patients, normetanephrine was elevated during the ischemic event without an accompanying increment in norepinephrine or epinephrine. The ratio of normetanephrine to norepinephrine and epinephrine (thought to reflect newly released norepinephrine)[62] was not altered during ischemia.

Metoprolol therapy in this partial analysis appeared to reduce the frequency and duration of the silent ischemic episodes in hypertensive subjects with stable angina. This effect may be construed as evidence of neutralization of an important "demand" component of the ischemic event or of neutralization of excessive adrenergic overdrive by blockade of presynaptic facitatory receptors of the coronary vasculature mediating constriction—the "supply" component. However, evidence is accumulating that beta-receptor blockers may stimulate synthesis of local vascular eicosanoids (prostacycline) and thereby shift vasomotion to a pattern of vasodilation.[63]

Our preliminary findings suggest that noradrenergic hyperactivity may play an important role in "silent" coronary ischemia in addition to its important role in the genesis of left ventricular hypertrophy. Thus, therapy that neutralizes sympathetic tone as well as decreasing blood pressure should be of special value to the patient with hypertension and coronary atherosclerosis.

Acknowledgment: We gratefully acknowledge the assistance of Alan Rozanski, MD, and Noel Bairey, MD, Cedars-Sinai Medical Center, Los Angeles, California.

REFERENCES

1. Roberts WC: Frequency of systemic hypertension in various cardiovascular diseases. *Am J Cardiol* 1987;60:1E–8E.
2. Messerli FH, Ventura HO, Elizardi DJ, Dunn FG, Frohlich ED: Hypertension and sudden death: Increased ventricular ectopic activity in left ventricular hypertrophy. *Am J Cardiol* 1984;77:18–22.
3. Strauer BE: Myocardial oxygen consumption in chronic heart disease: Role of wall stress, hypertrophy and coronary reserve. *Am J Cardiol* 1979;44:730–740.
4. Nademanee K, Intarachot V, Josephson MA, Rieders D, Mody FV, Singh BN: Prognostic significance of silent myocardial ischemia in patients with unstable angina. *J Am Coll Cardiol* 1987;10:1–9.
5. Gottlieb SO, Weisfeldt ML, Ouyang P, Mellits ED, Gertenblith G: Silent ischemia as a marker for early unfavorable outcomes in patients with unstable angina. *N Engl J Med* 1986;314:1214–1219.
6. DeQuattro V, Chan S: Raised plasma-catecholamines in some patients with primary hypertension. *Lancet* 1972;1:806–809.
7. Bairey CN, Rozanski A, Friedman JD, Bietendorf J, Hestin L, Cramty D, Berman DF: Characteristic of silent myocardial ischemia during mental stress: Laboratory assessment using equilibrium radionuclide ventriculography. *J Am Coll Cardiol* 1987;9:5A.
8. Tamada K, Ito Y, Fukzaki H: Autonomic hyperactivity in patients with vasospastic angina. *Jap Heart J* 1985;26:715–726.
9. Jenkins CD, Rosenman RH, Zysanski SJ: Prediction of clinical coronary heart disease by a test for the coronary-prone behavior pattern. *N Engl J Med* 1974;290:1271–1275.
10. Gambrill ED, Richey LA: An assertion inventory for use in assessment and research. *Behavior Therapy* 1975;6:550–561.
11. Harburg E, Erfurt JC, Hauenstein LS, Chape C, Schull WJ, Schork MA: Socioecological stress, suppressed hostility, skin color, and black and white male blood pressure: Detroit. *Psychosomatic Med* 1973;35:276.
12. Buss AH: *The Psychology of Aggression*. New York, Wiley, 1961, pp 169–181.
13. Spielberger CD, Gorsuch RL, Lushene RE: *Manual for the State-Trait Anxiety Inventory*. Palo Alto, California, Consulting Psychology Press, 1970.
14. Beck AT: Measuring depression: The depression inventory, in Williams T, Katz MM, Shield JA (eds): *Recent Advances in the Psychobiology of the Depressive Illnesses*. Washington, DC, US Government Printing Office, 1972.
15. Sahn DJ, DeMaria A, Kisslo J, Weyman A and The Committee on M-Mode Standardization of the American Society of Echocardiography: Recommendations regarding quantitation in M-mode echocardiography: Results of a survey of echocardiographic measurements. *Circulation* 1978;58:1072–1083.
16. Devereux RB, Alonso DR, Lutas EM, Gottleib GJ, Campo E, Sachs I, Reichek N: Echocardiographic assessment of left ventricular hypertrophy: Comparison with necropsy findings. *Am J Cardiol* 1986;57:450–458.
17. Foti A, Kimura S, DeQuattro V, Lee D: Liquid-chromatographic measurement of plasma and urine catecholamines and metabolites. *Clin Chem* 1987;33:2209–2213.
18. Rozanski, A, Elkayam U, Berman D, Diamond G, Prause J, Swan HJC: Improvement of resting asynergy with cessation of upright bicycle exercise. *Circulation* 1983;67:529–535.
19. Stern S, Tzivoni D: Diagnostic accuracy of ambulatory ECG monitoring in ischemic heart disease. *Circulation* 1975;52:1045.
20. Crawford MH, Mendoza CA, O'Rourke RA, White DH, Boucher CA, Gorwit J: Limitations of continuous ambulatory electrocardiogram monitoring for detecting coronary artery disease. *Ann Intern Med* 1978;89:1.
21. Deanfield JE, Shea M, Ribiero P, deLandsheere CM, Wilson RA, Horlock P, Selwyn AP: Transient ST segment depression as a marker of myocardial ischemia during daily life. *Am J Cardiol* 1984;54:1195.
22. Strauer BE, Bayer F, Brecht H, et al: The influence of sympathetic nervous activity on regression of cardiac hypertrophy. *J Hypertension* 1985;(Suppl 4):S39–S44.
23. Feigl EO: Coronary physiology. *Physiol Rev* 1983;63:1–205.

24. Kurita A, Satomura K, Takase B, Sugawara H, Hosono K: Effects of treadmill and pacing stress testing on peripheral arterial thromboxane, platelet function and catecholamine activities in patients with chronic coronary artery disease. *Jpn J Med* 1987;26:7–14.
25. Matsuguchi T, Araki H, Anan T, Hayata N, Nakagaki O, Takeshita A, Nakamura M: Provocation of variant angina by alcohol ingestion. *Eur Heart J* 1984;5:906–912.
26. Daughtery A, Frayn KN, Redfern WS, Woodward B: The role of catecholamines in the production of ischemia-induced ventricular arrhythmias in the rat in vivo and in vitro. *Br J Pharmacol* 1986;87:265–277.
27. Haneda T, Arai T, Kanda H, Ikeda J, Takishima T: Reduction of plasma norepinephrine levels in response to brief coronary occlusion in experimental dogs. *Am Heart J* 1985;109:1264–1268.
28. McGrath BP, Lim SP, Laversha L, Shanahan A: Myocardial and peripheral catecholamine response to acute coronary artery constriction before and after propranolol treatment in the anaesthetised dog. *Cardiovasc Res* 1981;15:28–34.
29. Oguma M, Tsuiki K, Kaminishi T, Ohta I, Yasui S: Hyperkinetic contraction of a non-ischemic segment of ischemic left ventricle in anesthetized dogs. *Heart Vessels* 1985;1:145–151.
30. Fujita T, Ajisaka R, Matsumoto R, Iida K, Iida K, Sugishita Y, Ito I, Takeda T, Akisada M: Variable neurohumoral and hemodynamic responses to exercise in patients with exertional angina: Influence of the severity of coronary artery disease. *Clin Cardiol* 1987;10:99–103.
31. Robertson RM, Bernard Y, Robertson D: Arterial and coronary sinus catecholamines in the course of spontaneous coronary artery spasm. *Am Heart J* 1983;106:901–906.
32. Marcella JJ, Nichols AB, Johnson LL, Owen J, Reison DS, Kaplan KL, Cannon PJ: Exercise-induced myocardial ischemia in patients with coronary artery disease: Lack of evidence for platelet activation or fibrin formation in peripheral venous blood. *Am J Coll Cardiol* 1983;1:1185–1193.
33. Williford DJ, Zavadil AP, Walsh RA, Weise V, Kopin IJ, Gillis RA: Influence of vagotomy on changes in feline plasma catecholamine levels induced by occlusion of either the left or right coronary vessel. *Cardiovasc Res* 1983;17:568–576.
34. Carlsson L, Abrahamsson T, Almgren O: Local release of myocardial norepinephrine during acute ischemia: An experimental study in the isolated perfused rat heart. *J Cardiovasc Pharmacol* 1985;7:791–798.
35. DeQuattro V, Hamad R: The role of stress and the sympathetic nervous system in hypertension and ischemic heart disease: Advantages of therapy with beta-receptor blockers. *Clin Exp Hypertens* 1985;7:907–932.
36. DeQuattro V, Loo R, Foti A: Sympathoadrenal responses to stress: The linking of type A behavior pattern to ischemic heart disease. *Clin Exp Hypertens* 1985;7:469–481.
37. Case records of the Massachusetts General Hospital. Weekly clinicopathological exercises. Case 18–1986. A 44-year-old woman with substernal pain and pulmonary edema after severe emotional stress. *N Engl J Med* 1986;314:1240–1247.
38. Bayliss J, Canepa-Anson R, Norell M, Poole-Wilson P, Sutton G: The renal response to neuroendocrine inhibition in chronic heart failure: Double-blind comparison of captopril and prazosin. *Eur Heart J* 1986;7:877–884.
39. Myers MG, Norris JW, Hachniski VC, Sole MJ: Plasma norepinephrine in stroke. *Stroke* 1981;12:200–204.
40. Little RA, Frayn KN, Randall PE, Stoner HB, Morton C, Yates DW, Laing GS: Plasma catecholamines in the acute phase of the response to myocardial infarction. *Arch Emerg Med* 1986;3:20–26.
41. Sakaguchi K, Hattori R, Yui Y, Takatsu Y, Susawa T, Yui N, Nonogi H, Tamaki S, Kawai C: Altered platelet alpha 2 adrenoceptor in acute myocardial infarction and its relation to plasma catecholamine concentrations. *Br Heart J* 1986;55:434–438.
42. Randall DC, Evans JM, Billman GE, Ordway GA, Knapp CF: Neural, hormonal and intrinsic mechanisms of cardiac control during acute coronary occlusion in the intact dog. *J Auton Nerv Syst* 1981;3:87–99.
43. Emanuelsson H, Hjalmarson A, Holmberg S, Waagstein F, Waldenstrom A: Effects of

nifedipine on arterial concentration and myocardial extraction of catecholamines during pacing-induced angina pectoris. *J Cardiovasc Pharmacol* 1984;6:224–232.
44. Renard M, Liebens I, Waterschoot P, Bernard R: Central inhibition of sympathetic overdrive by clonidine in acute myocardial infarction with systolic hypertension. Haemodynamic study. *Angiology* 1986;37:633–641.
45. Zochowski RJ, Lada W: Intravenous clonidine treatment in acute myocardial infarction (with comparison to a nitroglycerin-treated and control group). *J Cardiovasc Pharmacol* 1986;8(Suppl 3):S41–S45.
46. Kakihana M, Noda H, Ohtsuka S, Sugishita Y, Ito I: Significant role of alpha 2-adrenoceptors in coronary artery spasm. *Jpn Circ J* 1985;49:108–118.
47. Coker SJ, Dean HG, Kane KA, Parratt JR: The effects of ICS 205–930, a 5-HT antagonist, on arrhythmias and catecholamine release during canine myocardial ischemia and reperfusion. *Eur J Pharmacol* 1986;127:211–218.
48. Polwin W, McDonald FM, Brinkman C, Hirche H, Addicks K: Effects of lidocaine on catecholamine release in the ischemic rat heart. *J Cardiovasc Pharmacol* 1987;9:6–11.
49. DeQuattro V, Miura Y: Neurogenic factors in hypertension: Mechanism or myth? *Am J Med* 1973;55:362–378.
50. DeQuattro V, Miura Y, Lurvey A, Cosgrove M, Mendez R: Increased plasma catecholamines and vas deferans norepinephrine biosynthesis in men with elevated blood pressure. *Circ Res* 1975;36:118–126.
51. Esler M, Julius S, Sweifler A, Randall O, Harburg E, Gardiner H, DeQuattro V: Mild high-renin essential hypertension: A neurogenic human hypertension? *N Engl J Med* 1977;296:405–511.
52. Esler M, Zweifler A, Randall O, DeQuattro V: Pathophysiologic and pharmacokinetic determinants of the antihypertensive response to propranolol. *Clin Pharmacol Ther* 1977;22:299–308.
53. DeQuattro V, Sullivan P, Minagawa R, Kopin I, Bornheimer J, Foti A, Barndt R: Central and peripheral noradrenergic mechanisms in primary hypertension. *Fed Proc* 984;43:47–51.
54. Sullivan PA, DeQuattro V, Foti A, Curzon G: Effects of clonidine on central and peripheral nerve tone in primary hypertension. *Hypertension* 1986;8:611–617.
55. deOrtiz HK, DeQuattro V, Schoentgen S, Stephanian E: Raised plasma catecholamines in old and young patients with disproportionate systolic hypertension. *Clin Exp Hypertens* 1982;A4:1107–1120.
56. Goldstein DS: Plasma norepinephrine in essential hypertension: A study of the studies. *Hypertension* 1981;3:48–52.
57. Folkow B: Introductory remarks. *Acta Physiol Scand* (Suppl) 1984;527:7–9.
58. DeQuattro V, Lee D, Shkvatsabaya IK, Yurenev AP, Salenko B, Allen J, Azen S, Barndt R, Foti A, Davison G: Primary hypertension: Left ventricular mass and function, sympathetic nervous system activity and therapy. *Health Psychology* 1988 (in press).
59. Corea L, Bentivoglio M, Verdecchia, et al: Plasma norepinephrine and left ventricular hypertrophy in systemic hypertension. *Am J Cardiol* 1984;53:1299–1303.
60. Masoro EJ: Lipids and lipid metabolism. *Ann Rev Physiol* 1977;39:301–321.
61. Kobayashi K, Kolloch R, DeQuattro V, Miano L, Dugger R, Van der Meulen J: Raised cerebrospinal fluid noradrenaline in some patients with primary hypertension. *Hypertension* 1979;1:255–260.
62. Kopin IJ, Gordon EK: Metabolism of norepinephrine 3H released by tyramine and reserpine. *J Pharmacol Exp Ther* 1962;138:351.
63. Daniell HB, Webb JG, Walle T, Oatis JE, Gaffney TE: Inhibitors of prostaglandin synthesis reverse the effects of chronic beta receptor blockade to attenuate adrenergic neurovascular transmission in dogs. *J Cardiovasc Pharmacol* 1988 (submitted).

CHAPTER 11

Silent Myocardial Ischemia in the Diabetic Patient

Richard W. Nesto, MD and Kevin J. Kett, MD

Diabetic patients represent an important subgroup of those with coronary artery disease and silent myocardial ischemia. The use of angina as an index of the clinical activity of coronary artery disease in diabetic patients may be of particular importance given the recognized influence of diabetes on the incidence and natural history of coronary heart disease and therapeutic outcomes in such patients. The Framingham Study, a longitudinal study of more than 5,000 patients with a minimum 20-year follow-up, documented the frequency of coronary disease and its consequences in the diabetic population.[1] Compared with nondiabetic patients, diabetic male and female patients have a 60 percent and 100 percent greater incidence of coronary artery disease, respectively. With regard to myocardial infarction, diabetic men have a 50 percent and diabetic women a 150 percent higher incidence of myocardial infarction than do nondiabetic men and women. Similarly, angina is much more common in diabetic than in nondiabetic persons with diabetic men and women having a 60 percent and 100 percent greater incidence of the symptoms of coronary artery disease. When compared with patients who have anginal symptoms of similar severity, patients with diabetes have more extensive coronary artery disease; however, the extent of disease is not clearly related to duration, extrapancreatic organ involvement, or type of treatment of diabetes.[2] This paper will discuss the prevalence and possible significance of silent myocardial ischemia in diabetic patients with coronary artery disease.

MYOCARDIAL INFARCTION IN DIABETIC PATIENTS

Myocardial infarction may be the cause of death in approximately 20 percent of diabetic patients because of more widespread coronary artery disease.[3] Patients with diabetes who have survived myocardial infarction appear to have a poorer short- and long-term prognosis than do nondiabetic patients, possibly because of greater left ventricular dysfunction despite similar size and site of infarction. The issue has been raised that diabetic patients may present with subclinical left ventricular dysfunction as a result of remote silent infarction.[4] Barring the direct deleterious effects of accelerated atherosclerosis, autonomic nervous system dysfunction due to diabetes appears to be a marker of increased cardiovascular mortality. Once autonomic nervous system dysfunction is clearly detected, 5-year survival is only 40 percent compared with 8 percent in age- and sex-matched diabetic patients without autonomic system dysfunction.[5] Most of these deaths are cardiac in origin. The causal relation between autonomic nervous system disease and risk of cardiac disease is not completely clear, however, but unrecognized extensive coronary artery disease and silent ischemia may partly be responsible. It is generally accepted that diabetic patients may not experience typical anginal symptoms despite significant myocardial ischemia or infarction, presumably because of the associated neuropathy. The clinical maxim that ischemia is silent in such patients is an extrapolation from studies that have examined the relation of anginal pain to myocardial infarction. This may not, however, be the most appropriate way to evaluate the significance of silent myocardial ischemia in the diabetic population. Reported studies examining the relation of angina to myocardial infarction in patients with diabetes have been largely retrospective, relying on chart review that employs loosely defined criteria for myocardial infarction and ischemia.

In 1962, Bradley and Schoenfield[6] described the presence and severity of symptoms in 100 diabetic and 100 nondiabetic patients who presented with myocardial infarction at the Joslin Diabetes Center. The study revealed that severe pain, characteristic of angina, was nearly three times as frequent among nondiabetic patients as it was among diabetic patients. Chest pain limited to mild to moderate intensity was twice as common in the diabetic group. Forty-two diabetic patients presented with symptoms such as nausea, fatigue, and dyspnea compared to only six nondiabetic patients who presented with atypical symptoms in the setting of myocardial infarction. In 1975, Soler et al[7] reported on 285 diabetic patients with myocardial infarction, and 33 percent of these patients had no complaints suggestive of typical angina. Consistent with the previous results of Bradley and Schoenfeld,[6] patients in this study complained of worsening congestive heart failure, symptoms of hyperglycemia or hypoglycemia, gastrointestinal distress, hypotension, confusion, or transient cerebral ischemia instead of typical angina at presentation. These patients had a higher mortality rate than did a nondiabetic cohort. It is unclear whether the higher mortality was the result of less specialized care (because of the atypical presentation at infarction) or an indication that the diabetic and nondiabetic groups were not suitably matched. Nonetheless, the importance of the immediate and accurate diagnosis of myocardial infarction cannot be overemphasized.

Data from the Framingham Study indicate that 60 of 259 (23%) electrocardiographically demonstrated myocardial infarctions were discovered only on routine biennial electrocardiograms.[8] Diabetic patients tended to experience more of these electrocardiographically diagnosed infarcts. Patients with silent myocardial infarction also demonstrated a similar prognosis as that of patients with symptomatic and clinically recognized infarction.

An autopsy series performed in the late 1950s at the New England Deaconess Hospital revealed that 33 of 77 diabetic patients who died of acute myocardial infarction had evidence of at least one healed myocardial infarction that was not related to the patient's clinical history.[9] Autopsy studies have also documented a high incidence of myocardial scar and severe coronary artery disease in diabetic patients who die of noncardiac causes. Thus, the available data clearly indicate that as a group, diabetic patients have a high incidence of coronary artery disease with a significant potential for silent myocardial infarction.

SILENT ISCHEMIA IN DIABETIC PATIENTS WITH ASYMPTOMATIC CORONARY ARTERY DISEASE

To evaluate the relation of angina to reversible ischemia, Bellet and Roman[10] using a two-step exercise tolerance test assessed 85 diabetic patients who were clinically free of coronary artery disease. Within this group, 22 percent displayed ischemic ST-segment changes, whereas only 8 percent of matched controls showed a similar ischemic response.

In a more recent investigation, using a standard Bruce protocol and thallium-201 scintigraphy, Abenavoli et al[11] studied exercise capacity, maximum oxygen consumption, ST-segment depression, and thallium perfusion in 16 asymptomatic diabetic males and 12 nondiabetic controls. The duration of exercise was longer in control subjects than in diabetic patients (663 vs 519 seconds) and maximum oxygen consumption was greater in the nondiabetic group. Diabetic patients also demonstrated significantly greater aerobic impairment (10.4 vs −7.8%). Significant ST-segment depression was found in two diabetic patients and one control patient. Although the incidence of ST-segment depression between the two groups was not statistically significant, 5 of the 12 diabetic patients compared with only 1 nondiabetic patient had focal abnormalities by thallium perfusion scintigraphy. Echocardiography revealed no significant differences between the diabetic and nondiabetic group in left ventricular end-diastolic or end systolic dimensions. There was a statistically significant decrease in the fractional circumferential fiber shortening in the diabetic group.

It should be noted that not all published studies show a clearly increased incidence of silent ischemia in diabetic patients. For example, Hume et al[12] compared a group of 30 diabetic patients with demonstrated neuropathy but without known coronary artery disease to a cohort of 30 asymptomatic age-matched diabetic controls without neuropathy. There were 14 exercise tests that were positive for ischemia; however, these were equally distributed between the two groups. Although this study demonstrated a surprisingly high incidence of asymptomatic ischemia, diabetic patients with neuropathy who were presumed to be at a higher risk for sensory dysfunction did not have a higher incidence of coronary artery disease. Furthermore, during a mean follow-up of 50 months, an abnormal exercise tolerance test result was associated with a high risk of developing clinical coronary disease.

Campbell et al[13] also reported on diabetic patients who, after autonomic neuropathy was confirmed by abnormal autonomic function tests, developed symptoms of angina during myocardial infarction. This population, although small in number, demonstrates a significant population of patients who maintain at least some anginal mechanism.

CORONARY ANGIOGRAPHIC EVALUATION OF DIABETIC PATIENTS WITHOUT CLINICAL CORONARY ARTERY DISEASE

The incidence of unsuspected coronary artery disease in diabetic patients with significant renal and vascular disease has been defined utilizing coronary angiography in a totally asymptomatic population. Weinrauch et al[14] reported on 21 juvenile diabetic patients who underwent catheterization before renal transplantation. Although none of the 21 had clinical evidence of coronary artery disease, angiographically severe disease was demonstrated in 9 patients (defined as greater than 50% stenosis in a major vessel). Although the patients with coronary artery disease were demographically similar to those without coronary disease, the 2-year survival rate was increased in those with coronary disease (73 vs 22%). Outcome following renal transplantion was primarily related to the extent of coronary disease. Braun et al,[15] in a study of 100 diabetic patients with end-stage renal disease, found a 39 percent incidence of severe coronary disease. Within this group, only 25.6 percent (10 of 39) had typical angina pectoris. These two studies of diabetic patients with severe vascular or renal disease demonstrated a high prevalence of coronary disease despite the absence of angina.

SILENT ISCHEMIA IN DIABETIC PATIENTS WITH CLINICAL CORONARY ARTERY DISEASE

Although the studies just reviewed clearly document the presence of subclinical coronary disease in diabetic patients, the prevalence of asymptomatic ischemia in diabetic patients with established coronary disease is still largely unknown. Once a diagnosis of coronary disease has been made, the character and frequency of symptoms are used as an index of the activity of disease and as a potential means of guiding therapy. Because latent coronary disease may be more prevalent in the diabetic population and because myocardial infarction may occur in the absence of recognizable anginal symptoms and is associated with a poor prognosis, it is understandably important to assess the prevalence of asymptomatic ischemia in diabetic patients with coronary artery disease. The presence of silent ischemia in this context might have incremental prognostic significance with a significant bearing on therapy. As in other subsets of patients, silent ischemia in these patients may be detected either by stress testing with/without radionuclide techniques or by continuous ambulatory ECG monitoring.

FINDINGS ON EXERCISE STRESS TESTING

We recently (1984–1986) studied the relation of angina to ischemia in 50 consecutive diabetic and 50 consecutive nondiabetic persons using exercise thallium-201 scintigraphy.[16] The indications for the test in each group were as follows: a history of chest pain typical of angina pectoris, postinfarction evaluation, coronary angioplasty, coronary bypass surgery, and atypical chest pain, or as a screening test in a patient with multiple risk factors for coronary disease. The frequency of each indication was also similar in both groups. There was no difference between the two study groups with respect to age, sex, incidence of prior infarction, tobacco use, hyperlipidemia, and number of antianginal medications (Table 11.1). Test parameters included exercise capacity as well as severity of and time to ST-segment depression; thallium segment scoring was used to determine the extent of ischemia and infarction. In this study, angina was present in only 14 of 50 diabetic patients with ischemia defined as a reversible perfusion defect on exercise thallium scintigraphy. In the nondiabetic group, 34 of 50 experienced angina, a frequency of angina on exercise tolerance testing similar to that of other large previously published series. This difference between diabetic and nondiabetic groups was highly significant ($p < 0.01$). There was no difference between the diabetic and nondiabetic groups with regard to the extent of infarction or ischemia, exercise capacity, submaximal or peak double products, time

Table 11.1. Comparison of Diabetic Patients with and without Angina on Exercise Treadmill Testing*

	No. of Patients:		
	With Angina	Without Angina	*P* Value
Sex			
Men	10	29	NS†
Women	4	9	NS
Mean age (yr)	61	56	NS
Hypertension	7	22	NS
Smoking	7	16	
Family history of coronary artery disease	9	23	NS
Hyperlipidemia	4	10	NS
Neuropathy	3	7	NS
Nephropathy	0	1	NS
Retinopathy	2	5	NS
Vasculopathy	2	8	NS
Q waves on electrocardiogram	7	16	NS
Anterior‡	1	9	NS
Inferior	6	7	NS
Mean duration of diabetes (yrs)	12	13	NS
Treatment of diabetes			
Insulin	10	28	NS
Oral	4	8	NS

* Fourteen patients had angina; 36 did not.

† Not significant ($p > 0.05$).

‡ Anterior = Q waves in leads I and a VL and/or V_2–V_6; inferior = Q waves in at least two of the following leads: II, III, and aVF.

Reproduced from Nesto et al[16] with the permission of the authors and the *Annals of Internal Medicine*.

to ST-segment depression, or maximum ST-segment depression. Within the diabetic population the duration and treatment of diabetes as well as the presence of diabetic induced retinopathy, nephropathy, peripheral neuropathy, and vasculopathy were noted. No difference in extrapancreatic manifestations of diabetes was noted between diabetic patients with and those without angina. The data indicate that angina is frequently absent in the diabetic patient despite evidence of myocardial ischemia documented on stress thallium-201 scintigraphy. However, not all studies are concordant in this regard. For example, Chipkin et al[17] reviewed 211 exercise tolerance tests that were positive for exercise-induced ischemia. Although there was a high incidence of silent myocardial ischemia, diabetic patients did not seem to experience a greater frequency of silent exertional ischemia (54 vs 47%; p = NS). Although the duration of exercise was shorter in patients with diabetes, there was no significant difference in age, gender, medical regimen, or prior myocardial infarction between the two groups. Chipkin et al[17] came to opposite conclusions to ours regarding the relation of angina to ischemia in diabetic and nondiabetic patients. However, the differences in the patient populations and methodology between the two studies should be emphasized. The discrepancies in the data also emphasize the need for further controlled studies to quantify the prevalence and significance of silent myocardial ischemia in the diabetic patient.

DETECTION OF SILENT ISCHEMIA IN THE DIABETIC PATIENT BY AMBULATORY ECG MONITORING

Despite its known limitations, ambulatory monitoring of the ST segment provides another approach to the quantification of the "total ischemic burden" in diabetic patients with known coronary artery disease. Numerous studies in nondiabetic patients have shown that most episodes of ST-segment depression detected by Holter are asymptomatic and not associated with activities requiring excessive myocardial oxygen demand.[18] In diabetic patients, the overall data are limited, Chiariello et al[19] evaluated 51 diabetic and 70 nondiabetic patients with coronary artery disease and 40 nondiabetic patients without coronary artery disease. Thirty-eight of the 51 diabetic patients had evidence associated with coronary artery disease, and 19 of these patients had evidence of previous myocardial infarction. Ambulatory monitoring revealed that significantly more diabetic patients (18 of 51; 35%) experienced asymptomatic episodes of ST-segment depression than did matched nondiabetic controls (12 of 70; 17%). The number of episodes of ST-segment depression was also greater in diabetic patients (93 of 129; 72%) than in nondiabetic patients (48 of 80; 60%). At the New England Deaconess Hospital we are evaluating diabetic patients with documented coronary artery disease and angina in a protocol with 48-hour Holter monitoring during out-of-hospital activities to determine the ratio of asymptomatic to symptomatic ischemic episodes. Our preliminary findings suggest that only 3 to 5 percent of ischemic events are associated with chest pain recorded in patients' diaries.

In a recent study, Hume et al[20] performed ambulatory monitoring for ischemia in 27 diabetic men without evidence of peripheral neuropathy and in 28 age-matched diabetic patients with evidence of peripheral neuropathy. Asymptomatic ST-segment depression was more common in the diabetic population but was not related to the presence of peripheral neuropathy. The prevalence of ST-segment depression was slightly higher in the diabetic group with peripheral neuropathy. However, peripheral neuropathy was not an independent risk factor for the development of asymptomatic ST-segment depression. Hume et al[20] also showed that the presence of ST-segment depression in both groups increased the risk of subsequent clinical coronary disease.

SOME PATHOPHYSIOLOGIC CONSIDERATIONS

No single pathophysiologic basis has proved a sufficient explanation for the lack of angina with ischemia among diabetic patients with coronary artery disease. The relation between diabetes-induced autonomic nervous system dysfunction, peripheral nervous system dysfunction, and angina has been explored, as neuropathy is a well-known sequela of diabetes and is associated with abnormalities of cardiac function such as orthostatic hypotension, resting tachycardia, and loss of heart rate variability on cardiovascular reflex testing. Peripheral neuropathy is manifested by pain and paresthesias in the extremities, whereas physical examination reveals decreased sensation to pinprick and vibration.

Although a detailed description of the neuropathways responsible for transmission of cardiac pain is beyond the scope of this chapter, it is clear that the afferent (sensory) fibers running through the cardiac sympathetic nerves form the essential pathway for the transmission of cardiac pain. From the heart, afferent nerve fibers run to the spinal cord via the upper five sympathetic ganglia, the white rami communicantes, the grey rami, and the upper five dorsal thoracic roots. It is reasonable to assume that diabetic neuropathy may interfere with impulse transmission via afferent cardiac sensory fibers given the recognized disturbance in sympathetic and parasympathetic control of cardiac function due to diabetes-induced neuropathy of efferent (motor) fibers.

Data on the histology of autonomic nervous system dysfunction are limited. Using histologic techniques, Fearman et al[21] studied sympathetic and parasympathetic nerve fibers within the myocardium of diabetic and nondiabetic patients who had died of myocardial infarction. In all five diabetic patients who had died of painless myocardial infarction, the sympathetic and parasympathetic nerves showed morphologic alteration of diabetic neuropathy consisting of (1) beaded thickenings within the nerves, (2) spindle-shaped nerve fibers, (3) fragmentation of nerve fibers, and (4) a decrease in the actual number of neurons. The five diabetic patients with painful infarction were not found to have these neuropathic alterations. It should be noted, however, that peripheral neuropathy, retinopathy, and the duration of the treatment of diabetes did not correlate with the presence of cardiac autonomic neuropathy.

To further evaluate the relation between silent myocardial ischemia and autonomic neuropathy, Niakan et al[22] evaluated 73 consecutive diabetic patients with peripheral neuropathy for evidence of autonomic neuropathy and myocardial infarction. Twenty-five (43%) of the 73 patients demonstrated autonomic nervous system dysfunction. Within this group of 25 patients, 5 (20%) demonstrated ECG evidence of a myocardial infarction without antecedent clinical history. Only two controls (4.2%) without evidence of autonomic neuropathy had a silent Q-wave infarction. Thus, these data suggest but do not conclusively establish the role of autonomic neuropathy as a basis for the high incidence of silent ischemia in diabetic patients.

CONCLUSIONS

The data reviewed herein indicate that the frequency of anginal symptoms may not accurately reflect the degree of myocardial ischemia in patients with diabetes mellitus. Angina, especially in the diabetic population, may be an insensitive indicator of coronary artery disease activity. Although the prognostic implications of these findings are uncertain, information obtained with ECG monitoring in large numbers of patients followed in a controlled fashion for long periods of time may help determine the prognostic significance of asymptomatic ischemic episodes. However, potential applications for ambulatory ECG monitoring in this setting include (1) its use in lieu of exercise tolerance testing for establishing a diagnosis of coronary artery disease, and (2) its value in providing objective evidence of therapeutic efficacy and in assessing the relation of symptoms, often atypical in nature, to electrocardiographic evidence of ischemia. However, the limitation of the approach to completely asymptomatic patients with its low sensitivity and specificity in this subset of patients should not be ignored. Its overall utility should clearly be evaluated against that of exercise testing in combination with noninvasive techniques which provide adjunctive information on segmental wall abnormalities and perfusion deficits. Such data will be of much clinical importance in evaluating the need for aggressive therapy for silent ischemia in diabetic patients with or without known coronary disease.

REFERENCES

1. Shurtleff D: Some characteristics related to incidence of C-V disease and death: Framingham Study 18 year follow-up. Washington, DC, US Government Printing Office, 1974, p 30.
2. Dortimer AC, Shenoy PN, Shiroff RA, et al: Diffuse coronary artery disease in diabetic patients: Fact or fiction? *Circulation* 1978;57:133–136.
3. Smith JW, Marcus FI, Serokman R, with the Multicenter Postinfarction Research Group: Prognosis of patients with diabetes mellitus after acute myocardial infarction. *Am J Cardiol* 1984;54:718–721.
4. Kannel WB, Abbott RD: Incidence and prognosis of unrecognized myocardial infarction: An update on The Framingham Study. *N Engl J Med* 1984;311:1144–1147.
5. Ewing DJ, Campbell IW, Clarke BF: The natural history of diabetic autonomic neuropathy. *Q J Med* 1980;149:95–108.
6. Bradley RF, Schoenfield A: Diminished pain in diabetic patients with acute myocardial infarction. *Geriatrics* 1962;17:322–326.
7. Soler NG, Bennett MA, Pentecost BL, Fitzgerald MG, Malins JN: Myocardial infarction in diabetics. *Q J Med* 1975;44:125–132.
8. Margolis JR, Kannel WB, Feinleib M, Dawber TR, McNamara PM: Clinical features of unrecognized myocardial infarction-silent and symptomatic: Eighteen-year follow-up: The Framingham Study. *Am J Cardiol* 1973;32:1–7.
9. Bradley RF, Partamian JO: Coronary heart disease in the diabetic patient. *Med Clin North Am* 1963;1093–1104.
10. Bellet S, Roman L: The exercise test in diabetic patients as studied by radioelectrocardiography. *Circulation* 1967;36:245–254.
11. Abenavoli T, Rubler S, Fisher VJ, Axelrod HI, Zuckerman KP: Exercise testing with myocardial scintigraphy in asymptomatic diabetic males. *Circulation* 1981;63:56–64.
12. Hume L, Oakley GD, Boulton AJM, Hardisty C, Ward JR: Asymptomatic myocardial ischemia in diabetes and its relationship to diabetic neuropathy: An exercise electrocardiography study in middle-aged diabetic men. *Diabetes Care* 1986;9:384–388.
13. Campbell IW, Ewing DJ, Clarke BF: Painful myocardial infarction in severe diabetic autonomic neuropathy. *Acta Diabetol Lat* 1978;15:201–204.
14. Weinrauch L, D'Elia JA, Healy RW, Gleason RE, Christlieb AR, Leland OS Jr: Asymptomatic coronary artery disease: Angiographic assessment of diabetics evaluated for renal transplantation. *Circulation* 1978;58:1184–1189.
15. Braun WE, Phillips DF, Vidt DG, Novick AC, Nakamoto S, Popowniak KL, Paganini E, Magnusson M, Pohl M, Steinmuller DR, Protiva D, Bustza C: Coronary artery disease in 100 diabetics with end-stage renal failure. *Transplant Proc* 1984;XVI:603–607.
16. Nesto RW, Phillips RT, Kett KG, et al: Angina and exertional myocardial ischemia in diabetic and nondiabetic patients: Assessment by exercise thallium scintigraphy. *Ann Int Med* 1988;108:170–175.
17. Chipkin SR, Frid D, Albert JS, Baker SP, Dalen JE, Aronin N: Frequency of painless myocardial ischemia during exercise tolerance testing in patients with and without diabetes mellitus. *Am J Cardiol* 1987;59:61–65.
18. Nesto RW, Phillips RT: Asymptomatic myocardial ischemia in diabetic patients. *Am J Med* 1986;80:40–47.
19. Chiariello M, Indolfi C, Cotecchia MR, Sifola C, Romano M, Condorelli M: Asymptomatic transient ST changes during ambulatory ECG monitoring in diabetic patients. *Am Heart J* 1985;110:529–534.
20. Hume L, Oakley GDG, Boulton AJM, Peach M, Hardisty CA, Wart JD: Ambulatory monitoring of the ST segment in diabetic men with and without peripheral neuropathy. *Diabetes Med* 1986;3:545–548.
21. Fearman I, Faccio E, Melei J, et al: Autonomic neuropathy and painless myocardial infarction in diabetic patients: Histologic evidence of their relationships. *Diabetes* 1977;26:1147–1158.
22. Niakan E, Harati Y, Rolak LA, Comstock JP, Rokey R: Silent myocardial infarction and diabetic cardiovascular autonomic neuropathy. *Arch Intern Med* 1986;146:2220–2230.

CHAPTER 12

Angiographic Correlates of Silent Myocardial Ischemia Documented by Ambulatory ECG Monitoring in Chronic Stable Angina

Freny Vaghaiwalla Mody, MD,
Koonlawee Nademanee, MD,
and Bramah N. Singh, MD, DPhil

Spontaneous episodes of asymptomatic transient myocardial ischemia have now been well documented by Holter recordings in unstable as well as stable coronary syndromes.[1-6] Such episodes of "silent" ischemia have been reasonably well characterized with respect to prevalence,[1-6] hemodynamic correlates,[7] associated perfusion deficits,[1] variability, and reproducibility.[8-10] However, their prognostic and therapeutic significance in coronary artery disease has not been clearly established. It is nevertheless known that persistent silent myocardial ischemia in unstable angina despite medical therapy is a predictor of adverse short-term clinical outcomes,[11-13] being associated with angiographic severity of coronary lesions.[11,13] This relation in stable coronary artery disease has not been tested; however, a correlation of silent ischemic episodes to the parameters of exercise stress testing that are important determinants of prognosis has been demonstrated.[14,15]

Because it is known that angiographic severity of coronary artery disease and the severity of ischemia judged by exercise stress testing are important prognostic determinants,[16] the occurrence of silent myocardial ischemia during Holter monitoring is of obvious clinical interest. In recent years, studies have examined the issue of whether ambulatory ECG monitoring provides adjunctive data on the risk profile in a subset of patients among the large heterogeneous population presenting with the initial diagnosis of coronary artery disease. This chapter will review the findings from these studies and provide some new data from our own laboratory that bear on the issue of the clinical use of ambulatory ECG monitoring in defining the significance of silent ischemia in patients with chronic stable angina.

PREVIOUS OBSERVATIONS

Data from three studies will be discussed. The earliest study was that of Kunkes et al[17] who obtained Holter recordings in 50 patients scheduled for diagnostic coronary angiography for symptoms suggestive of ischemic heart disease. Of importance, Holter monitors were attached for 24 hours but recordings were made for only 97 periods of random 6-second recordings at 15-minute intervals for a total of 9.67 hours per patient. In addition, patients continued to take antianginal medications during these recordings. They correlated the number of episodes of silent ST-segment deviations with the extent of coronary artery disease as judged by the number of vessels with stenotic lesions. The essential data are graphically summarized in Figure 12.1. Patients with multivessel coronary artery disease had a higher frequency of silent ischemic episodes than did patients with one-vessel disease.

Quyyumi et al[18] examined the morphology of ambulatory ST-segment changes in patients with varying severity of coronary artery disease in 100 patients (74 men and 26 women; mean age 53.2 years) presenting with chest pain and undergoing diagnostic coronary angiography. In all patients, antianginal therapy was discontinued

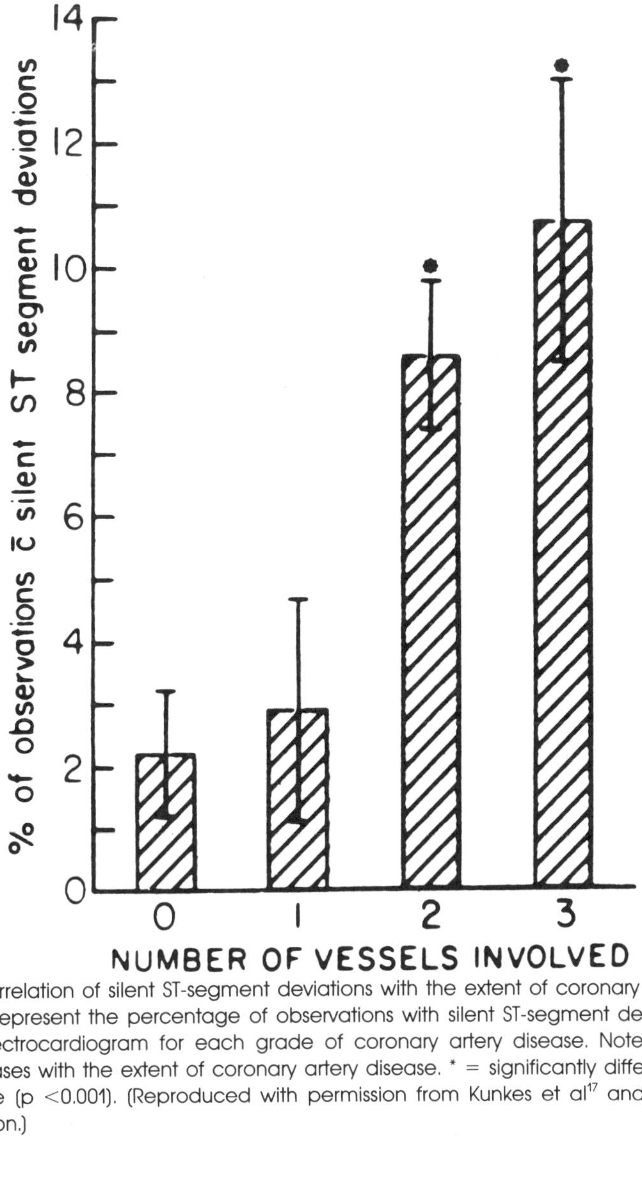

FIGURE 12.1. Correlation of silent ST-segment deviations with the extent of coronary artery disease. *Hatched bars* represent the percentage of observations with silent ST-segment deviations on the ambulatory electrocardiogram for each grade of coronary artery disease. Note how this percentage increases with the extent of coronary artery disease. * = significantly different from 0- to 1-vessel disease ($p < 0.001$). (Reproduced with permission from Kunkes et al[17] and the American Heart Association.)

for 48 hours before they were enrolled in the study. Ambulatory monitoring was carried out for 48 hours; exercise testing was performed and diaries were kept by all patients during the study. Of the 100 patients studied, 58 developed 294 episodes of transient myocardial ischemia during each 24 hours of ambulatory ECG monitoring. Angiography revealed that 25 patients had insignificant disease and one had normal coronary arteries subject to spasm. Seventy-four patients had a spectrum of varying severity of coronary artery disease.

Quyyumi et al[18] reported that the frequency and duration of the episodes of ST-segment deviation were generally greater in patients with more severe coronary artery disease. However, there was considerable overlap between the groups and a statistically significant correlation was not obtained. The correlative data are shown in Table 12.1. It is of interest that both exercise testing (not reproduced) and ambulatory ECG monitoring failed to accurately predict patients with normal coronary arteries. It should also be emphasized that in a significant number of patients, anatomically severe coronary artery disease was not associated with episodes of silent transient myocardial ischemia during Holter monitoring.

The findings of Nikutta et al[19] recently reported are also of practical importance. They studied 101 patients (84 men and 17 women; mean age 55 years) also undergoing diagnostic coronary angiography, all having had chest pain. The objective of the study was to correlate the findings on Holter recordings with those obtained at coronary angiography. Patients continued medical therapy during the investigation. Before angiography all patients also underwent an exercise stress testing using bicycle ergometry.

Holter recordings were obtained for 24 (61 patients), 48 (12 patients), or 72 (28 patients) consecutive hours. The episodes of ST-segment deviation were correlated with the diary of symptoms kept by the patients during the period of monitoring. It was of interest that the number of completely asymptomatic patients during the period of monitoring declined as the numbers of stenosed vessels increased (Figure 12.2). It was found that less than 20 percent of patients with ST-segment depression and three-vessel disease or left main stem stenosis were entirely asymptomatic during Holter monitoring. More than 80 percent of the patients with single-vessel disease had only asymptomatic episodes. However, there were no patients with single- or double-vessel disease who had exclusively symptomatic episodes of myocardial ischemia; four of the six patients with left stem main disease had only symptomatic disease. Figure 12.3 shows the relation between the total duration of transient ST-segment depression per day in patients with single-, double-, and triple-vessel (greater than 70% stenosis) disease and isolated left main stem stenosis. Considerable overlap is clearly apparent.

It must be emphasized that these data reported by Nikutta et al[19] should be interpreted in light of the fact that all patients studied were on continuous medical therapy and the data from this study cannot be compared without qualification to those in other studies in which antianginal therapy had been withdrawn before Holter monitoring was performed.

OUR OBSERVATIONS

We undertook a prospective study to define the correlative relation between the results of ambulatory Holter monitoring, exercise stress testing, and coronary angiography in 102 patients (100 men and 2 women; mean age 64 years) consecutively

Table 12.1. Frequency, Duration, and Magnitude of Episodes of ST-segment Change During Ambulatory Electrocardiographic Monitoring in 100 Patients with Varying Severity of Coronary Artery Disease and Nocturnal Angina*

	Coronary artery disease						
	Not significant	Spam only	1 vessel	2 vessel	3 vessel	Left main stem stenosis	Nocturnal angina
Total no. of patients	25	1	22	22	30	7	12
with ST-segment changes (%)	5(19)	1	11(50)	17(77)	24(80)	7(100)	12(100)
Total no. of episodes	2(1.6)	1.8	2.9(1.9)	3.7(4.4)	7.3(9.2)	17(13)	12(8.6)
Duration of episodes	44(57)	7(4)	63(52)	59(73)	99(119)	174(65)	3.8(1.6)
Mean maximum ST change (mm)	1.5(0.5)	1.6(0.5)	1.1(0.3)	2.5(1.1)	2.3(1.5)	3.8(1.6)	3.4(1.4)

Values are mean (SD).
* Reproduced with permission from Quyyumi et al[18] and the *British Heart Journal*.

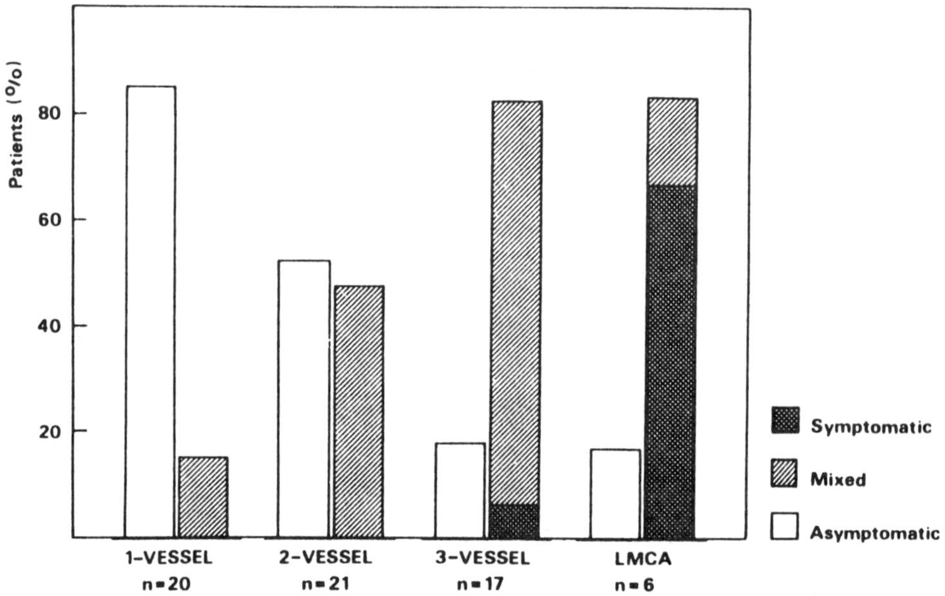

FIGURE 12.2. Patients with exclusively asymptomatic, mixed (asymptomatic and symptomatic), or exclusively symptomatic episodes of ST-segment depression during the recording period in single-, double-, and triple-vessel disease (1-, 2-, and 3-vessel stenoses greater than 70%) and isolated left main stem stenosis (LMCA). (Reproduced with permission from Nikutta et al[19] and Springer-Verlag, New York.)

scheduled for elective coronary angiography for the delineation of coronary anatomy. Forty-two normal volunteers in whom Holter monitoring and stress testing only were performed served to validate the Holter findings. All patients were in New York Heart Association Functional Class I–IIIA. All patients had their antianginal therapy discontinued before they were enrolled in the study. Sublingual nitroglycerin was permitted for chest pain. Antianginal medications were discontinued (mean 45.6 ± 22.8 hours) prior to Holter recordings in 79 patients; 23 patients either had never begun or were off medications for more than 5 days before Holter recording. Twenty-four hours before angiography, all patients underwent ambulatory Holter recordings which were analyzed using the compact analog technique[20] by a blinded technologist. All treadmill exercise tests (data not presented here) were performed using a standard Bruce protocol with a Marquette Case II computerized system.

The coronary angiograms were read and analyzed by the cardiac catheterization teams unaware of Holter recording results. Two indices were used to score the extent of coronary artery disease in the manner described by Rinquist et al[21]: (1) the score based on the number of major coronary vessels with lesions, and (2) the score based on the site (proximal) of the lesion.

Detection of Myocardial Ischemia by Ambulatory Electrocardiographic Monitoring

Ninety-seven patients underwent 2,503 hours of monitoring (mean 25.8 ± 1.6 hours). A total of 159 episodes of ischemia were identified; 10 percent were associated with angina. The mean duration of the ischemic episodes was 22.7 ± 147 minutes (range 1–234). Of note, only 26 of the 70 patients with one- to three-vessel stenosis greater

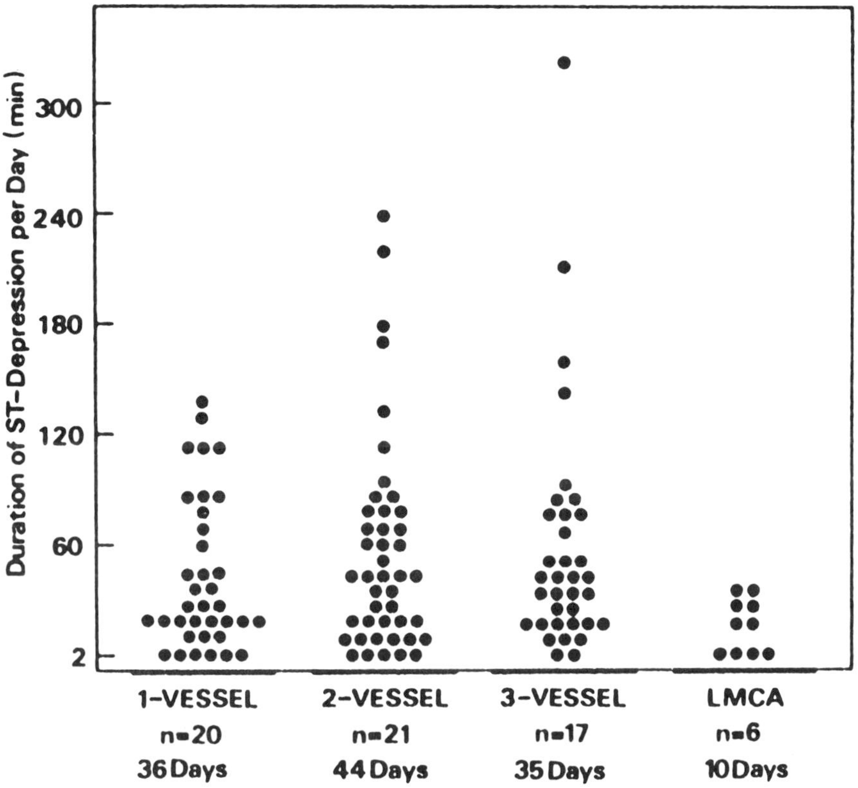

FIGURE 12.3. Total duration of transient ST-segment duration per day in patients with one-, two-, or three-vessel disease and isolated left main stem stenosis (LMCA). Same source as Figure 12.2.

than 70 percent on coronary angiography had ischemia on ambulatory ECG monitoring despite the discontinuation of antianginal therapy. Of additional interest, only 4 Holter recordings in the 23 patients without vessel disease had myocardial ischemia. Similarly, Holter recordings from the normal volunteers demonstrated only one subject as having ischemia in addition to the ECG changes noted during exercise treadmill testing. Thus, when the data from our study groups (patients and volunteers) were pooled, the specificity was 92 percent and positive predictive value 80 percent for the ambulatory ECG monitoring, but the sensitivity and negative predictive value were 37 and 27 percent, respectively.

Relation of Ambulatory Electrocardiographic Monitoring to Coronary Angiography

Figures 12.4 and 12.5 graphically depict the frequency distribution of total ischemia duration on ambulatory ECG recordings in relation to the number of vessels and proximal artery score index derived from coronary angiography. Figure 12.4 demonstrates the high frequency of a Holter recording with greater than 60 minutes per 24 hours of ischemia, indicating patients with multivessel or left main coronary artery disease versus with no-vessel disease (72 versus 10%). Of note, however, is the reasonably even distribution of negative Holter recordings (Group I) in all categories of angiographic severity of coronary artery disease (28% in no-vessel disease, 24% in one-vessel disease, 26% in two-vessel disease, and 22% in three-vessel or left

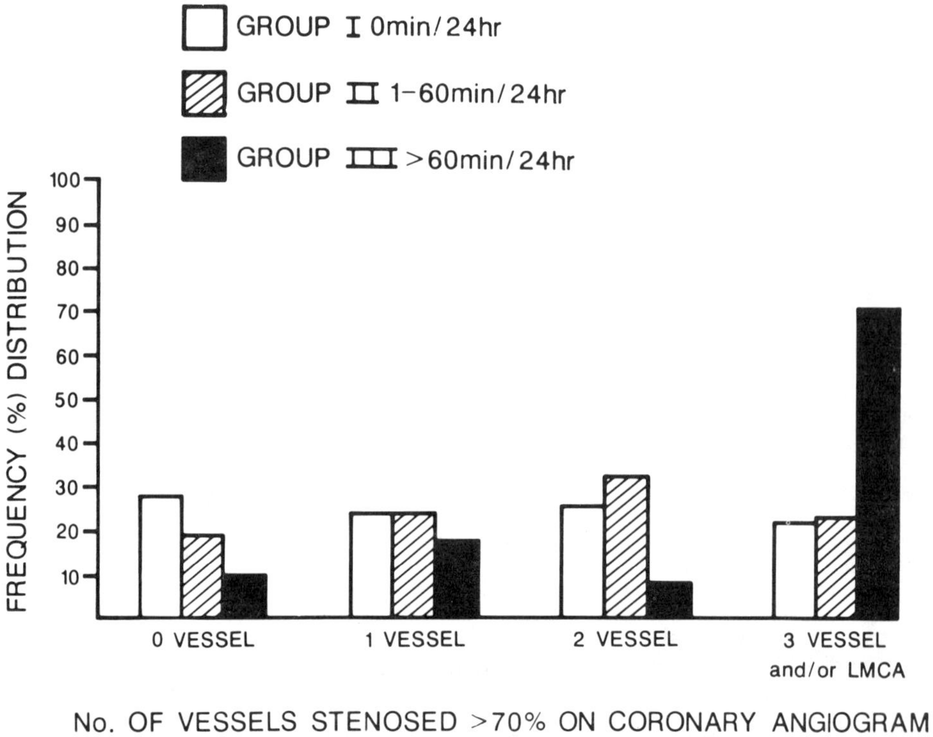

FIGURE 12.4. Relation of total cumulative duration (in minutes per hours) of ischemia on ambulatory ECG recordings to the angiographic severity of coronary artery disease in terms of the numbers of vessels having ≥70 percent stenosis. Note that irrespective of the angiographic abnormalities, ischemia was absent in about 25 percent of Holter recordings. However, the longer duration of ischemia was associated with a greater frequency of three-vessel disease or left main stem lesions. (See text.)

main coronary artery disease). A similar relation between Holter recordings and proximal coronary artery score indexes was demonstrated (Figure 12.5). In addition, the data suggested that proximal artery score rather than the number of stenosed vessels (Figures 12.4 and 12.5) was more closely correlated with the duration of ischemia on ambulatory ECG recordings.

Table 12.2 presents the overall data on the frequency distribution of total ischemia duration on ambulatory ECG recordings relative to the predictive probability (odds ratio) of severity of angiographic coronary artery disease. Contingency tables with Ridit odds-ratio analysis were used to test if the distribution of angiographic score indices were shifted based on parameters on Holter recordings.[22] Thus, a patient with greater than 60 minutes per 24 hours of total ischemia duration was found to have 3.48 and 6.75 times greater probability of having a greater number of stenosed coronary vessels ($p < 0.003$) and a higher proximal coronary artery stenosis index score ($p < 0.0001$), respectively, compared to the patient with no ischemia on Holter recordings.

DISCUSSION AND COMMENTS

There is now a large body of data that indicates that the presence and duration of myocardial ischemia documented on ambulatory ECG recordings bear a correlation with the angiographic severity of coronary artery disease in patients with a diagnosis

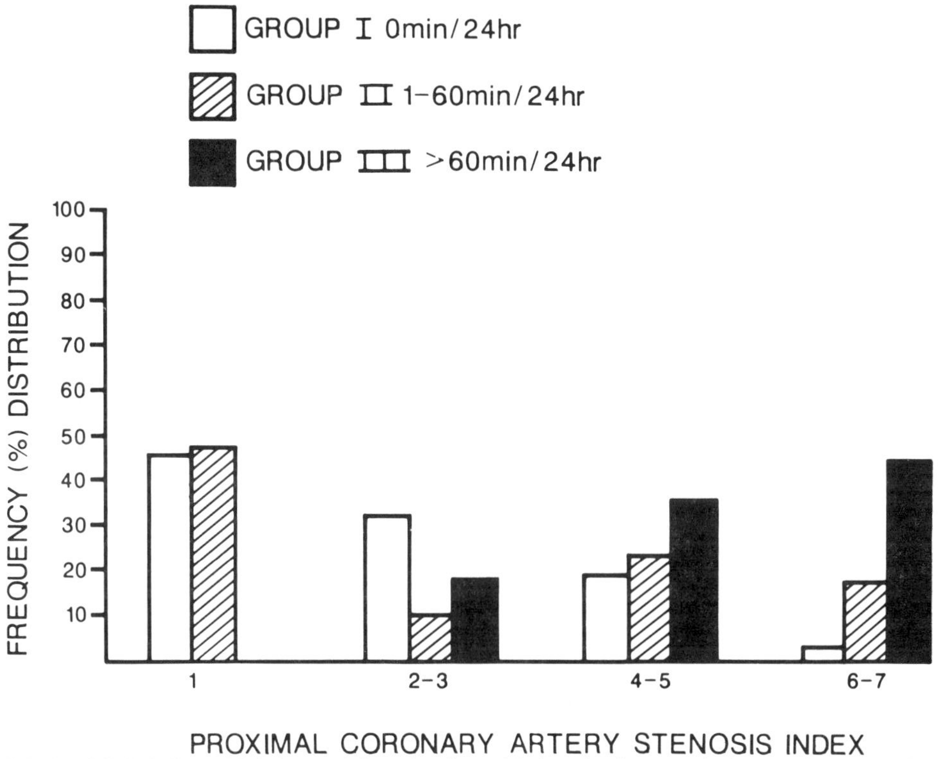

FIGURE 12.5. Relation of total cumulative duration of ischemia documented on ambulatory ECG recordings to angiographic severity of coronary artery disease as graded by proximal coronary artery score index. Note the decreasing frequency of negative Holter recordings (Group I) as the severity of coronary disease increases. Also, prolonged duration of ischemia (Group III) is markedly increased in patients with severe coronary disease (score 6–7) versus those with score 1.

of chronic stable angina.[17–19] A significant correlation between ambulatory ECG recordings with prolonged ischemia and angiographically severe coronary artery disease was demonstrated. As indicated, such a trend has also been reported recently by Quyyumi et al[18] whose study population was equivalent to ours in size and character. In addition, Kunkes et al[17] reported similar findings, demonstrating a linear increase in the magnitude of silent ischemia as a function of the number of diseased vessels; however, their patient population was considerably smaller and more heterogeneous than ours. Furthermore, their patients did not undergo continuous am-

Table 12.2. Predictive Probability (Using Ridit's Odds-Ratio Analysis) of Having More Severe Coronary Artery Disease on Angiography for a Given Total Duration of Ischemia on Holter Monitor Recording

Total Duration of Ischemia/24 Hours on Holter Recordings	Odds for More Vessel Stenosis	p Value	Odds for Higher PASI Score	p Value
1–60 min vs Ø min	1.21	NS	1.27	NS
>60 min vs Ø min	3.48	<0.003	6.75	<0.0001
>60 min vs 1–60 min	2.69	<0.02	4.32	<0.004
No. of ischemic episodes (>Ø episodes vs Ø episodes)	1.67	<0.04	2.0	<0.006

NS = not significant; PASI = proximal coronary artery stenosis index.

bulatory ECG monitoring and were taking antianginal therapy during the monitoring period. In this regard, the observations of Nikutta et al[19] are of particular interest. Although all their patients remained on medical therapy during the period of Holter monitoring, the data showed significant silent ischemia, the distribution of which, while increasing in density as a function of the number of vessels that were involved, demonstrated considerable overlap over the entire spectrum of coronary artery disease severity.

In our own study, 23 patients with prolonged cumulative duration of ischemia (>60 minutes/24 hours) had approximately a three times higher probability of having three-vessel or left main coronary artery disease and a four to seven times higher probability of having more proximal segment coronary stenosis. The ischemia documented on ambulatory ECG recordings was predominantly (90%) asymptomatic or silent; the findings further extend and confirm previous observations.[1–6] The striking feature in all of these studies, however, is the considerable overlap in the density of ischemia per day relative to the number of vessels demonstrating significant arterial stenoses. Although the overall findings reveal a high specificity and positive predictive value of the ambulatory ECG recording for the presence of severe coronary artery disease, our data indicated that only 37 percent of patients with one- to three-vessel coronary artery stenosis on angiography had evidence of ischemia on the Holter recording at a time when they were not on antianginal therapy. Thus, although prolonged ischemia on ambulatory ECG recording increases the likelihood of multivessel coronary disease and the consequent adverse influence on prognosis, its absence is of little predictive significance.

It is noteworthy that our data are similar to those reported previously by Nademanee et al[13] in patients with unstable angina. Residual prolonged cumulative ischemia was significantly more frequent in patients with a larger number of stenosed vessels and with higher proximal coronary artery stenosis indices. It was also of prognostic significance. However, our current data in chronic stable angina clearly indicate that the absence of prolonged episodes of myocardial ischemia on Holter recordings does not exclude the presence of severe multivessel coronary artery disease.

THERAPEUTIC IMPLICATIONS AND CONCLUSIONS

These data form the basis for a number of conclusions on the overall utility of Holter monitoring in the evaluation of chronic stable angina. The results of our study establish that although ambulatory monitoring detects silent and symptomatic episodes of ischemia with a high degree of specificity (over 90%), the sensitivity and predictive accuracy of coronary artery disease are low. Thus, quantification of the total ischemia burden by ambulatory Holter recordings is of little *diagnostic* value in identifying the presence of coronary artery disease. Although data directly comparing ambulatory ECG monitoring with exercise stress testing have not been discussed, as a screen test for coronary artery disease, stress testing with or without adjunctive radionuclide techniques might be preferable and more practical. However, Holter monitoring may provide valuable information on the activity of coronary disease as gauged by the frequency and severity of silent ischemia in patients with a positive exercise test results but without pain. However, the significant positive correlation between the cumulative duration of ischemia on Holter recordings and the angiographic extent and severity of coronary artery disease found herein may provide an indirect inferential link between myocardial ischemia on ambulatory ECG recordings and prognosis. Whether the magnitude of ischemia documented on Holter recordings may constitute an index of prognosis as in unstable angina[11–13] is not known, but it clearly merits further investigation by controlled studies of adequate sample size. Such studies will be crucial in determining if the elimination of silent and symptomatic ischemia on Holter recordings should constitute a therapeutic end point in patients with chronic stable angina.

Acknowledgment: This work was done during the tenure of a Research Fellowship of the American Heart Association, Greater Los Angeles Affiliate (Grant #839F1–2), by one of the authors (FVM).

REFERENCES

1. Deanfield JE, Shea M, Ribiero P, de Landsheere CM, Wilson RA, Horlock P, Selwyn AP: Transient ST-segment depression as a marker of myocardial ischemia during daily life. *Am J Cardiol* 1984;54:1195–1212.
2. Schang SJ, Pepine CJ: Transient asymptomatic ST-segment depression during daily activity. *Am J Cardiol* 1977;39:396–402.
3. Deanfield JE, Selwyn AP, Chierchia S, Maseri A, Ribeiro P, Krikler S: Myocardial ischemia during daily life in patients with stable angina: Its relation to symptoms and heart rate changes. *Lancet* 1983;2:753–758.
4. Cecchi AC, Dovellini EV, Marchi F, Pucci P, Santoro GM, Fazini F: Silent myocardial ischemia during ambulatory electrocardiographic monitoring in patients with effort angina. *J Am Coll Cardiol* 1983;1:934–939.
5. Stern S, Tzivoni D: Early detection of silent ischemic heart disease by 24-hour electrocardiographic monitoring of active subjects. *Br Heart J* 1974;36:481–490.
6. Allen RD, Gettes LS, Phalan C, Avington D: Painless ST-segment depression in patients with angina pectoris. *Chest* 1976;69:467–472.
7. Figueras J, Singh BN, Ganz W, Charuzi Y, Swan HJC: Mechanisms of rest and nocturnal angina: Observations during continuous hemodynamic and electrocardiographic monitoring. *Circulation* 1979;59:955–962.
8. Rocco MB, Barry J, Campbell S, Nabel E, Cook EF, Goldman L, Selwyn AP: Circadian variation of transient myocardial ischemia in patients with coronary artery disease. *Circulation* 1987;75:395–400.
9. Nademanee K, Intarachot V, Josephson MA, Singh BN: Circadian variation in the occurrence of transient overt and silent myocardial ischemia in chronic stable angina and comparison with Prinzmetal angina in men. *Am J Cardiol* 1987;60:494–499.
10. Nademanee K, Intarachot V, Robertson HA, Mody Vaghaiwalla F, Singh BN: Variability of parameters of myocardial ischemia: A comparison of exercise treadmill tests, ambulatory ECG monitoring, and symptoms of myocardial ischemia. *Circulation* 1987;76(Suppl II):IV–390.
11. Johnson SM, Mauritson PR, Winniford MD, Willerson JT, Firth BG, Cary JR, Hillis LD: Continuous electrocardiographic monitoring in patients with unstable angina pectoris: Identification of high-risk subgroup with severe coronary disease, variant angina and/or impaired early prognosis. *Am Heart J* 1982;103:4–12.
12. Gottlieb SO, Weisfeldt ML, Ouyang P, Mellits ED, Gerstenblith G: Silent ischemia as a marker for early unfavorable outcomes in patients with unstable angina. *N Engl J Med* 1986;314:1214–1219.
13. Nademanee K, Intarachot V, Josephson MA, Rieders D, Mody Vaghaiwalla F, Singh BN: Prognostic significance of silent myocardial ischemia in patients with unstable angina. *J Am Coll Cardiol* 1987;10:1–9.
14. Nademanee K, Intarachot V, Piontek M, Mody Vaghaiwalla F, Josephson MA, Singh BN: Relationship of myocardial ischemia detected by compact Holter analog technique to that induced by exercise treadmill testing. *Circulation* 1984;70(Suppl II):451.
15. Campbell S, Barry J, Rocco MB, Nabel EG, Mead-Walters K, Rebecca GS, Selwyn

AP: Features of the exercise test that reflect the activity of ischemic heart disease out of hospital. *Circulation* 1986;74:72–80.
16. C.A.S.S. Principal Investigators and their associates: Coronary Artery Surgery Study (CASS). A randomized trial of coronary artery bypass surgery. Survival data. *Circulation* 1983;68:939–950.
17. Kunkes SH, Pichard AD, Smith H, Gorlin R, Herman MV, Kupersmith J: Silent ST-segment deviations and extent of coronary artery disease. *Am Heart J* 1980;100:813–820.
18. Quyyumi AAQ, Mockus L, Wright C, Fox KM: Morphology of ambulatory ST-segment changes in patients with varying severity of coronary artery disease. *Br Heart J* 1982;53:186–193.
19. Nikutta PD, Hausmann D, Daniel WG, Wenzlaff P, Hartwig CA, Lichtlen PR: Silent ischemia and coronary anatomy, in Arnim TV, Maseri A (eds): "Silent Ischemia." New York, Springer-Verlag, 1987, pp 131–139.
20. Nademanee K, Singh BN, Guerrero J, Hendrickson JA, Intarachot V, Baky S: Accurate rapid compact analog method for the quantification of frequency and duration of myocardial ischemia by semi-automated analysis of 24-hour Holter ECG recordings. *Am Heart J* 1982;103:302–312.
21. Rinquist I, Fisher LD, Mock M, et al. Prognostic value of angiographic indices of coronary artery disease from the coronary artery surgery study (CASS). *J Clin Invest* 1983;71:1854–1864.
22. Miller RG, Jr: Normal univariate techniques, in *Simultaneous Statistical Inference*. New York, Springer-Verlag, 1981, pp 34–47.
23. Mody VF, Nademanee K, Intarachot V, Josephson MA, Robertson HJA, Singh BN: Severity of silent myocardial ischemia on ambulatory electrographic monitoring in patients with stable angina pectoris: Relation to prognostic determinants during exercise stress testing and coronary angiography. *J Amer Coll Cardiol* (in press, 1988)

PART C

Prognostic Significance

CHAPTER 13

Silent Myocardial Ischemia as an Index of Adverse Prognosis in Patients with Unstable Angina

Koonlawee Nademanee, MD and
Bramah N. Singh, MD, D Phil

For many years it was widely accepted[1,2] that the syndrome of unstable angina complicating coronary artery disease was associated with a poor prognosis. Gazes et al[1] reported that ST-T-wave changes on 12-lead electrocardiograms during episodes of chest pain in unstable angina identified patients as having a poor long-term prognosis. Subsequently, Papapietro et al[3] showed that the magnitude of such ECG changes during or immediately after painful episodes correlated with the angiographic extent of coronary artery disease in unstable angina.

Numerous reports[4–6] documented that most transient myocardial ischemic episodes associated with unstable angina are clinically silent. As indicated elsewhere in this monograph, such silent ischemic episodes do not differ from symptomatic episodes with respect to ECG manifestations, perfusion deficits, severity of ischemic ventricular dysfunction, or hemodynamic changes. Therefore, patients who experience silent ischemic episodes should have a prognosis similar to that of patients with symptomatic ones. Study of the role of Holter monitoring in assessing the prognosis of patients with unstable angina by Johnson et al[7] clearly shows two clinically significant features. First, patients who exhibited ST-T wave changes on 24-hour Holter recordings had a higher incidence of advanced coronary artery disease than did those who did not. Second, these same patients had a worse short-term prognosis with respect to infarction and sudden death than did those who did not have ST-segment changes. Recently, our study[8,9] and that of Gottlieb et al[10] confirm the findings of Johnson et al[7] that patients with unstable angina and persistent myocardial ischemia have a high risk for subsequent cardiac events.

This chapter will review the current data from both our own laboratory and others which indicate that the persistence of silent myocardial ischemia is of prognostic significance.

OBSERVATIONS OF OTHERS

Johnson et al[7] evaluated 116 patients (60 men and 56 women, mean age 55 years) with unstable angina who were admitted to the coronary care unit (CCU). The mean period of two-channel Holter monitoring was 27 ± 7 hours (range 12 to 50). Twenty-four of these patients developed acute myocardial infarction. Holter monitoring revealed transient ST-segment changes indicative of ischemia in 21 of the remaining 92 patients. Seventy-one (77%) had no ST-segment changes, and four patients were lost to follow-up. Coronary angiography was undertaken in 43 of the remaining 67 patients. A comparison of angiographic findings in patients who had ST-segment changes on Holter monitoring versus those who did not is shown in Figure 13.1. Patients who had ST-segment changes on Holter monitoring had a greater incidence of either three-vessel or left main coronary artery stenosis.

Figure 13.2 summarizes the Holter findings in this study. At 3-month follow-up, 50 of the 63 patients (83%) without ST-segment changes were alive and well on medical therapy, whereas only 3 of the 12 (25%) with ST-segment changes were alive and well. This difference is highly significant ($p < 0.001$). Seventeen percent of the patients (10 of 60) without ST-T wave changes had major cardiac events: two deaths, three myocardial infarctions, and five worsening of angina. In contrast, 58 percent of patients with ST-T wave changes (7 of 12 patients) had major cardiac events: one death, three myocardial infarctions and three worsening of angina. Although the different outcomes of the two groups were only of borderline significance, the trend for the unfavorable outcome in the group with ST-T wave changes on Holter monitoring was striking.

The study by Gottlieb et al[10] indicated that silent myocardial ischemia is a marker for an early unfavorable prognosis in patients with unstable angina. They used Holter monitoring in 70 patients with unstable angina. These patients had been on study

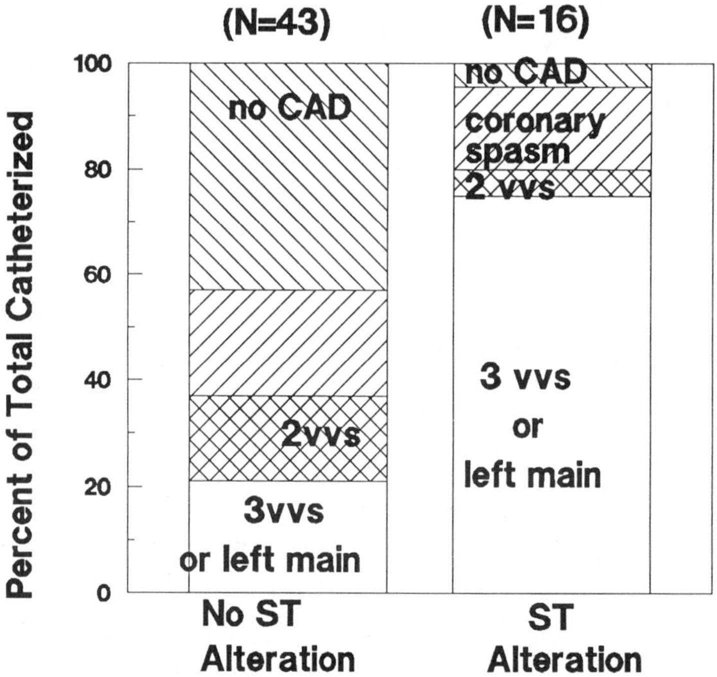

FIGURE 13.1. Comparison of findings at angiography in patients without ST-segment alterations on Holter monitoring (*left*) and those with ST-segment alterations (*right*) expressed as a percentage of each group. Note the high incidence of triple-vessel disease and left main stem stenosis in the group with ST-segment alterations. (Reproduced with permission from Johnson et al[7] and the American Heart Association.)

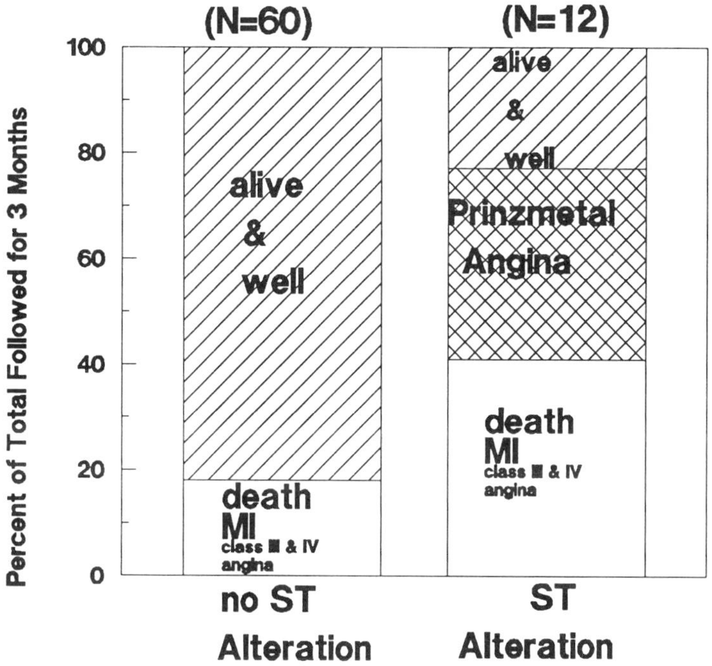

FIGURE 13.2. Comparison of the clinical course over 3 months after Holter monitoring in patients with unstable angina without ST-segment alterations (*left side*) and those with ST-segment alterations, expressed as a percentage of each group. Note that most patients without ST-segment deviations had a good prognosis and the converse was true for those who did have abnormal ST-segment deviations on Holter monitoring. Source as for Figure 13.1.

protocols in which they had received triple therapy (including nitrates, beta-blockers, and calcium channel-blockers).

Of the 70 patients, 37 (Group 1) had at least one episode of silent myocardial ischemia and 33 (Group 2) had no ischemia. Table 13.1 clearly shows the differences between the occurrence of myocardial infarction and the need for myocardial revascularization or percutaneous transluminal coronary angioplasty between the two groups at 1-month follow-up. Similarly, Kaplan-Meier analysis showed a significantly higher cumulative probability of infarction or the need for revascularization ($p < 0.002$) in Group 1 (Figure 13.3). The authors have recently published a long term outcome of the same patients.[18] Interestingly, Group 1 patients whose cumulative silent ischemic

Table 13.1. Clinical Outcomes During One Month Among Patients with (Group 1) and without (Group 2) Silent Ischemia*

Outcome	Total No.	Group 1 (n = 37)	Group 2 (n = 33)	p Value
Myocardial infarction	7	6	1	0.005
CABG or PTCA† for symptoms	13	10	3	0.02
Total	20	16	4	0.01

* Adapted from Gottlieb et al.[10]

† CABG = coronary artery bypass surgery; PTCA = percutaneous transluminal coronary angioplasty.

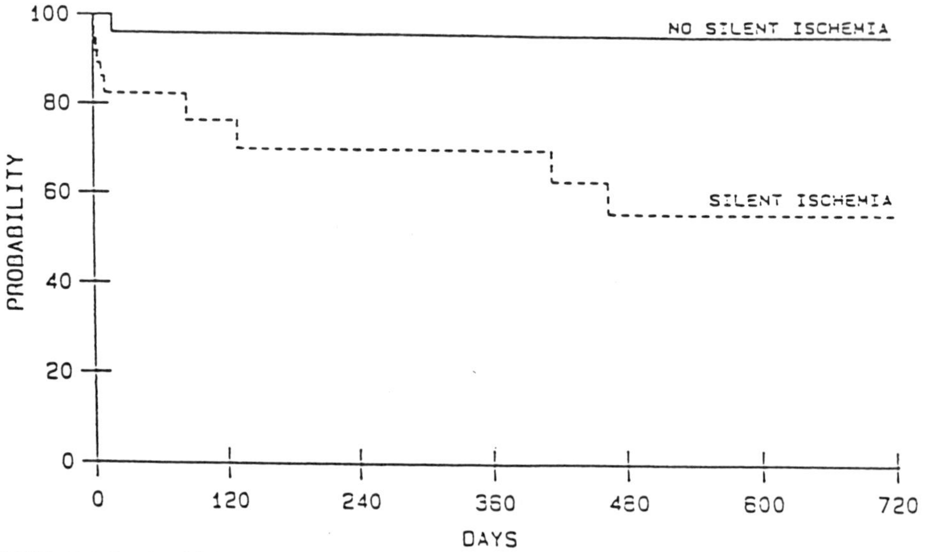

FIGURE 13.3. Kaplan-Meier curves comparing the cumulative probabilities of not experiencing myocardial infarction or death in the 37 patients from the silent ischemia group and the 33 patients without it, as detected by continuous ECG monitoring. (Reproduced from Gottlieb et al[18] with the permission of the authors and the *Journal of the American College of Cardiology*.)

episodes following medical therapy exceeded 60 minutes per 24 hours had a less favorable outcome than did those who had less ischemia ($p < 0.05$). The authors concluded that silent myocardial ischemia occurred in over 50 percent of patients with unstable angina treated intensively with medical therapy. In addition, the presence of ischemia, especially that of longer duration, was highly predictive of an unfavorable outcome.

OBSERVATIONS IN OUR LABORATORY

We recently investigated the significance of the frequency and duration of residual silent myocardial ischemia determined by compact analog analysis[11] of 24-hour Holter recordings.

We prospectively studied 81 male patients (mean age 59 years) admitted to the CCU for control of severe anginal symptoms. Twenty-nine patients (Group 1) were excluded from analysis because their symptoms could not be stabilized with therapy and they required emergency intervention. Of the 27 who had emergency coronary angiography, 4 had left main disease, 10 had three-vessel disease, 8 had two-vessel disease, 3 had one-vessel disease, and 2 had normal coronary arteries. Two patients died of acute myocardial infarction.

The remaining 52 (Group 2), after stabilization, underwent 24-hour ambulatory ECG monitoring in the hospital. Patients were considered to be in stable condition if in the opinion of the attending physician the chest pain had been controlled to the extent that the patients were deemed safe to be discharged from the hospital. The Holter recordings were scanned by blinded observers using the compact analog technique.[11]

Forty-two patients in Group 2 underwent coronary angiography, 25 electively and 13 on an emergency basis; in 4 the indication could not be determined. The coronary angiograms were interpreted by the cardiac catheterization teams who were unaware of the results of Holter monitoring with respect to the severity of myocardial ischemia. We used two indices for scoring the extent of coronary artery disease as described by Rinquist et al[12]: (1) the score based on the number of coronary vessels with lesions, and (2) the score based on the site (proximal) of the lesion.

Duration of Silent Ischemia as a Basis for Analysis of Prognosis

The number of patients who had coronary angiograms relative to the cumulative duration of ischemia per 24 hours is shown in Table 13.2. Of the 49 patients who had ST-segment analysis for transient myocardial ischemia, 20 (Group 2A) had no ST-T wave changes positive for myocardial ischemia. In 11 (Group 2B) of the remaining 29, the cumulative duration of ischemia per 24 hours did not exceed 60 minutes (mean 23 ± 16); in the other 18 (Group 2C) of the 29, the cumulative duration of ischemia exceeded 60 minutes per 24 hours (mean 282 ± 241). In Group 2B (range of transient myocardial ischemia 4 to 53 min/24 h), 70 percent (7 of 10: one lost to follow-up) remained well during follow-up. In contrast, in Group 2C (transient myocardial ischemia 60 to 786 min/24 h) only 1 in 18 (6%) remained well. Therefore, it appeared reasonable to use transient myocardial ischemia of 60 minutes per 24 hours as an arbitrary basis for separating the prognostic groups. (The possibility exists that a different figure other than 60 minutes derived from a larger population sample might constitute a more reliable prognostic index.) Details of the overall data have been reported elsewhere.[9]

Silent Ischemia and Severity of Coronary Disease

Of the 42 patients undergoing coronary angiography, 14 were in Group 2A, 8 in Group 2B, and 17 in Group 2C (three whose Holter tapes could not be analyzed were excluded). Data comparing the severity of coronary artery disease with respect to the number of affected vessels and the score of proximal stenoses are presented in Figures 13.4 and 13.5.

Only one patient in Group 2A (no transient ischemia) and two in Group 2B (with transient ischemia not exceeding 60 min/24 h) had three-vessel coronary artery disease. In contrast, 10 patients in Group 2C (transient ischemia exceeding 60 min/24 h) had three-vessel coronary artery disease. Ridit analysis[13] was used to determine the odds that a patient from one group would have more affected vessels than would a patient from another group. Based on the data (Figure 13.2), the odds were 3.7 to 1 that a Group 2B patient might have more affected vessels than a patient from

Table 13.2. Subgrouping of 52 Study Patients Relative to the Duration of Transient Myocardial Ischemia

Group	No. of Patients	Coronary Angiograms	Lost to Follow-up or Excluded from Analysis
No TMI (Group 2A)	20	14	1
TMI <60 min/24 h (Group 2B)	11	8	1
TMI >60 min/24 h (Group 2C)	18	17	0
Unanalyzable tapes	3	3	3*
Total	52	42	5*

* Three patients excluded from analysis.

TMI = transient myocardial ischemia.

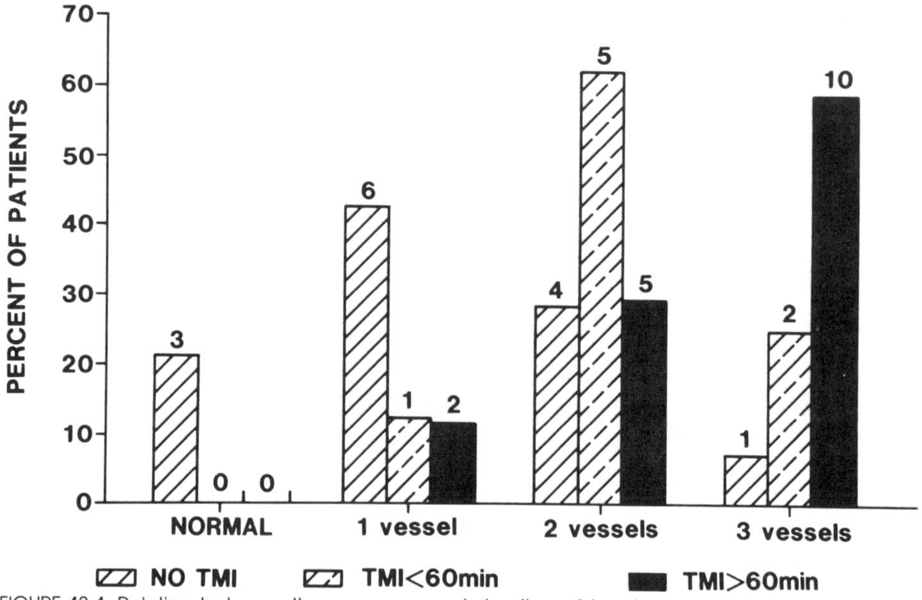

FIGURE 13.4. Relation between the presence and duration of transient myocardial ischemia (TMI) demonstrated on Holter recordings and the number of diseased coronary vessels found at angiography. The numbers at the top of each histogram bar refer to the number of patients. Note that the severity of transient myocardial ischemia as judged by its duration increases as a function of numbers of diseased vessels. Patients were subgrouped as: 2A = no TMI; 2B = TMI <60 min/24 hours; and 2C = TMI >60 min/24 hours. (See text.)

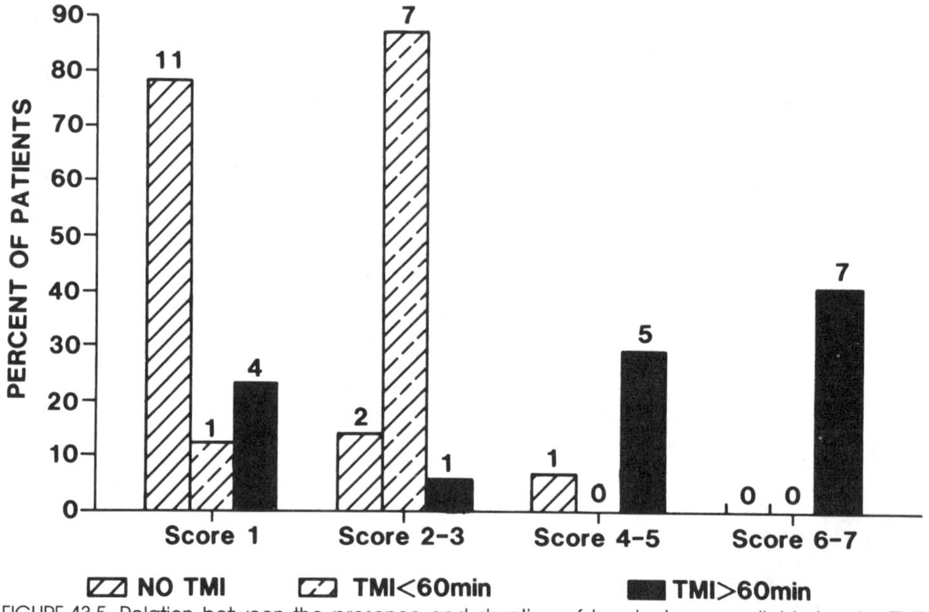

FIGURE 13.5. Relation between the presence and duration of transient myocardial ischemia (TMI) on Holter recordings and the severity of coronary artery disease estimated on the basis of derived proximal coronary artery stenosis score from angiographic data. Note that most patients with high proximal scores had TMI exceeding 60 minutes per 24 hours (Group 2C). See text for details.

Group 2A (p = 0.03) and 5.6 to 1 that a patient from Group 2C would have a greater number of affected vessels than one from Group 2A (p <0.01). However, a patient from Group 2B had about an equal probability of having more or fewer affected vessels than did a patient from Group 2C (p = 1.3).

Eleven of the 14 patients (80%) in Group 2A had no proximal stenoses (score 1), whereas one in Group 2B (12%) and 4 in Group 2C (23%) had a score of 1. Two patients in Group 2A, two in Group 2A, and one in Group 2C had scores between 2 and 3. Only one patient in Group 2A had a score between 4 and 5 compared to none in Group 2B and five in Group 2C. None of the patients in Group 2A or 2B had a score between 6 and 7, indicating the presence of either left main coronary artery disease or severe proximal stenosis of all three coronary vessels. Ridit analysis[17] indicated that the odds were 4 to 1 (p <0.02) for a patient from Group 2B to have a higher score than one from Group 2A. The odds for a Group 2C patient to have a higher score that one from Group 2A was 3.4 to 1 (p <0.01). By Ridit analysis, a patient in Group 2B had an equal chance to have a score either higher or lower than one in Group 2C (p = 0.81). However, when the Group 2C patients had a higher score, it was substantially so, over 70 percent of them scoring 4 or above, whereas none in Group 2B did. The difference by Fisher's exact test (pairwise comparison) was significant (p <0.001).

Silent Ischemia and Clinical Outcome

In a group of 20 patients who had no transient myocardial ischemia (Group 2A), there was one death from myocardial infarction, one patient was lost to follow-up and the remainder continued to do well without clinical incidents during the follow-up period as shown in Figure 13.6. In the 21 patients who had transient ischemia

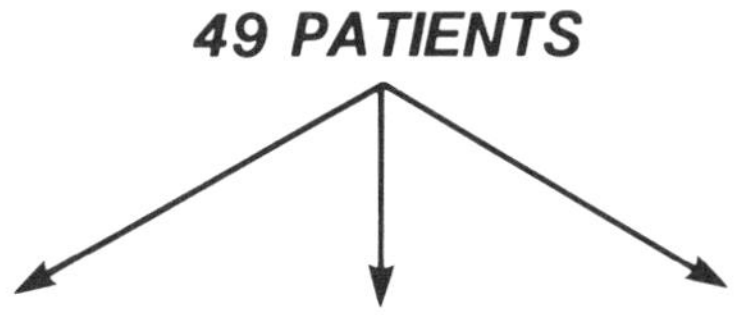

	2A (n=20)	2B (n=11)	2C (n=18)
LOST FOLLOW-UP	1	1	0
ALIVE & WELL	18	7	1
CABG	0	2	11 (NO DEATHS)
ANGIOPLASTY	0	1	1
ACUTE MI	1	0	5 (2 Deaths, 2 CABG, one well)

2A = NO TMI

2B = TMI <60min/24hours

2C = TMI >60min/24hours

FIGURE 13.6. Flow diagram demonstrating the clinical outcome of 49 patients with unstable angina relative to the presence and duration of transient myocardial ischemia (TMI) in patients with unstable angina. (See text.) CABG = coronary artery bypass surgery; MI = myocardial infarction.

on Holter monitoring not exceeding 60 minutes per 24 hours (Group 2B), one was lost to follow-up, two required coronary artery bypass grafts, one required angioplasty, and the seven remaining patients are alive and well. Of the 18 patients with evidence of transient myocardial ischemia exceeding 60 minutes per 24 hours (Group 2C), despite medical therapy during the follow-up period, only one continued to do well with stable angina. Eleven required coronary artery bypass surgery and one had coronary angioplasty. Five patients developed acute myocardial infarction, two of these died from severe left ventricular dysfunction, two required emergency bypass surgery for postinfarction angina, and one survived acute infarction on conservative management. Fisher's exact test using pairwise comparison was used to determine the differences in the frequency of favorable outcomes among the three groups of patients studied. For Group 2C, the favorable outcome occurred in 6 percent; this was significantly less ($p < 0.001$). However, there was statistically no significant difference between Group 2A and 2B (95% versus 70%) in this regard.

COMMENTS AND DISCUSSIONS

Numerous studies involving stress tests in patients with known as well as latent coronary artery disease show that evidence of ischemia is associated with an increased risk for the development of morbid coronary events.[14,15] Furthermore, recent data indicate that ischemia developing during exercise treadmill testing has the same prognostic significance whether or not it is associated with symptoms.[16] These overall findings suggest that ischemia whatever its manifestation should be expected to be associated with similar prognostic import. Although not subjected to critical analysis, symptomatic spontaneous ischemia in unstable angina has been thought to be of prognostic significance. The data discussed in this chapter clearly suggest that following reasonably intense medical therapy of unstable angina, a significant number of patients continue to experience silent episodes of myocardial ischemia documented by continuous Holter recordings. Such silent episodes, especially if the cumulative duration over 24 hours is sufficiently long, are associated with an increased incidence of myocardial infarction and recurrence of severe angina over 1 to 6 months of follow-up.

In the study reported by Gottlieb et al,[10] the silent ischemia detected on Holter recordings in patients undergoing therapy in the CCU was the most powerful predictor of the clinical outcome at 30 days. Angiographic studies by Johnson et al[7] revealed that patients with unstable angina who had ST-segment deviations generally tended to have a greater incidence of triple-vessel or left main coronary artery disease than did those who did not have ischemic abnormalities on Holter monitoring. In our own studies,[8,9] it is noteworthy that analysis of data from subsequent coronary angiographic studies showed that the score based on the number of coronary vessels involved showed a significant correlation with the duration of silent myocardial ischemia found on Holter monitoring. That is, the greater the number of diseased coronary vessels and the higher the score for proximal coronary stenoses, the longer was the cumulative duration of ischemia documented on 24-hour Holter recordings in individual patients. Our data agree with the findings of Papapietro et al[3] who reported that the magnitude of ST-segment shifts in patients with unstable angina was greater in triple-vessel disease than in those with either double- or single-vessel disease. These data suggest a relation between the persistence of transient ischemia on Holter recordings and the patients' subsequent clinical outcome.

We found that patients who either had no ischemia (n = 20) or had a cumulative duration of ischemia not exceeding 60 minutes per 24 hours (n = 11) had a relatively favorable clinical course over a 6-month follow-up. For example, of these patients in the two categories, only one died of acute infarction and three others required coronary artery bypass surgery or angioplasty. The remaining five developed acute myocardial infarction. Our data thus support the observations of Johnson et al[7] who reported on the use of Holter monitoring in the CCU for identifying a high-risk group of patients with coronary artery disease presenting with unstable angina. Transient ST-segment changes were specific predictors of a "high-risk" subgroup of unstable patients with advanced multivessel disease or variant angina. This subgroup had a poor 3-month prognosis.

Our data and those of Gottlieb et al[10] suggest that in patients with unstable angina, persistence of silent episodes of ischemia on Holter monitoring despite the initial near complete elimination of symptoms by medical therapy is associated with advanced severe coronary artery disease. It also identifies a subset of patients in whom there is a major incidence of recurrent symptoms, development of infarction, and occasionally sudden death *despite continued therapy*. The number of deaths in these studies was small and did not permit the authors to evaluate the role of persistent silent ischemia in the genesis of sudden death in coronary artery disease. Nevertheless, when these deaths are considered together with other morbid events such as acute infarction and recurrent unstable angina, they clearly suggest that persistent silent ischemia following amelioration of symptoms by antianginal therapy is of prognostic significance.

THERAPEUTIC IMPLICATIONS AND CONCLUSIONS

The potential practical value of silent ischemic episodes as an end point for judging the adequacy of therapy indicated by the observations discussed in this chapter merits emphasis and further investigation. In the past, symptomatic control of unstable angina was the main objective of initial medical therapy. However, whether the elimination by medical therapy of *all* episodes of ischemia, symptomatic as well as asymptomatic, might have a significant impact on morbidity and mortality from unstable angina is not known. In patients in our series[8,9] in whom Holter recordings were obtained before and after myocardial revascularization or angioplasty, transient ischemic episodes were abolished in all. For the present, it is not known whether different pharmacologic and nonpharmacologic regimens might exert varying effects on the frequency and duration of silent myocardial ischemia and whether such differences might be of clinical significance in altering prognosis. It is also not known to what extent silent myocardial ischemia in unstable angina needs to be reduced to alter prognosis. It must be emphasized that although the frequency and duration of myocardial ischemia documented on Holter recordings may serve as an objective index for determining the risk profile as well as the adequacy of therapy in patients with unstable angina, the validity of this approach in clinical practice will require controlled clinical observations in larger populations of patients. It should also be noted that although silent myocardial ischemia persisting after medical therapy as a marker of poor short-term prognosis is reasonably secure, its application in other subsets of coronary artery disease (eg, chronic stable angina) remains to be demonstrated.

REFERENCES

1. Gazes PC, Mobley EM Jr, Faris HM Jr, Duncan RC, Humphries GB: Preinfarction (unstable) angina—a prospective study and ten year follow-up. *Circulation* 1973;48:331–338.
2. Conti R, Brawley R, Pitt B, Ross R: Unstable angina: Morbidity and mortality in 57 consecutive patients evaluated angiographically. *Am J Cardiol* 1973;32:745–752.
3. Papapietro SE, Niess GS, Paine TD: Transient electrocardiographic changes in patients with unstable angina: Relation to coronary artery anatomy. *Am J Cardiol* 1980;46:28–36.
4. Chierchia S, Brunelli C, Simonetti I, Lazzari M, Maseri A: Sequence of events in angina at rest: Primary reduction in coronary flow. *Circulation* 1980;61:659–667.
5. Biagini A, Mazzei MG, Carpeggiani C, Testa R, Antonelli R, Michelassi C, L'Abbate A, Maseri A: Vasospastic ischemic mechanism of frequent asymptomatic transient ST-T changes during continuous electrocardiographic monitoring in selected unstable angina patients. *Am Heart J* 1980;103:13–20.
6. Nademanee K, Intarachot V, Josephson MA, Singh BN: Characteristics and clinical significance of silent myocardial ischemia in unstable angina. *Am J Cardiol* 1986;58:26B–33B.
7. Johnson SM, Mauritson DR, Winniford MD, Willerson JT, Firth BG, Carg JR, Hillis LD: Continuous electrocardiographic monitoring in patients with unstable angina pectoris: Identification of high-risk subgroup with severe coronary disease, variant angina, and/or impaired early prognosis. *Am Heart J* 1982;103:4–16.
8. Nademanee K. Intarachot V, Piontek M, Mody FV, Josephson MA, Singh BN: Silent myocardial ischemia on Holter: Has it clinical significance? (abstract). *Circulation* 1984;70:Sup III p, 452.
9. Nademanee K, Intarachot V, Josephson MA, Rieders D, Mody Vaghaiwalla F, Singh BN: Prognostic significance of silent myocardial ischemia in patients with unstable angina. *J Am Coll Cardiol* 1987;10:1–9.
10. Gottlieb SO, Weisfeldt ML, Ouyand P, Mellits ED, Gerstenblith G: Silent ischemia as a marker for early unfavorable outcomes in patients with unstable angina. *N Engl J Med* 1986;314:1214–1219.
11. Nademanee K, Singh BN, Guerrero J, Hendrickson JA, Intarachot V, Baky S: Accurate rapid compact analog method for the quantification of frequency and duration of myocardial ischemia by semi-automated analysis of 24-hour Holter ECG recordings. *Am Heart J* 1982;103:802–812.
12. Rinquist I, Fisher LD, Mock M, Davis KB, Wedel H et al: Prognostic value of angiographic indices of coronary artery disease from the coronary artery surgery study (CASS). *J Clin Invest* 1983;71:1854–1864.
13. Fleiss JL: Comparing proportions from independent samples, in *Statistical Methods for Rates and Proportions,* 2nd ed. New York, John Wiley and Sons, 1981, p 150.
14. Uhl GS, Froelicher VF: Screening for asymptomatic coronary artery disease. *J Am Coll Cardiol* 1983;3:946–953.
15. Bonow RO, Kent KM, Rosing DR et al: Exercise-induced ischemia in mildly symptomatic patients with coronary-artery disease and preserved left ventricular function. Identification of subgroups at risk of death during medical therapy. *Circulation* 1984;311:1339–1345.
16. Weiner DA, Ryan TJ, McCabe CH et al: Significance of silent myocardial ischemia during exercise testing in coronary artery disease. *Am J Cardiol* 1987;59:725–729.
17. Miller RG Jr: Normal Univariate Techniques, in: *Simultaneous Statistical Inference*. New York: Springer-Verlag 1981; pp 36–47.

CHAPTER 14

Transient Myocardial Ischemia in Survivors of Acute Myocardial Infarction

Prakash C. Deedwania, MD

In the United States each year, 1.5 million Americans experience acute myocardial infarction (MI). Of these, approximately 800,000 patients survive the acute event. Because infarction predicts a poor prognosis for life, survivors of the acute event comprise a large, readily identifiable group of patients with a relatively high short-term mortality rate.[1–7] Most recent studies indicate a 1-year mortality of 10 to 20 percent in these patients. The delineation of the clinical features, which allows the identification of a high-risk versus low-risk potential for morbid coronary events in survivors of acute infarction, is clearly of importance. This chapter will determine the clinical significance of silent myocardial ischemia in these patients.

PROGNOSIS AFTER ACUTE MYOCARDIAL INFARCTION

Prognosis after MI was shown to correlate closely with the initial clinical course, the size and location of the infarct, the status of left ventricular function and the presence or absence of ventricular arrhythmias and transient myocardial ischemia.[4–16] Comparison of various prognostic factors among survivors of acute MI clearly indicates that the presence of left ventricular (LV) dysfunction as suggested by a low LV ejection fraction (EF) or clinical findings of congestive heart failure (CHF) is the most important predictor of subsequent outcome.[5,6] More recently, several studies evaluating the prognostic significance of residual myocardial ischemia in these patients showed that transient myocardial ischemia occurs frequently and may be of prognostic significance in survivors of acute MI. This issue will be discussed at length herein. However, a distinction will be made between ischemia documented by stress testing and that recorded by ambulatory monitoring. The role of symptoms, exercise stress testing with and without associated radionuclide techniques as well as ambulatory ECG monitoring to detect myocardial ischemia in survivors of infarct will be discussed and the prognostic significance of the findings will be placed in perspective.

PREVALENCE OF TRANSIENT MYOCARDIAL ISCHEMIA IN SURVIVORS OF ACUTE MYOCARDIAL INFARCTION

Transient myocardial ischemia in survivors of acute MI indicates the presence of jeopardized myocardium supplied by the diseased coronary arteries. Residual myocardial ischemia may involve viable myocardium in the infarct zone or it may occur in other areas (ischemia at a distance) supplied by coronary arteries with significant narrowing.[12] Transient myocardial ischemia in these patients may occur spontaneously as manifested by post-MI angina or it may be diagnosed by silent ST-segment changes recorded during ECG monitoring.[12] In others, it may be detected during the exercise tolerance test. A significant proportion of these patients may have silent myocardial ischemia, because they do not experience chest pain during induced or spontaneous ST-segment changes suggestive of myocardial ischemia. The presence of transient myocardial ischemia, whether spontaneous or provoked, has been closely correlated with evidence of significant multivessel coronary artery disease in a vast majority of survivors of acute MI.

The exact prevalence of transient myocardial ischemia in survivors of acute MI is unknown. However, it is estimated that between 15 and 50 percent of the survivors of acute MI have evidence of residual myocardial ischemia.[12–24]

POSTINFARCTION ANGINA AS AN INDICATOR OF TRANSIENT MYOCARDIAL ISCHEMIA

In a study of approximately 400 patients with myocardial infarction, Schuster and Bulkley[12] identified 70 patients with early postinfarction angina, an incidence of 17 percent. Of these 70 patients, 43 (61%) had ischemia at a distance and 27 (38%) had ischemia in the infarct zone. There were no significant clinical differences between the two groups. However, patients with ischemia in the infarct zone were more likely to have anterior infarct (21 of 27 vs 20 of 43; $p < 0.01$) and seemed to have a higher prevalence of non-Q-wave infarcts (12 of 27 [44%] vs 10 of 43 [23%]). Twenty-six patients (30%) had reciprocal ECG changes in leads facing the infarcted segment of the heart. The presence of these reciprocal changes was predictive of ischemia at a distance and subsequent poor prognosis. Angiographic findings revealed that patients with ischemia at a distance mostly had total occlusion of the artery in the distribution of the infarct, whereas patients with ischemia in the infarct zone were more likely to have diseased but still patent coronary arteries. Overall, 86 percent of the patients had three-vessel coronary artery disease, and there was no difference in this regard between the two groups.

In a more recent study of 449 patients who survived MI and were hospitalized in the coronary care unit (CCU) until discharge, Bosch et al[13] demonstrated early postinfarction angina with associated ST-segment changes in 79 (18%). The detection was optimized by the prospective nature of the study, a high degree of awareness by the staff involved, and the recording of a 12-lead electrocardiogram before nitroglycerin administration during episodes of chest pain. In contrast to Schuster and Bulkley,[12] these investigators demonstrated that patients with early ischemia had a higher prevalence of three-vessel disease (39% vs 21%) as well as multivessel coronary artery disease (CAD) (74% vs 53%). These findings led Bosch et al[13] to conclude that early ischemia, as diagnosed by the presence of angina and ST-segment changes after MI appears to be a good clinical indicator of the presence of multivessel disease with a specificity of 90 percent. Like Schuster and Bulkley, these investigators also found the presence of non-Q-wave infarction and a history of previous angina as independent predictors of postinfarction angina.

In the Multicenter Post Infarction Program (MPIP), Bigger[14] demonstrated that 33 percent of 867 patients had early angina pectoris between 2 days and hospital discharge 17 ± 9 days after infarction. These investigators also demonstrated that 47 percent of the patients with anginal symptoms before the index infarct had angina during the postinfarction period. In contrast, 25 percent of patients without a history of angina pectoris had postinfarction angina. In about half the patients who had anginal symptoms before acute MI this symptom disappeared after the infarction. These studies demonstrated that postinfarction angina is a specific indicator of residual myocardial ischemia in the survivors of acute MI. However, these data also point out that many patients with ischemia may not experience anginal symptoms after their MI. These studies did not address the issue of differences in prognostic significance between symptomatic and asymptomatic myocardial ischemia following MI nor did they evaluate the frequency of silent ischemia in the survivors of acute infarcts.

EXERCISE-INDUCED ISCHEMIA IN SURVIVORS OF ACUTE MYOCARDIAL INFARCTION

Exercise testing in the immediate postinfarction period is now considered to be a safe procedure.[15–22] It has the potential to document the presence of residual ischemia associated with an increased risk of subsequent coronary events and increased mortality.[20–26] Most of the currently available data on the incidence and significance of inducible transient myocardial ischemia in survivors of acute MI is based on the information from these studies using exercise testing. Data from recent studies will be discussed briefly. Sami et al[15] evaluated the prognostic significance of serial exercise testing after uncomplicated acute MI in 200 patients. These investigators demonstrated a 22-percent incidence of ST-segment depression, many essentially silent. In a recent study of 210 patients with uncomplicated acute MI at Montreal Heart Institue, Theroux et al[23] performed a submaximal exercise test 1 day before hospital discharge (average 11 days after MI). ST-segment changes indicative of myocardial ischemia were noted in 64 patients (34%). When the presence of ST-segment abnormalities was correlated with associated exercise-induced angina, only 27 patients (42%) had symptomatic ischemia, whereas 37 patients (58%) had silent myocardial ischemia. More recently, Jespersen et al[24] evaluated the role of the maximal exercise test performed in the third to fourth week after acute MI in 126 consecutive patients with no evidence of prior MI, unstable angina pectoris, or severe heart failure. Forty-six patients (37%) had ST-segment depression during exercise. Like Theroux et al,[23] these investigators found that only 11 of the 46 patients (24%) had associated anginal symptoms, whereas others (76%) had silent myocardial ischemia.

In the most recent data from the Multicenter Post Infarction Research Group, Krone et al[25] evaluated the role of low level exercise testing in enhancing the clinical risk stratification of 866 patients enrolled in the study. Of the 667 patients who were able to perform the low level exercise test, 167 patients (25%) had ST-segment depression greater than 1 mm and in 62 patients (9%) it was 2 mm or greater. In updating the experience from the Montreal Heart Institute, Waters et al[26] recently reported the results of a predischarge limited exercise test in 225 survivors of acute MI all of whom were subsequently followed up for at least 5 years. Sixty-nine patients (31%) had ST-segment depression and 28 (12%) had ST-segment elevation. A comparison of the QRS score, a rough estimate of infarct size, between those with ST-segment depression and those with elevation, revealed that the QRS score was significantly higher in those with ST-segment elevation. Thus, the investigators concluded that exercise-induced ST-segment elevation is probably caused more often by LV dysfunction than by ischemia.

These results of early exercise testing showing ST-segment depression were correlated with subsequent angiographic findings in some studies.[13,27] Weiner[27] correlated the results of three studies comprised of 145 patients. Eighty percent of the 77 patients with exercise-induced ST-segment depression had multivessel coronary artery disease and 59 percent had three-vessel coronary artery disease. In contrast, 40 of the 68 patients without ST-segment changes had multivessel disease and only 19 percent had three-vessel coronary artery disease. Because prognosis after MI correlates with the extent of coronary artery disease, the associated presence of multivessel coronary artery disease with ST-segment depression further establishes the value of ST-segment depression in the diagnosis of residual ischemia in survivors of acute MI.

All of these studies demonstrated that exercise testing soon after MI is safe and useful in stratifying the survivors of acute MI into high- and low-risk groups. Both the low-level predischarge as well as the symptom-limited maximal exercise test performed after discharge accurately detect the presence of residual myocardial ischemia. These studies demonstrate that exercise-induced transient myocardial ischemia occurs frequently (Table 14.1) and correlates well with the presence of multivessel coronary artery disease in the survivors of acute MI.[20–28] However, no studies have addressed the issue of the potential difference in the prognostic significance of silent versus symptomatic myocardial ischemia in the survivors of acute MI. On general grounds, it is unlikely that a difference will be found (discussion follows).

DETECTION OF ISCHEMIA BY MYOCARDIAL PERFUSION (THALLIUM-201) SCINTIGRAPHY AND EXERCISE RADIONUCLIDE VENTRICULOGRAPHY

In a recent study, Dunn et al[29] showed that of 37 patients with MI and thallium-201defects in more than one specific vascular area, 92 percent had multivessel coronary artery disease compared with 72 percent of the 39 patients who had a postive exercise electrocardiogram. Similarly, Turner and associates[30] evaluated the role of thallium-

Table 14.1. Sharing Prevalence of Exercise-Induced Ischemia in Survivors of Acute Myocardial Infarction (MI)

Reference	Sample Size	Average Time after MI	Percentage with: ST-Segment Depression (1 mm or >)	Percentage with: Angina
Krone et al[25]	667	15 days	25	17
Waters et al[26]	225	11 days	31	NR
Jespersen et al[24]	126	3–4 wk	37	9
Theroux et al[23]	210	11 days	34	20
Starling et al[22]	130	15 days	32	27
Davidson and DeBusk[21]	195	3 wk	22	15
Markiewicz et al[20]	46	3–11 wk	45	NR

201 scintigraphy to detect residual jeopardized myocardium in 32 patients with acute MI. All patients underwent limited submaximal exercise testing and thallium-201 scintigraphy performed 3 weeks after MI. Of the 32 patients, 14 had a positive exercise test and 13 had reversible ischemia by thallium-201 scintigraphy. A total of 19 patients had either positive exercise tests or reversible ischemia by thallium-201 scintigraphy. Sixteen patients had significant multivessel coronary artery disease and 13 of these (81%) had either a positive exercise test or a reversible thallium-201 defect, or both. These investigators found that multiple thallium defects and significant ST-segment depression or angina pectoris during exercise testing identified 95 percent of patients with multivessel coronary artery disease. Results of these and other studies suggest that thallium-201 scintigraphy during exercise testing is highly sensitive and specific for detection of multivessel disease. Gibson et al[31] evaluated the role of predischarge exercise thallium-201 scintigraphy in 140 patients with uncomplicated acute MI and compared these results with those obtained during submaximal exercise treadmill test and coronary angiography. Multiple perfusion defects or increased lung uptake of thallium, both indicative of multivessel coronary artery disease were seen in 71 of the 140 patients. In comparison, only 47 patients (34%) had ST-segment depression and 22 (16%) had exercise-induced angina pectoris. Increased lung thallium uptake was correlated with a higher prevalence of ST-segment depression and/or angina on the exercise test (53% vs 36%; $p = 0.05$) and a greater number of scan segments with redistribution, angiographic evidence of multivessel disease, and a lower ejection fraction.

In another study Abraham and associates[32] evaluated the predictive accuracy of exercise ECG changes and thallium-201 scintigraphic abnormalities in detecting multivessel coronary artery disease in 103 patients. All patients performed symptom-limited exercise tests on a treadmill or upright bicycle ergometer. The sensitivity, specificity, and predictive accuracy in detecting multivessel coronary artery disease were 64, 77, and 64 percent, respectively, for a positive exercise ECG response; 64, 88, and 80 percent, respectively, for a remote thallium defect; and 42, 96, and 88 percent, respectively, for a combination of the two tests. If the findings on both tests were negative, the probability of multivessel coronary disease was only 13 percent.

In a more recent study, Gibson and associates[33] evaluated the prevalence of residual myocardial ischemia 2 weeks after uncomplicated non-Q-wave infarction and compared it to the prevalence of similar abnormalities in those with Q-wave infarctions. Compared to patients with Q-wave MI, those with non-Q-wave infarctions showed a higher prevalence of reversible defects (36% vs 60%; $p = 0.007$). Moreover, as expected, in comparison with patients with Q-wave infarct, fewer patients with non-Q-wave infarct had a persistent defect (92% vs 64%; $p < 0.0001$).These data suggest a higher prevalence of jeopardized myocardium at the risk of subsequent infarction in patients with non-Q-wave infarction. These data support the belief that patients with subendocardial infarction have a higher incidence of residual myocardial ischemia in the infarct zone and thus require an aggressive approach to prevent recurrent infarction and death.

DETECTION OF RESIDUAL ISCHEMIA BY RADIONUCLIDE VENTRICULOGRAPHY

Corbett et al[34] performed submaximal exercise testing with radionuclide ventriculography in 61 patients at 3 weeks after acute MI. Exercise response during ventriculography was considered abnormal if LVEF failed to increase by at least 5 percent. Patients were followed up to a mean of 9.6 months to correlate the incidence of subsequent events with abnormal response during exercise radionuclide ventriculography. By 6 months, 37 patients had subsequent cardiac events. Stepwise discriminant analysis revealed that the change in LVEF and LV end-systolic volume index during exercise were the most important prognostic indicators of subsequent cardiac events with a sensitivity of 95 percent and a specificity of 96 percent in predicting postinfarction complications.

Hung et al[35] recently compared the value of maximal treadmill testing, thallium scintigraphy, and exercise radionuclide ventriculography in 117 men with uncomplicated acute MI. These and other investigators[34–36] demonstrated that compared to thallium scintigraphic abnormalities and ECG changes, the peak treadmill workload and the abnormal LVEF response were better and independent predictors of subsequent hard medical events. These results suggest that exercise testing with radionuclide ventriculography is a highly sensitive test for classifying the survivors of acute MI into high- and low-risk subsets and helps to predict serious cardiac events in the postinfarction period.

CONTINUOUS HOLTER ELECTROCARDIOGRAPHIC MONITORING FOR DETECTION OF SPONTANEOUS TRANSIENT MYOCARDIAL ISCHEMIA

Holter monitoring has been used extensively to detect ventricular arrhythmia in the survivors of acute MI.[4–6] Recently, continuous ECG monitoring was used to evaluate ST-segment changes associated with transient myocardial ischemia. Several recent studies showed that when proper equipment is used with careful hook-up techniques and an adequate calibration signal, ST-segment depression can be detected and correlated with the presence of myocardial ischemia.[127–42] Figure 14.1 shows our findings in a patient who demonstrated simultaneous ST-segment depression on 12-lead ECG recordings and the Holter monitor strips recorded during a treadmill exercise test.[42] The ECG changes correlated well with the presence of reversible perfusion defects noted on the thallium-201 scintigram performed during the same test.

Holter monitoring has the advantage of providing continuous ECG monitoring during ambulatory activities and thus may be the most appropriate test for the detection of spontaneous transient myocardial ischemia whether accompanied by anginal symptoms or totally silent. Little data are currently available on the use of Holter monitoring to detect transient myocardial ischemia in survivors of acute MI. Recently, we evaluated the incidence and clinical significance of transient myocardial ischemia detected by continuous ECG monitoring in patients with acute MI.[43] Twelve consecutive patients with a confirmed diagnosis of acute MI were enrolled; six had anterior MI and six had inferior wall MI. Continuous ECG monitoring was

FIGURE 14.1. (A) Summary of EKG changes in the 12-lead electrocardiogram during the treadmill exercise test. Left side of the panel shows EKG at baseline, and right side shows ST-segment depression in inferior, septal, and lateral leads at peak exercise. (B) Evidence of reversible ischemia in inferior (*top*), septal (*middle*), and lateral walls of the heart on thallium scintigraphic images obtained during the same exercise test. Left side of the panel shows images obtained immediately after exercise, and right side shows redistribution images 4 hours later. (C) Electrocardiographic changes recorded in lead V_5 position on the Holter monitor during the same exercise test. These changes show good correlation with the ECG changes noted in regular treadmill tracings (*A*) and findings on the thallium images.

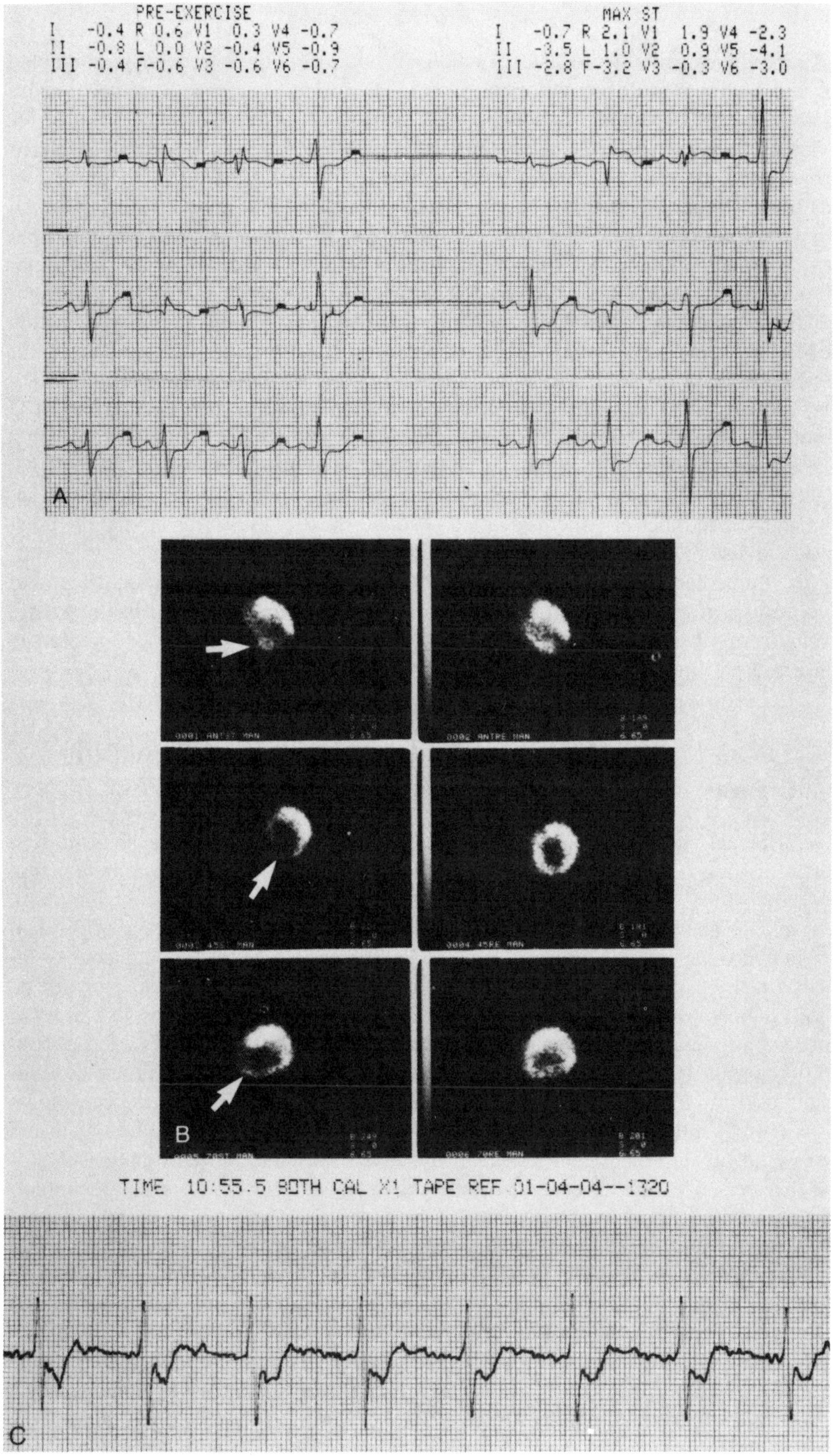
PRE-EXERCISE
I -0.4 R 0.6 V1 0.3 V4 -0.7
II -0.8 L 0.0 V2 -0.4 V5 -0.9
III -0.4 F-0.6 V3 -0.6 V6 -0.7
MAX ST
I -0.7 R 2.1 V1 1.9 V4 -2.3
II -3.5 L 1.0 V2 0.9 V5 -4.1
III -2.8 F-3.2 V3 -0.3 V6 -3.0
A
B
TIME 10:55.5 BOTH CAL X1 TAPE REF 01-04-04--1320
C

performed during the acute phase (within 72 hours), using a frequency-modulated (Oxford Medilog) Holter monitoring system. The monitoring leads were specifically selected to exclude the areas showing ECG changes of acute MI and to evaluate for ischemia at a distance. The Holter data were initially stored and analyzed in a blinded fashion after all clinical follow-up data had been obtained. Analysis of the Holter data revealed that ST-segment depression occurred for 2,375 minutes during a total monitoring period of 18,352 minutes amounting to 13 percent of the total time. Seventy-seven percent of such ST-segment changes were not associated with chest pain. All of the patients demonstrating predominantly silent ischemic ST-segment changes had developed postinfarction angina during the same hospitalization period or within the first 4 weeks. Six patients were referred by their primary care physician for angiographic evaluation and revascularization because of persistent angina. Of these, four patients had evidence of silent myocardial ischemia during continuous ECG monitoring. Coronary angiography revealed significant (greater than 70%) occlusion of the vessels corresponding to the areas showing ST-segment changes in all patients. Eighty percent of these patients had evidence of multivessel coronary artery disease. Although the number of patients studied is small, these results indicate that the presence of transient myocardial ischemia detected by continuous ECG monitoring during the immediate postinfarction period is highly suggestive of additional areas of myocardium at risk. Owing to the small number of patients enrolled in this study, results from other clinical trials involving larger numbers of patients are needed to confirm these findings before definite conclusions can be drawn.

PROGNOSTIC SIGNIFICANCE OF TRANSIENT MYOCARDIAL ISCHEMIA IN SURVIVORS OF ACUTE MYOCARDIAL INFARCTION

Several recent studies showed a mortality rate of 10 to 20 percent during the first year following acute MI.[1–7] Whereas the presence of left ventricular dysfunction (LVEF $< 40\%$) and complex ventricular arrhythmia correlates with poor long-term survival, the short-term prognosis is more closely related to the presence of residual myocardial ischemia.[12,13] Transient myocardial ischemia, whether spontaneous or induced, in the survivors of acute MI indicates the presence of residual jeopardized myocardium supplied by critical stenosis of the infarct-related vessel as well as other coronary arteries. Most patients with transient myocardial ischemia in the postinfarction period have angiographic evidence of multivessel coronary artery disease. As discussed in the preceding section, transient myocardial ischemia has been shown to occur frequently in the survivors of acute MI.[12–26] Several recent studies evaluated the prognostic significance of transient myocardial ischemia in these patients.

Schuster and Bulkley[12] evaluated the prognostic significance of early postinfarction angina in 70 patients with acute MI followed an average of 6 months. Forty-three patients had ischemia at a distance, and 27 had ischemia in the infarct zone. Mortality in the entire group was 50 percent. The patients with ischemia at a distance had a significantly higher mortality (72%) than did those with ischemia in the infarct zone (33% mortality). In a more recent study of 449 survivors of acute MI, Bosch et al[13] identified 79 patients (18%) who had evidence of early ischemia. All patients were hospitalized in the CCU until discharge and were subsequently followed for a mean period of 14 ± 8 months (range 2 to 28). During hospitalization, 31 patients were diagnosed to have extension of their infarction. Twenty-two of these 31 patients had experienced early ischemia, whereas nine had not ($p < 0.0001$). The sensitivity of early ischemia in predicting infarct extension was 71 percent and the specificity was 81 percent. By stepwise logistic regression, only early ischemia was retained as a significant predictor ($p < 0.001$, odds ratio 15.4) of infarct extension. During postdischarge follow-up (14 ± 8 months), 38 patients died, 41 had nonfatal recurrent MI, and six others were rehospitalized. The survival rates in those with and without early ischemia were compared using Kaplan-Meir survival curves. After 24 months, the survival rate was 83 percent in patients with early ischemia compared with 92 percent in those without it ($p = 0.01$). Similar results were found when survival without MI was analyzed: 67 vs 81 percent ($p < 0.001$). In the Multicenter Post Infarction Program (MPIP), Bigger[14] evaluated the prognostic significance of early angina pectoris in 867 patients with acute MI. Early angina was observed in 33 percent of the patients between 2 days and hospital discharge 17 ± 9 days after infarction. Early postinfarction angina was not significantly associated with cardiac death during the 2.5 years of follow-up. However, patients with early postinfarction angina were one and a half times as likely to experience recurrent nonfatal MI during the year after their index MI. Figueras and associates[44] also showed no worsening of prognosis due to early spontaneous angina during a follow-up of 26 months. Table 14.2 summarizes the results of several studies demonstrating increased 1-year mortality in patients who showed ST-segment depression during exercise testing performed after acute MI. Markiewicz et al[20] evaluated the prognostic significance of exercise-induced ischemia in 46 men under 70 years of age with uncomplicated acute MI. During a median follow-up period of 18 months, two patients died suddenly, one had an episode of ventricular fibrillation, and four had recurrent MI. All of these patients had ST-segment depression during exercise tests performed between 3 and 11 weeks after infarction. In contrast, none of the 25 patients without ST-segment changes experienced a coronary event during the follow-up.

Davidson and DeBusk[21] found that ST-segment depression greater than 2 mm and a maximal workload less than 4 METs were highly predictive of subsequent cardiac events. Starling and associates[22] evaluated the prognostic significance of treadmill-induced abnormalities in 130 patients with uncomplicated MI. Forty-two patients (32%) had execise-induced ST-segment depression. Compared with patients showing no ST-segment depression, patients with ST-segment depression were identified to have a significantly greater incidence of future cardiac events ($p < 0.001$). Twenty-four patients (60%) with ST-segment depression compared with only 14 percent (7 of 48) without any abnormality experienced cardiac events. The overall incidence of recurrent MI and death was small during the follow-up period and showed a significant difference ($p < 0.01$) only when patients with exercise-induced ST-segment depression and angina were combined.

Sami and coworkers[15] evaluated the prognostic significance of serial exercise testing in 200 male patients with uncomplicated acute MI. Their results demonstrate that exercise-induced ST-segment depression greater than 2 mm was significantly more prevalent in patients with subsequent cardiac arrest (100%) or coronary artery bypass surgery (64%) than in patients without subsequent events within 2 years of infarction ($p < 0.05$). It is also interesting to note that in this study, exercise-induced ventricular arrhythmia was a less powerful predictor of early fatal events in these patients than was exercise-induced ischemia. The overall risk of a coronary event was twofold greater in patients with greater than 2-mm ST-segment depression. Later studies[24,26] yielded similar prognostic data. The foregoing data, although not completely con-

Table 14.2. Prognostic Significance and 1-Year Mortality Rate in Patients with ST-Segment Depression During Exercise Testing after Acute Myocardial Infarction

Reference	Total Patients	Median Follow-Up (Mo.)	No. of Patients with ST-Segment Depression	1-Year Mortality Rate During Follow-Up		p Value
				With ST-Segment Depression	Without ST-Segment Depression	
Theroux et al[23]	210	12	64 (34%)	17 (27%)	3 (2%)	<0.001
Markiewicz et al[20]	42	18	17 (40%)	2 (12%)	0 (0%)	<0.01
Starling et al[22]	130	11	42 (32%)	4 (10%)	6 (7%)	<0.01
Sami et al[15]	85	19	18 (22%)	4 (22%)	0 (0%)	<0.01
Jespersen et al[24]	126	12	46 (37%)	6 (13%)	3 (4%)	<0.01

cordant,[45] leave little doubt on the prognostic significance of exercise-induced transient myocardial ischemia in the survivors of acute MI.

PROGNOSTIC SIGNIFICANCE OF ISCHEMIA DETECTED BY THALLIUM-201 SCINTIGRAPHY AND EXERCISE RADIONUCLIDE VENTRICULOGRAPHY

The prognostic significance of predischarge thallium-201 was compared to that of coronary angiography by Gibson et al[31] in 140 patients with uncomplicated acute MI. High risk was assigned if scintigraphy detected thallium-201 defects in more than one discrete vascular region, redistribution, or increased lung uptake, if exercise testing caused ST-segment depression ($\geq$1 mm), or angina, or if angiography revealed multivessel disease. Lack of these findings identified patients as a low-risk subset. By 15 $\pm$ 12 months, 50 patients had experienced a cardiac event; seven died (five suddenly), nine had recurrent MI, and 34 developed severe class III or IV angina pectoris. Compared with that of patients at low risk, the cumulative probability of a cardiac event was greater in high-risk patients identified by scintigraphy ($p < 0.001$). Also, thallium-201 scintigraphy predicted low-risk status better than did exercise testing ($p = 0.01$) or angiography ($p = 0.05$). Although each of the three variables predicted mortality risk equally, scintigraphy was more sensitive in detecting patients who experienced reinfarction or developed severe angina pectoris. When all 50 patients with cardiac events were combined, scintigraphy identified 47 (94%) of these, whereas exercise-induced ST-segment depression or angina detected only 28 (56%) patients ($p < 0.001$), and angiographic evidence of multivessel disease identified 9 more patients with cardiac events than did exercise testing ($p = 0.06$). These results indicate that submaximal exercise thallium-201 scintigraphy is useful in the detection of high- and low-risk patients, and scintigraphic findings suggestive of multivessel involvement are more sensitive predictors of subsequent cardiac events than is ST-segment depression, angina, or the extent of angiographic disease.[31]

Recently, Abraham et al[32] also compared exercise electrocardiography and myocardial perfusion scanning with thallium-201 in predicting multivessel coronary artery disease and prognosis early after infarction. In this study, 103 patients performed exercise testing with thallium-201 scintigraphy at a mean of 24 days after uncomplicated MI. Of the three predictive variables, the positive exercise ECG response, the remote thallium defect, and the presence of multivessel coronary artery disease, the relative risk of combined events was 2.5 ($p < 0.05$) for a positive exercise ECG response, 1.8 (NS) for a remote thallium defect, 2.6 ($p < 0.05$) for multivessel coronary artery disease, and 3.1 ($p < 0.025$) for both positive ECG response and remote defect. Thus, in contrast to Gibson et al,[31] these investigators demonstrated a greater chance of identifying patients at greatest risk of subsequent events when the combination of positive ECG response and thallium perfusion abnormalities was utilized. Because patients with non-Q-wave infarction were shown to be at increased risk of subsequent coronary events, Gibson et al[33] recently reported on the significance of residual myocardial ischemia detected by exercise thallium-201 scintigraphy. In this study of 241 consecutive patients with uncomplicated MI, 87 with non-Q-wave infarcts and 154 with Q-wave infarcts, the significance of clinical variables, the size of the infact (evaluated by creative kinase levels), left ventricular function (LVEF), the presence of ventricular arrhythmia, and residual myocardial ischemia detected by thallium-201 were compared. Their findings demonstrated that patients with non-Q-wave infarction have a higher rate of reinfarction, anginal symptoms, and the need for bypass surgery than do those with Q-wave infarcts during the 30-month follow-up period. Comparison of thallium-201 scintigraphic findings showed that patients with non-Q-wave infarcts had a higher prevalence of thallium-201 redistribution in the infarct zone ($p < 0.007$). This finding also correlated with a large percentage of patent infarct-related arteries in patients with non-Q-wave infarcts than in those with Q-wave infarcts (54% vs 25%; $p < 0.0001$). These findings further confirm the previous reports showing a higher incidence of spontaneous as well as inducible myocardial ischemia with an associated increased risk of coronary events in patients with non-Q-wave infarcts.[12,13]

Several recent studies have focused attention on the prognostic value of exercise radionuclide ventriculography in predicting postinfarction events.[34–36] Corbett and associates[31] evaluated the prognostic value of submaximal exercise testing with radionuclide ventriculography before hospital discharge in 61 patients with recent MI. Patients were followed up a mean of 9.6 months to determine the incidence of cardiac death, recurrent MI, unstable angina, medically refractory angina, or congestive heart failure. By 6 months, 37 patients had one of these complications, 4 patients died, and 5 patients had recurrent infarction. Exercise response during ventriculography was considered abnormal if LVEF failed to increase by at least 5 units. Radionuclide ventriculography during exercise had a sensitivity of 95 percent and a specificity of 96 percent in predicting these important postinfarction complications. These results suggest that submaximal exercise testing with radionuclide ventriculography is highly sensitive in classifying patients at the time of hospital discharge after myocardial infarction and helps to predict serious cardiac events. In a study of 117 men tested 3 weeks after a clinically uncomplicated MI, Hung et al[35] evaluated the comparative value of maximal treadmill testing, exercise thallium scintigraphy, and exercise radionuclide ventriculography in distinguishing high- and low-risk subsets.[36] During a mean follow-up period of 11.6 months, 8 men experienced "hard" events, fibrillation, or recurrent MI and 14 were hospitalized for unstable angina pectoris, congestive heart failure, or coronary bypass surgery (a total of 22 combined events). By multivariate analysis (Cox proportional hazards model), peak treadmill workload and the change in LVEF during exercise were significant ($p < 0.01$) predictors of hard medical events; these two risk factors and recurrent ischemic chest pain in the CCU were also significantly predictive ($p < 0.0001$) of combined events. A peak treadmill workload of 4 METs or less or a decrease in EF of 5 percent or more below the value at rest during submaximal effort distinguished 22 high-risk patients (20% of the study population) from 89 low-risk patients. The rate of hard medical events within 12 months was 23 percent (5 of 22 patients) versus 2 percent (2 of 89 patients) in the high- and low-risk patient subsets, respectively ($p < 0.001$). Thus, in patients who undergo evaluation 3 weeks after a clinically uncomplicated MI, exercise radionuclide ventriculography contributes independent prognostic information in addition to that provided by symptom-limited treadmill testing and was superior to exercise thallium scintigraphy for this purpose.

All of these studies evaluating the prognostic value of exercise thallium-201 scintigraphy and exercise radionuclide ventriculography have shown that both of these tests are sensitive and reliable in the identification of high- and low-risk subsets of patients with acute MI. The distinct abnormalities (as discussed herein) observed during either of these tests are associated with a subsequent poor prognosis. Additionally, some of these studies have shown that these tests may be complementary to the findings observed during routine exercise testing.[32,36]

SILENT (PAINLESS) MYOCARDIAL ISCHEMIA IN THE SURVIVORS OF ACUTE MYOCARDIAL INFARCTION

Silent myocardial ischemia has been shown to occur more frequently than ischemia associated with anginal symptoms in patients with chronic stable angina.[37–42,46] It has been suggested that patients with acute MI may have a significantly higher incidence of silent myocardial ischemia, because sensory nerve endings may be damaged during the infarction process.[47] Data from the Framingham Study (see Chapter 15) showed that as many as one third of patients may have total absence of symptoms during acute MI.[48]

The exact prevalence of silent myocardial ischemia in suvivors of acute MI is not known. Based on the available data, it can be estimated that of the 250,000 patients with uncomplicated acute MI who are presumably asymptomatic at the time of discharge from the hospital, approximately 20 percent (50,000 patients) will have silent myocardial ischemia.[23–26,47] Because most of the available data regarding the incidence of silent myocardial ischemia have been derived from exercise testing performed soon after acute MI, these will be discussed.

In the study from the Montreal Heart Institute, Theroux et al[23] reported that of the 210 patients with uncomplicated acute MI, predischarge exercise testing identified 64 patients with ST-segment depression indicative of myocardial ischemia. Of these 64 patients, 27 patients (42%) had associated exercise-induced angina pectoris, whereas 37 patients (58%) had silent myocardial ischemia. Patients with asymptomatic transient myocardial ischemia represent 18 percent of their total population. During the 1-year follow-up period, the mortality rate among the 146 patients without ST-segment changes was 2.1 percent compared with 27 percent (17 of 64) in patients with ST-segment changes ($p < 0.001$). The presence or absence of angina during exercise testing did not affect the subsequent mortality rate. Seven of the 27 patients with both exercise-induced angina and ST-segment depression died, compared with 10 of 37 patients with silent myocardial ischemia. These results suggest that silent myocardial ischemia may occur in as many as 20 percent of patients, and when present it is predictive of poor prognosis during the follow-up period.

In the Multicenter Post Infarction Program, Krone et al[25] evaluated the incidence of exercise-induced myocardial ischemia in 866 patients with acute MI. Of the 667 patients who performed exercise tests before discharge, 167 patients (25%) had ST-segment depression greater than 1 mm and 61 patients (9%) had 2 mm or greater ST-segment depression. Exercise-induced angina occurred in 115 patients (17% of total patients), but both exercise-induced angina and ST-segment depression were noted in only one third of the patients with evidence of myocardial ischemia. Thus, two thirds of their patients had silent myocardial ischemia induced during the predischarge treadmill exercise test. Similar to these data, the study of Jespersen et al[24] demonstrated that exercise testing performed during the third or fourth week after acute MI in 126 patients identified 46 patients (37%) with ST-segment depression indicative of myocardial ischemia. Only 11 of the 46 patients (24%) had associated anginal symptoms, whereas others (76%) had silent myocardial ischemia.

Recently, Gibson et al[49] evaluated the prevalence and clinical significance of painless ST-segment depression during early postinfarction exercise testing. Of the 190 patients studied, 100 (53%) had a negative exercise test response, 43 (23%) exhibited painless ST-sgment depression, and 47 patients (25%) experienced angina (n = 21) with ST-segment depression. Comparison of coronary angiographic findings in those with silent or symptomatic ischemia versus those with negative exercise test results revealed a higher prevalence of multivessel coronary artery disease with significant stenosis (>50% narrowing). In patients with ischemia, the ECG data were then compared with the scintigraphic findings in the three groups, revealing that the number of segments showing redistribution were similar in asymptomatic patients and in those with negative test results. In contrast, patients with angina had a higher prevalence of redistribution and more extensive evidence of ischemia than did the other two groups. These data suggest that despite similar angiographic findings in the two groups, those with associated angina have a larger amount of hypoperfused myocardium. During follow-up, there was a trend toward a higher cardiac event rate in patients with painless ST-segment depression and thallium-201 redistribution. However, because painless ST-segment depression by itself did not correlate with evidence of extensive residual myocardial ischemia, these investigators suggest that evidence of redistribution in thallium-201 scintigraphic findings would enhance the prognostic value of conventional exercise tests in survivors of acute MI.

In a more recent study, Ouyang et al[50] compared the angiographic findings and prognostic significance of silent versus symptomatic ischemia in 60 consecutive patients with positive predischarge exercise test findings. Ischemia was silent in 63 percent (38 of 60) of patients. Age, sex, and the use of antianginal drugs did not differ in the two groups. The severity of coronary artery disease on angiography was also comparable in the two groups. Over a 1-year follow-up of 92 percent of patients, four patients (11%) with silent ischemia and only one (5%) with symptomatic ischemia had cardiac death or recurrent MI (p = NS). Seventeen patients with silent ischemia and 13 with symptomatic ischemia required revascularization (p = NS). These data led the investigators to conclude that silent ischemia occurs frequently during early predischarge exercise testing and has prognostic significance similar to that of symptomatic exercise-induced ischemia.

Although Holter monitoring has been frequently used to detect myocardial ischemia during daily activity, there is little available data on evaluation of transient myocardial ischemia by this technique in survivors of acute MI.[38–42] As already discussed, we recently evaluated the prevalence and clinical significance of silent myocardial ischemia in 12 patients with acute MI.[43] During a total monitoring period of 18,352 minutes, ST-segment changes indicative of transient myocardial ischemia were observed for 2,375 minutes. A total of 34 transient ischemic events were noted and 68 percent of these were asymptomatic, accounting for 1,830 minutes (77% of total ischemic time) of ischemic changes noted during the monitoring period. Subsequent follow-up of these patients revealed that all patients showing predominantly silent ST-segment shifts had developed postinfarction angina during the 4 to 6 weeks of the initial follow-up period. Six patients were referred by their primary care physician for angiographic evaluation because of persistent angina; four of these patients had evidence of silent ischemia during the initial monitoring period in the CCU. Coronary angiographic findings revealed multivessel coronary artery disease in 80 percent of the patients. These data tend to suggest that silent myocardial ischemia as detected by Holter monitoring occurs frequently in patients with acute MI and appears to be associated with angiographic evidence of multivessel coronary artery disease. These preliminary data also suggest that silent ischemia in these patients may have prognostic significance similar to that observed in patients with unstable angina.[51,52]

CONCLUSIONS AND THERAPEUTIC IMPLICATIONS

The available data from relatively uncontrolled studies indicate that spontaneous as well as exercise-induced transient myocardial ischemia is relatively common in the survivors of acute MI. Whether such episodes of ischemia are symptomatic or silent, evidence for the occurrence of silent ischemia has been obtained from ambulatory ECG monitoring and from early and late treadmill exercise testing with or without associated measurements on thallium perfusion scintigraphy or radionuclide ventriculography. Although not entirely uniform, evidence is reasonably compelling that the presence and severity of ischemia are associated with multivessel coronary disease and with generally adverse prognosis in terms of the occurrence of infarction, sudden death, or the development of unstable angina. Formal prospective studies addressing the issue of a difference between silent ischemia and symptomatic ischemia have not been reported. Uncontrolled observations indicate however that the prognostic implications of silent and symptomatic ischemic episodes in the suvivors of acute MI are essentially the same. Thus, treatment regimen designed to alter the adverse consequences of persistent myocardial ischemia following MI should not distinguish between symptomatic and asymptomatic ischemia. However, controlled clinical trials will be needed to determine whether the elimination of persistent asymptomatic myocardial ischemia in the survivors of acute myocardial ischemia will reduce short- and long-term morbidity and mortality.

REFERENCES

1. Pitt B: Natural history of myocardial infarction and its prodromal syndromes. *Circulation* 1976;53(Suppl 1):132.
2. Norris RM, Caughey DE, Deeming LW, et al: Coronary prognostic index for predicting survival after recovery from acute myocardial infarction. *Lancet* 1970;11:485.
3. Taylor G, Humphries JO, Mellits ED, et al: Predictors of clinical course, coronary anatomy and left ventricular function after recovery from acute myocardial infarction. *Circulation* 1980;62:960.
4. Bigger JT Jr, Heller CA, Wenger TL, et al: Risk stratification after acute myocardial infarction. *Am J Cardiol* 1978;42:202.
5. Moss AJ, Bigger JT, Odoroff CL: Post infarct risk stratification. *Prog Cardiol Dis* 1987;29:389.
6. The Multicenter Postinfarction Research Group: Risk stratification and survival after myocardial infarction. *N Engl J Med* 1983;309:331.
7. Kannel WB, Sorlie P, McNamara PM: Prognosis after initial myocardial infarction: The Framingham Study. *Am J Cardiol* 1979;44:53.
8. Peel AAF, Semple T, Wang I, et al: A coronary prognostic index for grading the severity of infarction. *Br Heart J* 1962;24:745.
9. Forrester JS, Diamond G, Chatterjee K, et al: Medical therapy of acute myocardial infarction by application of hemodynamic subsets. *N Engl J Med* 1976;295:1356.
10. Fioretti P, Brower RW, Simoons ML, et al: Prediction of mortality in hospital survivors of myocardial infarction. Comparison of predischarge exercise testing and radionuclide ventriculography at rest. *Br Heart J* 1984;52:292.
11. Luria MH, Knocke JA, Wacks JS, et al: Survival after recovery from acute myocardial infarction: Two and five year prognostic indices. *Am J Med* 1979;67:7.

12. Schuster EH, Bulkley BH: Early post-infarction angina, ischemia at a distance and ischemia in the infarct zone. *N Engl J Med* 1981;305:1101.
13. Bosch X, Theroux P, Waters DD, et al: Early post-infarction ischemia: Clinical, angiographic, and prognostic significance. *Circulation* 1987;75:988.
14. Bigger JT Jr: Angina pectoris early after myocardial infarction: Clinical experience of the multicenter postinfarction program. *E Heart J* 1986;7(suppl c):37.
15. Sami M, Kraemer H, DeBusk RF: The prognostic significance of serial exercise testing after myocardial infarction. *Circulation* 1979;60:1238.
16. DeFeyter PJ, Van Eenige MJ, Dighton DJ, et al: Prognostic value of exercise testing, coronary angiography and left ventriculography 6–8 weeks after myocardial infarction. *Circulation* 1982;66:527.
17. Turner JD, Schwartz KM, Logic JR, et al: Detection of residual jeopardized myocardium 3 weeks after myocardial infarction by exercise testing with thallium-201 myocardial scintigraphy. *Circulation* 1980;61:729.
18. Dunn RF, Freedman B, Bailey IK, et al: Noninvasive prediction of multivessel disease after myocardial infarction. *Circulation* 1980;62:726.
19. Turner JD, Rogers WJ, Mantle JA, et al: Coronary angiography soon after myocardial infarction. *Chest* 1980;77:58.
20. Markiewicz W, Houston N, DeBusk R: Exercise testing soon after myocardial infarction. *Circulation* 1977;56:26.
21. Davidson DM, DeBusk R: Prognostic value of a single exercise test 3 weeks after uncomplicated myocardial infarction. *Circulation* 1980;61:236.
22. Starling M, Crawford MH, Kennedy GT, et al: Exercise testing early after myocardial infarction: Predictive value for subsequent unstable angina and death. *Am J Cardiol* 1980;46:909.
23. Theroux P, Waters DD, Halphen C, et al: Prognostic value of exercise testing soon after myocardial infarction. *N Engl J Med* 1979;301:341.
24. Jesperson CM, Kassis E, Edeling CJ, et al: The prognostic value of maximal exercise testing soon after first myocardial infarction. *Eur Heart J* 1985;6:769.
25. Krone RJ, Gillespie JA, Weld FM, et al: Low level exercise testing after myocardial infarction: Usefulness in enhancing clincal risk stratification. *Circulation* 1985;71:80.
26. Waters DD, Bosch X, Bouchard A, et al: Comparison of clinical variables and variables derived from a limited predischarge exercise test as predictors of early and late mortality after myocardial infarction. *J Am Coll Cardiol* 1985;5:1.
27. Weiner DA: Predischarge exercise testing after myocardial infarction: Prognostic and therapeutic features. *Cardiovasc Clin* 1985;15:95.
28. DeBusk RF, Blomquist CG, Kouchoukos NT, et al: Identification and treatment of low-risk patients after acute myocardial infarction and coronary-artery bypass graft surgery. *N Engl J Med* 1986;314:161.
29. Dunn RF, Freedman B, Bailey IK, et al: Noninvasive prediction of multivessel disease after myocardial infarction. *Circulation* 1980;62:726.
30. Turner JD, Schwartz KM, Logic JR, et al: Detection of residual jeopardized myocardium 3 weeks after myocardial infarction by exercise testing with thallium-201 myocardial scintigraphy. *Circulation* 1980;61:729.
31. Gibson RS, Watson DD, Craddock GB, et al: Prediction of cardiac events after uncomplicated myocardial infarction: A prospective study comparing predischarge thallium-201 scintigraphy and coronary angiography. *Circulation* 1983;68:321.
32. Abraham RD, Freedman B, Dunn RF, et al: Prediction of multivessel coronary artery disease and prognosis early after acute myocardial infarction by exercise electrocardiography and thallium-201 myocardial perfusion scanning. *Am J Cardiol* 1986;58:423.
33. Gibson RS, Beller GA, Gheorghiade M, et al: The prevalence and clinical significance of residual myocardial ischemia 2 weeks after uncomplicated non-Q-wave infarction: A prospective natural history study. *Circulation* 1986;73:1186.
34. Corbett JR, Nicod P, Lewis SE, et al: Prognostic value of submaxial exercise radionuclide ventriculography after myocardial infarction. *Am J Cardiol* 1983;52:82A.
35. Hung J, Goris ML, Nash E, et al: Comparative value of maximal treadmill testing, exercise thallium myocardial perfusion scintigraphy and exercise radionuclide ventriculography for distinguishing high- and low-risk patients soon after acute myocardial infarction. *Am J Cardiol* 1984;53:221.

36. Hakki AH, Nestico PF, Heo J, et al: Relative prognostic value of rest thallium-201 imaging, radionuclide ventriculography and 24 hour ambulatory electrocardiographic monitoring after acute myocardial infarction. *J Am Coll Cardiol* 1987;10:25.
37. Schang SJ Jr, Pepine CJ: Transient asymptomatic ST-segment depression during daily activity. *Am J Cardiol* 1977;39:396.
38. Deanfield JE, Selwyn AP, Chierchia SL, et al: Myocardial ischemia during daily life in patients with stable angina: Its relation to symptoms and heart rate changes. *Lancet* 1983;1:753.
39. Nademanee K, Intarachot V, Piontek M, et al: Relationship of myocardial ischemia detected by compact Holter analog technique to that induced by exercise testing. *Circulation* 1984;70(Suppl 2):451.
40. Stern S, Tzivoni D: Early detection of silent ischaemic heart disease by 24-hour electrocardiographic monitoring of active subjects. *Br Heart J* 1974;16:481.
41. Pepine CJ: Asymptomatic myocardial ischemia during daily activities. Observations in persons with and without coronary artery disease, in Stern S (ed): *Ambulatory ECG Monitoring,* Chicago, Yearbook Medical Publisher Inc., 1978, p 107.
42. Deedwania PC: Silent myocardial ischemia and its relationship to acute myocardial infarction. *Cardiol Clin* 1986;4:643.
43. Deedwania P, Carbajal E, Golden P, et al: Clinical significance of silent myocardial ischemia detected during acute myocardial infarction. Proceedings of the X World Congress of Cardiology, Washington DC, 1986, p 565.
44. Figueras J, Cinca J, Valle V, et al: Prognostic implications of early spontaneous angina after acute transmural myocardial infarction. *Int J Cardiol* 1983;4:261.
45. Weld FM, Chu KL, Bigger JT, et al: Risk stratification with low-level exercise testing 2 weeks after acute myocardial infarction. *Circulation* 1981;64:306.
46. Singh BN, Nademanee K, Figueras J, et al: Hemodynamic and electrocardiographic correlates of symptomatic and silent myocardial ischemia: Pathophysiologic and therapeutic implications. *Am J Cardiol* 1986;58:3B.
47. Cohn P: Silent myocardial ischemia: Dimensions of the problem in patients with and without angina. *Am J Med* 1986;80(Suppl 4C):3.
48. Kannel WB, Abbott RD: Incidence and prognosis of unrecognized myocardial infarction. *N Engl J Med* 1984;311:1144.
49. Gibson RS, Beller GA, Kaiser DL: Prevalence and clinical significance of painless ST segment depression during early post-infarction exercise testing. *Circulation* 1987;75(Suppl II):II–36.
50. Ouyang P, Shapiro EP, Chandra NC, et al: Silent vs symptomatic ischemia in early post-infarction treadmill testing: Angiographic characterization and 1 year follow-up (Abstract). *J Am Coll Cardiol* 1987;9:223 A.
51. Nademanee K, Intarachot V, Josephson MA, et al: Prognostic significance of silent myocardial ischemia in patients with unstable angina. *J Am Coll Cardiol* 1987;10:1.
52. Gottlieb SO, Weisfeldt ML, Ouyang P, et al: Silent ischemia as a marker for early unfavorable outcomes in patients with unstable angina. *N Engl J Med* 1986;314:1214.

CHAPTER 15

Silent Myocardial Infarction

Incidence, Prevalence, and Prognostic Significance

William B. Kannel, MD, MPH
and L. Adrienne Cupples, PhD

Coronary heart disease is a common, highly lethal disease that often progresses from an inapparent state to an abrupt lethal outcome with little warning. One in five coronary attacks presents with sudden death as the first, last, and only symptom;[1] half of all deaths from coronary heart disease are sudden and half of these occur in persons without known coronary disease.[2,3] Only one in five myocardial infarctions is preceded by angina pectoris of any duration.

Although these attacks appear to occur unforeseen, they are often heralded by an adverse coronary risk profile and signs of silent myocardial ischemia.[1] There is actually a large reservoir of silent coronary disease in the general population from which most of these apparently unheralded coronary attacks evolve. It is estimated that some 2 to 4 percent of the asymptomatic general population have a compromised coronary circulation that can be detected by an exercise electrocardiogram or ambulatory ECG monitoring.[4,5] Also, 20 percent of persons surviving myocardial infarction without residual symptoms have positive exercise ECG tests that indicate residual ischemia. Even among persons with angina, ambulatory monitoring indicates that three of four episodes of transient ischemia during the day occur without pain.[6,7]

It is not surprising, therefore, that a substantial proportion of actual myocardial infarctions are silent or so atypical as to go unrecognized.[8] Silent or unrecognized myocardial infarction constitutes a substantial part of potentially lethal inapparent coronary disease.

INCIDENCE

The incidence of myocardial infarction reaches substantial proportions beyond age 45 years in men and age 55 in women. In the Framingham Study no infarctions occurred under age 45 in women, whereas they occurred at a rate of 3 per 1,000 in men (Figure 15.1). In men, the rate under age 65 (6 per 1,000) more than doubled (13 per 1,000) after that age. Women lagged men in incidence by about 20 years for symptomatic infarction, but by only 10 years for unrecognized MI.

Of the myocardial infarctions that evolved in the Framingham Study over 3 decades of biennial surveillance, more than 30 percent were discovered only by the new appearance of diagnostic evidence on routine ECG examinations.[8] The propor-

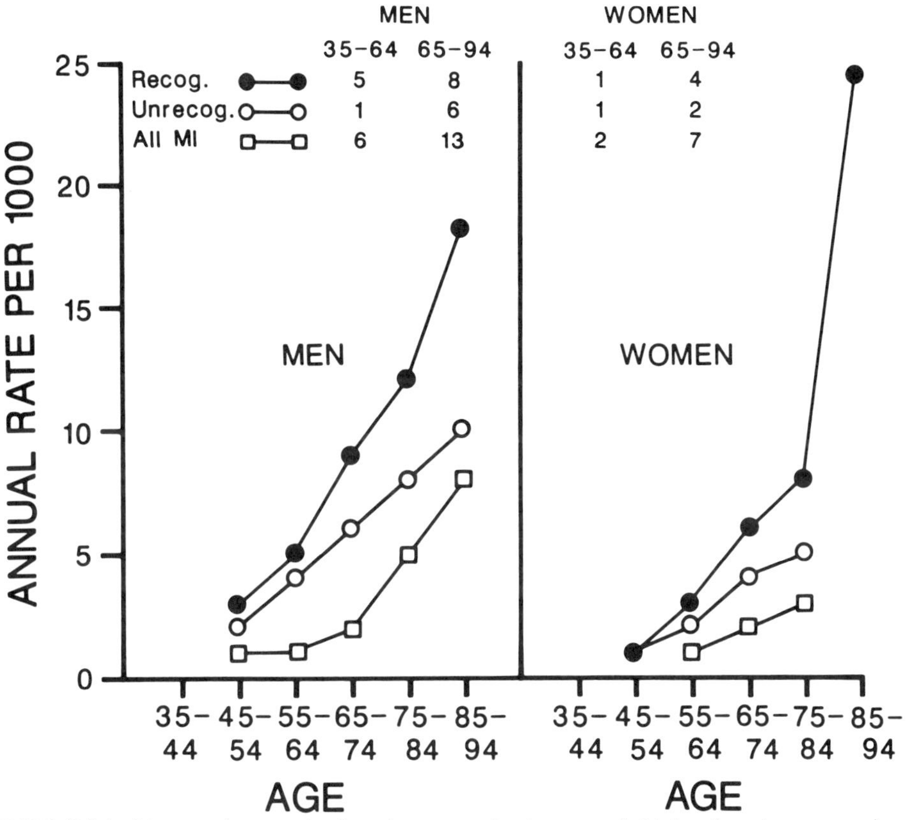

FIGURE 15.1. Incidence of recognized and unrecognized myocardial infarctions by age and sex. Framingham Study—30 year follow-up.

tion of all myocardial infarctions that went unrecognized was higher in women (35%) than in men (28%). The fraction of myocardial infarctions that are unrecognized tends to increase with age, particularly in men (Figure 15.2).

There is a possibility that the incidence of silent or unrecognized myocardial infarction is underestimated even by general population studies. Some 10 percent of anterior and 25 percent of inferior myocardial infarctions detected on ECG examination will revert to a nondiagnostic pattern within 2 years of acute MI. Also, some sudden deaths may be based on unrecognized MI.

SILENT INFARCTION

About half the myocardial infarctions that go unrecognized are completely silent, the subject recalling absolutely no symptoms that could be attributed to coronary disease (Table 15.1). The rest have symptoms that could be compatible with myocardial infarction, but that are attributed to some other condition such as a gallstone attack, hiatus hernia, or peptic ulcer, which may indeed be the case.[9]

ANGINA PECTORIS

Angina pectoris is a common accompaniment of myocardial infarction. About 20 percent of myocardial infarctions are preceded by angina pectoris of some duration. When infarctions are silent or unrecognized, only 5 percent are preceded by angina.

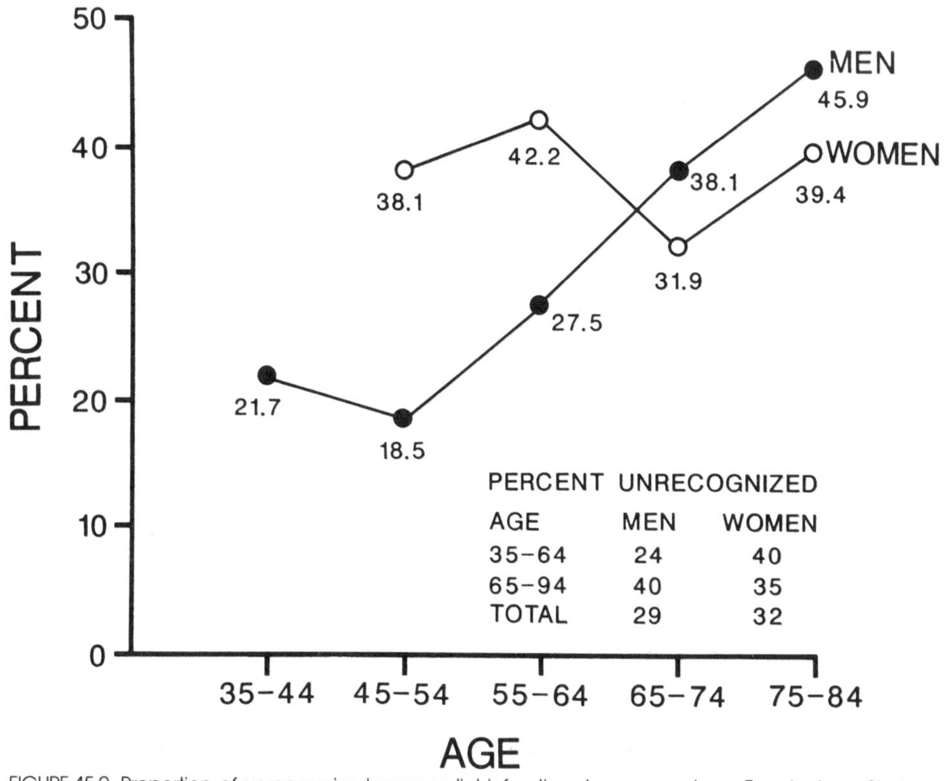

FIGURE 15.2. Proportion of unrecognized myocardial infarctions by age and sex. Framingham Study—30 year follow-up.

Angina develops less often after unrecognized infarctions; in fact, angina in these manifest half as often as in those who have recognized MI. Also, with time the incidence of angina increases steadily after recognized MI, but after unrecognized MI it plateaus after 6 years.

RISK FACTORS

The ECG location of the myocardial infarction is no different in unrecognized than in symptomatic myocardial infarction,[10] making an atypical pain referral pattern unlikely.

A poor cardiovascular risk profile predicts unrecognized myocardial infarction as well as recognized MI (Table 15.2). However, few risk factors specific for unrec-

Table 15.1. Proportion of Unrecognized, Silent Myocardial Infarctions in the Framingham Study: 22-Year Follow-up of Subjects 30 to 62 Years of Age at Entry

		Silent Infarctions	
Sex	Number	Number	Percent
Men	69	39	56
Women	39	13	33
Total	108	52	48

Table 15.2. Risk Factors for Unrecognized vs Recognized Myocardial Infarction in the Framingham Study: 30-Year Follow-up

	Myocardial Infarction			
	Unrecognized		Recognized	
Factors	35–64	65–94	35–64	65–94
Systolic BP	**	**	***	***
Diastolic BP	**	*	**	+
Serum cholesterol	*	+	***	+
Hematocrit	*	+	*	+
Glucose	*	+	+	**
MRW	+	+	+	+
Vital capacity	+	+	+	+
Heart rate	**	+	+	+
Cigarettes	***	+	***	+
CE X-Ray	**	***	+	*
ECG-LVH	***	***	+	*
I-V Block	+	+	+	+
NSA-ECG	+	+	+	+

KEY: + NS (not significant); $*p < 0.05$; $**p < 0.01$; $***p < 0.001$.

ognized as distinct from recognized myocardial infarction have been identified. Two notable exceptions are hypertension and diabetes. The incidence of unrecognized myocardial infarction is increased in persons with hypertension, much as it is in persons with overt symptomatic infarctions.[11] However, the fraction of myocardial infarctions that are unrecognized increases with the severity of hypertension (Table 15.3). Among persons with definite hypertension in the Framingham Study, 38.6 percent of MI's in men and 49.3 percent in women were silent or unrecognized. Thus, persons with hypertension are at increased risk of sustaining myocardial infarction, and despite close medical supervision, this is twice as likely to be an unrecognized MI as in normotensive persons. This predisposition to silent or unrecognized myocardial infarction persists on excluding all possible confounding factors such as diabetes, left ventricular hypertrophy, and antihypertensive treatment.[11]

Diabetes is also a recognized cause of silent myocardial infarction. This is confirmed in the Framingham Study but only for men. Among diabetic persons, women have little advantage over men against coronary disease, so that the incidence of myocardial infarction in diabetic women exceeds that of nondiabetic men. Women with diabetes have a three- to fourfold increased risk of myocardial infarction com-

Table 15.3. Proportion of Myocardial Infarctions Unrecognized by Hypertensive Status: 30-Year Follow-up*

	Age-Adjusted Percentage	
Hypertension	Men	Women
Normal	18.1	27.3
Mild	30.7	36.3
Definite	35.3**	49.3
Treated	38.6	37.5

* Framingham Study subjects aged 33 to 90 years.

pared with nondiabetic persons. In male diabetics, unrecognized, asymptomatic infarctions occurred at 3 times the rate in nondiabetic persons. In diabetic women, unrecognized MI occurred at only 1.7 times the rate in nondiabetic women. Whereas in diabetic men 37 percent of MIs went unrecognized, in women only 18 percent were silent (Table 15.4). Thus, there is a paradoxic difference in the sexes in that diabetes predisposes to silent or unrecognized MIs in men, but in women it makes for more symptomatic MIs. Women with diabetes, in contrast to men, are not predisposed to silent MIs.

PROGNOSIS

The surviving victim of myocardial infarction faces substantial risks of disability, recurrence, and premature death. Although unrecognized MIs appear to be benign, they are in the long-term just as lethal and disabling as symptomatic myocardial infarctions. Whether painful or not, ischemic myocardial damage is dangerous.

Mortality following unrecognized myocardial infarction is just as great as that after recognized MI (Table 15.5). In men in the Framingham Study, 71 percent of those with unrecognized MIs were dead at 10 years compared with 53 percent of those with recognized MIs. Adjusting for differences in age and comparing this risk to that of the general population, there is a 2.3-fold excess risk of death in recognized MI and a 2.5-fold excess risk for unrecognized MI. In women, the recognized MI carried a 63 percent mortality rate at 10 years and the unrecognized MI a 51 percent death rate. On age adjustment, the risk ratio is 3.7-fold for recognized MI versus 2.5-fold for unrecognized MI.

In both sexes cardiovascular, coronary, and sudden death mortality were also comparable for unrecognized and recognized MIs (Table 15.5). Various forms of cardiovascular mortality were increased 3.3- to 3.8-fold in men with unrecognized MIs; 2.4- to 6.5-fold in women.

Cardiovascular events in general are also substantially increased following unrecognized MI and are almost as great as those after symptomatic recognized MIs (Table 15.6). At 10 years, the risk of a cardiovascular event in men is increased 3.6-fold in recognized MI and 2.4-fold in unrecognized MI. In women, risk ratios are 4.8 and 3.2, respectively, compared to those of the general population of the same age. Only risks of recurrent MI and angina are substantially lower in unrecognized MI (Table 15.6). Also, a recurrent MI is less likely to be unrecognized or silent than is

Table 15.4. Unrecognized Myocardial Infarction and Glucose Intolerance: 26-Year Follow-up*

	Biennial Age-Adjusted Rate per 1,000			
	Women		Men	
	All MI	Unrecognized MI	All MI	Unrecognized MI
Glucose intolerance				
Absent	3.8	1.4	13.1	3.2
Present	13.8	2.4	24.8	9.7
Risk ratio	3.6	1.7	1.8	3.0
Percentage of unrecognized MIs				
Without glucose intolerance		37%		18%
With glucose intolerance		17%		39%

* Framingham Study Subjects 35 to 84 Years.

Table 15.5. Age-Adjusted Risk of Mortality after Recognized vs Unrecognized Myocardial Infarctions at 10 Years: 30-Year Follow-up*

	Standardized Mortality Ratios			
	Men		Women	
	Unrecognized	Recognized	Unrecognized	Recognized
All causes of mortality	245	229	245	366
Cardiovascular mortality	345	318	405	594
Coronary heart disease mortality	382	429	745	877
Sudden death	330	452	653	593

* Framingham Study subjects 35 to 94 years of age.

a first attack. About half of recurrent myocardial infarctions are fatal whether the prior MI is unrecognized or symptomatic. After an unrecognized MI, men are at a 3.6-fold increased risk of a stroke and 4.6-fold risk of cardiac failure; for women the corresponding risk ratios are 2.3 and 4.8 (Table 15.6).

SECULAR TRENDS

There is no indication that the proportion of myocardial infarctions that go unrecognized has decreased with time over the past 3 decades. Increased awareness of silent coronary disease and improved diagnostic capability have not greatly affected the results.[8] Clearly, closer monitoring of candidates for unrecognized MI is needed, particularly in those with hypertension and diabetes.

PATHOGENESIS

The mechanism whereby ischemic episodes occur without pain is obscure.[11,12] It is not clear why on ambulatory monitoring of patients with angina more transient ischemic attacks occur without pain than with it. Neither is it clear why ischemia to the point of infarction occurs without symptoms in some persons, with atypical symptoms in others, and with severe symptoms in most. Denial probably plays a role, as some people are unwilling to recognize a life-threatening situation. Cohn's

Table 15.6. Age-Adjusted Risk of Cardiovascular Events after Recognized vs Unrecognized Myocardial Infarctions: 30-Year Follow-up*

	Standardized Morbidity Ratio†			
	Men		Women	
Cardiovascular Event	Recognized MI	Unrecognized MI	Recognized MI	Unrecognized MI
Any coronary heart disease event	363	242	483	323
Coronary attack	368	254	690	397
Myocardial infarction	282	199	829	432
Angina	506	205	496	333
Stroke or transient ischemic attack	238	364	589	233
Cardiac failure	367	462	756	483

* Framingham Study subjects 35 to 94 years of age.
† At 10 years.

postulated defective anginal warning system is supported by the finding of less angina preceding and following unrecognized than recognized MI. Evidently these patients tend not to express ischemia with pain. Persons subject to silent MI may simply be less sensitive to pain in general, as they have been shown to possess a higher pain threshold,[12] possibly because of a more centrally located process of pain regulation and variable endorphin accumulation.

Because there is no difference in the ECG location of MIs that are silent or symptomatic, an atypical pattern of referred pain seems unlikely. Denervated hearts exhibit no pain after transplant, and sensory neuropathy has been incriminated, particularly in diabetic patients. However, this finding is not well documented in either the diabetic or the nondiabetic patient who is subject to silent coronary disease.

It is possible that the extent of ischemic involvement or the rapidity of its evolution may not be as great in painless infarction. Angina occurs late in the course of exercise-induced myocardial ischemia, following evidence of contractile abnormality and ECG changes. Pain may only be the tip of a dangerous iceberg of myocardial ischemia.

PREVENTIVE IMPLICATIONS

Silent coronary disease in general and unrecognized MI in particular present a common and potentially lethal situation that warrants greater attention. Actual myocardial infactions often are unrecognized and can be just as disabling as symptomatic infarctions. Persons with a poor cardiovascular risk profile in general and with hypertension and diabetes in particular need to be monitored by periodic ECG examination to detect silent myocardial infarction.

Because of the high incidence and serious prognosis associated with unrecognized MI, those that are detected deserve preventive management equivalent to that indicated for symptomatic MI. However, there are no controlled trial data to support any therapeutic recommendations, and decisions have to be made on rationale alone. Studies show that silent transient ischemic episodes respond to the same treatment as do symptomatic episodes. Hence, nitroglycerin, calcium antagonists, and beta blockers may all be useful. Ambulatory monitoring of patients with silent MI may indicate silent ischemia that may be controlled by such therapy. Beta blockers have been shown to reduce the risk of sudden death following symptomatic MI and possibly also after unrecognized MI that also imposes a substantial risk of sudden death.

Because the risk of cardiac failure and stroke is substantial following unrecognized MI, control of elevated blood pressure would seem prudent. There may also be a theoretic justification for low-dose aspirin or fish oil therapy to inhibit platelet aggregation.

Careful and vigorous control of cardiovascular risk factors appears prudent in a patient with an unrecognized, but potentially lethal MI. Because quitting cigarette smoking can halve the risk of having a recurrent symptomatic MI, it is reasonable to recommend this in patients with silent MI. Weight reduction in the obese can lessen the burden of all major risk factors and help slow the progression of atherosclerosis as well as improve tolerance for exercise without accompanying transient silent ischemia. A prudent diet and cholesterol-lowering drugs such as colestipol, nicotinic acid, and lovastatin may slow the progression of lesions and reduce the likelihood of lethal recurrences.

The role of surgery or angioplasty in silent myocardial infarction is particularly controversial as there are no symptoms to relieve. It is unlikely to improve the outlook unless there is demonstrated left main coronary artery disease or three-vessel disease with impaired left ventricular function.

In any event, patients with unrecognized MI should be sought out among high risk candidates for coronary disease by periodic ECG examination and carefully followed for evidence of transient silent ischemic attacks on ambulatory monitoring, signs of cardiac failure, and arrhythmia. When these signs appear, they should be corrected as they would be in symptomatic patients.

SUMMARY

Advanced occlusive coronary disease often exists without symptoms or overt clinical manifestations. In a third of those who experience myocardial infarction, it will be discovered only by the appearance of characteristic changes on routine periodic ECG examination. Of these unrecognized myocardial infarctions, 48 percent are completely silent. Women are more prone (32%) to silent infarctions than are men (29%). The fraction of infarctions that remain unrecognized increases with age in men, but not in women. Unrecognized MIs are infrequently preceded by angina and less often followed by angina.

Morbidity and mortality after unrecognized MI are substantial, and except for angina and recurrent MI are almost as great as those following symptomatic infarction. The risk factors for unrecognized and asymptomatic MI are similar, but hypertensive and diabetic persons are particularly likely to have the MI go unrecognized.

The proportion of unrecognized MIs has not decreased over the past 3 decades despite increased awareness of silent coronary disease and improved diagnostic capability. Periodic ECG surveillance of persons with an atherogenic cardiovascular risk profile appears indicated for this serious asymptomatic disease. Greater emphasis on vigorous secondary prevention is needed for this deceptively "benign" condition.

REFERENCES

1. Kannel WB: Epidemiologic insights into atherosclerotic cardiovascular disease from the Framingham Study, in Pollock ML, Schmidt DH (eds): *Heart Disease and Rehabilitation,* 2nd, ch 1. New York, John Wiley & Sons, 1986, pp 3–28.
2. Gordon T, Kannel WB: Premature mortality from coronary heart disease: The Framingham Study. *JAMA* 1971;215:1617–1625.
3. Kannel WB, Barry P, Dawber TR: Immediate mortality in coronary heart disease: The Framingham Study, in Proceedings of the IV World Congress of Cardiology, Mexico City, 1962. *Int Soc Cardiol* 1963;4B:176–188.
4. Erikssen J, Engle I, Forfang K, Storstein O: False positive diagnostic tests and coronary angiography findings in 105 presumably healthy males. *Circulation* 1976;54:371–376.
5. Froelicher VF, Thompson AJ, Long MR Jr, et al: Value of exercise testing for screening asymptomatic men for latent coronary artery disease. *Prog Cardiovasc Dis* 1976;18:265–276.
6. Schang SJ, Pepine CJ: Transient asymptomatic ST segment depression during daily activity. *Am J Cardiol* 1977;39:396–401.
7. Deanfield JE, Selwyn AP, Chierchia S, et al: Myocardial ischemia during daily life in patients with stable angina: Its relation to symptoms and heart rate changes. *Lancet* 1983;2:753–758.
8. Kannel WB, Abbott RD: Incidence and prognosis of unrecognized myocardial infarction: An update on the Framingham Study. *N Engl J Med* 1984;311:1144–1147.

9. Margolis JR, Kannel WB, Feinleib M, et al: Clinical features of unrecognized myocardial infarction—silent and symptomatic: Eighteen year follow-up: The Framingham Study. *Am J Cardiol* 1973;32:1–7.
10. Kannel WB, Dannenberg AL, Abbott RD: Unrecognized myocardial infarction and hypertension: The Framingham Study. *Am Heart J* 1985;109:581–585.
11. Droste C, Roskamm H: Experimental pain measurement in patients with asymptomatic myocardial ischemia. *J Am Coll Cardiol* 1983;1:940–945.
12. Cohn PF: Silent myocardial ischemia in patients with a defective anginal warning system. *Am J Cardiol* 1980;45:697–702.

CHAPTER 16

Exercise-Induced Painless Myocardial Ischemia in Patients Who Survived Out-of-Hospital Ventricular Fibrillation

Bimlendra Sharma, MD, and Richard P. Wyeth, MA

Sudden cardiac death, described over 2,000 years ago by Hippocrates,[1] continues as a major problem with over 300,000 deaths yearly in the United States alone.[2] Not surprisingly, out-of-hospital ventricular fibrillation (VF) is the leading cause of sudden death.[3] For example, of the 1,070 patients brought to the Hennipen County Medical Center Emergency Room between 1974 and 1979 after suffering out-of-hospital VF, 325 (30%) were successfully rescuscitated. One hundred fifty of these 325 patients (14% of the 1,070 brought to the emergency room) were discharged alive. Thirty of these 150 survivors (20%) had anoxic brain damage (unpublished observations, 1979).

The precise pathophysiologic aspects of out-of-hospital VF remain elusive, but in patients over the age of 40 years, myocardial ischemia due to coronary artery disease (CAD) is thought essential in precipitating most episodes of VF.[44–11] Nonetheless, approximately 25 percent of patients who survive VF have previously known evidence of neither CAD nor myocardial ischemia. Such circumstantial evidence suggests that painless myocardial ischemia is a contributory factor in the genesis of VF. This study investigates left ventricular (LV) functional, hemodynamic, and ECG evidence of painless myocardial ischemia during exercise and the effects of sublingual nitroglycerin on exercise-induced painless myocardial ischemia in patients who sustained and survived out-of-hospital VF.

MATERIALS AND METHODS

Patient Profile

Twenty-eight patients comprised the study population. There were 15 patients (14 men and 1 woman) who sustained and survived out-of-hospital VF. Nine of these survivors had no previous clinical evidence of CAD (Group A), whereas the remaining six clearly experienced angina, myocardial infarction or both before this episode of out-of-hospital VF (Group S). No patient had evidence of valvular heart disease or diabetes mellitus. Two patients in Group A had essential hypertension. Before this episode of out-of-hospital VF all patients in Group S were receiving vasodilators and beta blockers for angina. Within Group A, one patient was treated with procainamide because of a previous cardiac arrest. Two patients in Group A and two patients in Group S had unequivocal acute myocardial infarction concurrent with this episode of out-of-hospital VF.

Upon ambulation, 24-hour Holter monitoring showed episodes of ventricular tachycardia in four of nine patients in Group A and two of six patients in Group S. Frequent premature ventricular complexes, 30 or more per hour, were present in seven patients in Group A and four patients in Group S. It was technically impossible to ascertain the presence of myocardial ischemia before the onset of VF. Cardiac catheterization was performed as an essential part of the patient's diagnosis.

Thirteen patients who underwent exercise ventriculography for chest pain despite negative cardiac and other organ system workups serve as a normal control population (Group C) for this study.

Design of Investigation

One day before catheterization, each patient had a practice session to determine if they could perform supine ergometric bicycle exercise without chest pain for at least 6 minutes. On the day of catheterization, selective coronary angiography was performed first. After a 10- to 15-minute rest period, cardiac output and intracardiac and aortic pressures were measured and left ventriculography was performed at rest. After a 20-minute interval the patient was exercised with the supine ergometric bicycle (25 to 100 kW/min) for a total of 6 minutes. During the last 2 minutes of exercise, hemodynamics and ventriculography were repeated.

Sublingual Nitroglycerin

In six patients in Group A, the effects of sublingual nitroglycerin were tested. Twenty minutes were allowed to pass between the conclusion of exercise without nitroglycerin and a second identical submaximal exercise period with the same workload following a 20 mm Hg downward adjustment of LV peak systolic pressure with 150 $\pm$ 50 μg of sublingual nitroglycerin.

Informed Consent

Written informed consent was obtained from all patients. The project was approved by the appropriate human research advisory committees.

Hemodynamic and Angiographic Methods

Selective coronary angiography was performed using the standard Judkins technique. A Swan-Ganz thermodilution catheter was positioned in the right pulmonary artery. Aortic pressure was recorded with a 5 French catheter introduced percutaneously through the right brachial artery. Left heart catheterization was carried out with a 7 French pigtail catheter via the right femoral artery. Left ventriculography was performed at a 45 degree right anterior oblique projection.

Measurements and Calculations

ST-segment depression in chest lead V_5 of the electrocardiogram was measured from 80 ms after the J point to the isoelectric line joining two consecutive P-R intervals. Left ventricular end-diastolic pressure was measured at the nadir of the atrial wave just before systolic contraction. Cardiac output was determined by the thermodilution technique. Stroke volume was calculated as cardiac output divided by heart rate. The severity of coronary lesions was expressed as the maximum percentage of diameter narrowing in any standard projection (left or right anterior oblique or axial plane). Significant disease implies a $\geq$ 70% diameter stenosis. Diastolic and systolic volumes were calculated by the single plane area-length method.[12] Global LV ejection fraction was determined from ventriculographic volumes and reported as a percentage. Regional LV wall motion was assessed by methods previously described.[13,14] Volumetric measurements were divided by body surface area and are reported as the index. Data are expressed as the mean $\pm$ 1 standard deviation. Statistical significance was tested by paired and two-sample *t* tests or chi-square analysis as appropriate. The term "significant" implies a p value of < 0.05.

RESULTS

Coronary Angiography (Table 16.1)

Significant one-, two-, and three-vessel CAD was found in three, five, and one of the nine patients in Group A, respectively. Similar widespread CAD in Group S patients was found at coronary angiography; two-vessel CAD in two and three-vessel CAD in four. Coronary angiographic findings in both groups were statistically similar irrespective of the clinical manifestation of ischemia. No patient in Group C had angiographic evidence of coronary arterial disease.

Electrocardiographic ST-Segment Depression (Chest Lead V_5)

At rest, horizontal or down-sloping ST-segment depression was found in two Group A and four Group S patients (pns). During exercise, ST-segment depression significantly increased in both Group A and Group S, but although up-sloping ST-segment depression developed in four patients in Group C, it was not statistically significant (Figure 16.1). There was no statistically significant difference in ST-segment depression in Group A compared with Group S at rest or on exercise. When ST-segment depression in the control group was compared with that in both Group A and Group S, there were differences both at rest and on exercise that were, on the whole, significantly different (Table 16.2). In the six Group A patients given nitroglycerin, there was a significant reduction in the magnitude of ST-segment depression during exercise (Table 16.3 and Figure 16.1).

Hemodynamic Findings (Tables 16.2 and 16.3 and Figures 16.2 and 16.3)

At rest, the mean heart rate, aortic pressure, cardiac index, and stroke volume index were within normal limits and statistically similar in all groups. Left ventricular end-diastolic pressure in Group A and Group S was significantly increased compared with that in Group C. There was no statistical difference in filling pressure between Group A and Group S. On exercise, a comparison between Group C and Groups A and S indicated the development of severe systolic and diastolic dysfunction. When six Group A patients performed exercise after sublingual nitroglycerin, there was a significant improvement in most hemodynamic parameters compared with those after exercise without nitroglycerin.

Table 16.1. Coronary Angiographic Findings

Case #	% Stenosis LM	LAD	LCX	R	Others	Collateral*
			Group A			
1	N	95	N	75	N	————
2	N	100	99	50	N	R → LAD
3	N	80	N	70	N	————
4	N	100	N	N	70, LOM	R → LAD
5	N	99	50	50	95, D, LOM	R → LAD
6	N	70	70	70	N	————
7	N	80	70	N	90, LOM	————
8	N	70	90	50	N	LAD → LCX
9	N	75	N	N	N	————
			Group S			
10	N	90	100	95	70, D	LAD → LCX
11	N	90	30	100	50, LOM	LCX → R
12	N	75	80	50	75, D	————
13	50	50	80	100	50, D	LAD → R
14	N	100	95	80	N	R → LAD
15	N	100	N	70	N	LCX → LAD

* Arrow indicates flow direction.

D = diagonal; LAD = left anterior descending; LCX = left circumflex; LM = left main; LOM = left obtuse marginal; N = within normal limits; R = right.

Left Ventricular Volumes and Ejection Fraction (Table 16.2 and 16.3 and Figure 16.4)

The mean LV end-diastolic volume at both rest and exercise in Group C was significantly smaller than that in either Group A or Group S. When compared with the respective data at exercise, LV end-diastolic volume increased significantly during exercise in Group S but not in Group A. Conversely, in Group C, LV end-diastolic volume significantly decreased during exercise ($p < 0.001$). There was no significant difference between values for LV end-diastolic volume at rest and those during exercise in either Group A or Group S. Similarly, LV end-systolic volume increased during exercise in Group A ($p < 0.04$) and Group S ($p < 0.02$), whereas in the control group (Group C) it markedly decreased ($p < 0.01$). This abnormal increase in volume during exercise was similar in magnitude and not statistically different between Group A and Group S. Although ejection fraction increased during exercise in Group C ($p < 0.001$), no significant change occurred during exercise in either Group A or Group S and there was no statistical difference between Group A and Group S. In Group A patients given sublingual nitroglycerin and re-exercised, an improvement in global LV function was associated with a reduction in LV volume and a markedly improved ($p < 0.01$) ejection fraction. Individual data and statistical results for exercise following sublingual nitroglycerin in Group A patients are found in Table 16.3.

Regional Wall Motion Abnormalities (Figure 16.5)

From rest to exercise in both Group A and S either a new wall motion abnormality developed or a preexisting abnormality extended further (11 of 15 patients). Assessment of wall motion indicated that 56 percent of all LV segments measured

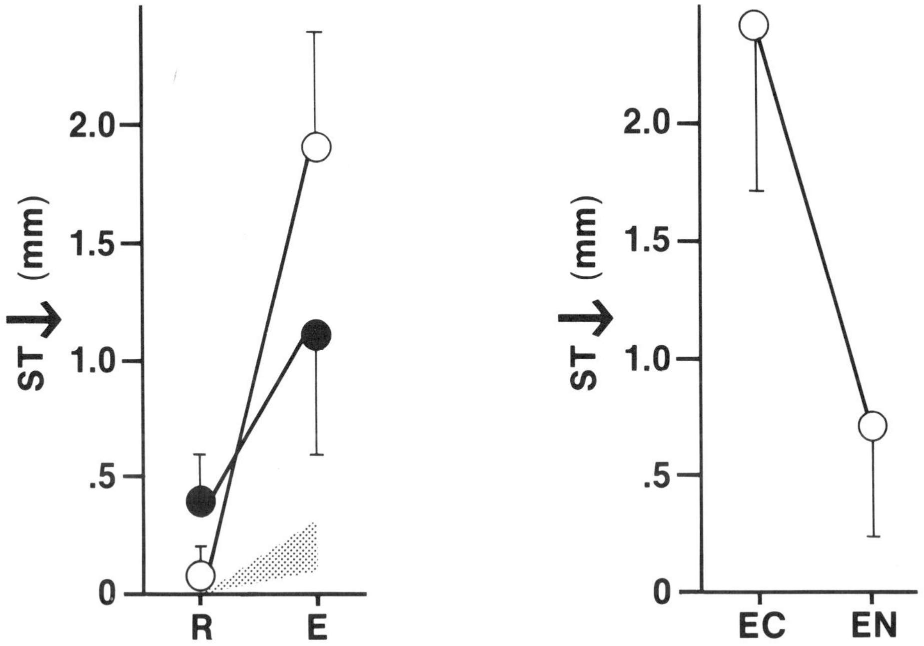

FIGURE 16.1. *Left,* there is a significant increase in ST-segment depression (ST) for Group A patients (*open circles;* $p < 0.01$) and a statistically nonsignificant increase for Group S (*closed circles*) patients from rest (R) to exercise (E). In Group C (*stippled area*) there is up-sloping ST-segment depression that did not reach significance. *Right,* a significant ($p < 0.01$) decrease in ST-segment depression after sublingual nitroglycerin. EC = exercise before nitroglycerin, EN = exercise after nitroglycerin. Data are shown as the mean ± the standard error of the mean. The *stippled area* represents upper and lower limits of the standard error of the mean in Group C.

(n = 27) in Group A patients and 72 percent of all segments (n = 18) in Group S patients showed abnormality at rest. During exercise 78 percent of all LV segments (n = 27) in Group A and 94 percent of all segments measured (n = 18) in Group S showed wall motion abnormality. The proportion of wall motion abnormalities at rest or on exercise was not significantly different between Groups A and S. In Group C all segments measured (n = 39) showed either normokinesia (87%) or slight hyperkinesia (13%). With exercise the control patients had a significant increase in the number of hypercontractile segments (51%; $p < 0.02$). In the six Group A patients given nitroglycerin and subsequent exercise the number of abnormal segments was reduced from 72 percent (n = 18) at exercise before nitroglycerin to 22 percent at exercise with sublingual nitroglycerin ($p < 0.01$). Figure 16.5 depicts representative regional wall motion data before and after sublingual nitroglycerin (case 1).

Left Ventricular Pressure/Volume Relationship (Figures 16.6 and 16.7)

Left ventricular end-diastolic volume in all patients in Groups A, S, and C was plotted against LV end-diastolic pressures. In both Groups A and S, LV end-diastolic pressure increased during exercise with a concurrent rise in LV end-diastolic volume. This contrasted markedly to that in Group C patients who, while having an increase in LV end-diastolic pressure associated with exercise, had a decline in LV end-diastolic volume. When LV end-diastolic volume at exercise was compared with and

Table 16.2. Hemodynamic Data

Groups	Heart Rate (beats/min)		CI (l/min/m^2)		SVI (ml/m^2)		SAP (mm Hg)		LVEDP (mm Hg)		LVEDVI (ml/m^2)		LVESVI (ml/m^2)		LVEF (%)		ST ↓ (mm)	
	R	E	R	E	R	E	R	E	R	E	R	E	R	E	R	E	R	E
Group C (Normal) (n = 13)	73 ± 8	112 ± 12	3.3 ± .5	5.7 ± 1.1	46 ± 5	50 ± 8	136 ± 18	175 ± 21	9.4 ± 2.2	14.9 ± 2.3	70 ± 8	63 ± 8	24 ± 7	14 ± 6	66 ± 8	79 ± 7	0 ± 0	.2 ± .2
Group A (asymptomatic) (n = 9)	80 ± 11	116 ± 19	2.9 ± 0.5	4.1 ± 1.5	42 ± 8	42 ± 11	136 ± 25	151 ± 23	19 ± 4	31 ± 8	83 ± 13	92 ± 23	39 ± 17	51 ± 22	55 ± 13	46 ± 13	0.1 ± 0.2	1.9 ± 1.4
Group S (symptomatic) (n = 6)	82 ± 11	106 ± 13	3.0 ± 0.6	3.8 ± 0.7	38 ± 10	37 ± 10	130 ± 19	148 ± 16	21 ± 9	37 ± 11	100 ± 25	107 ± 26	61 ± 25	65 ± 25	40 ± 13	42 ± 12	0.4 ± 0.4	1.1 ± 1.2
p values comparing Group C to:																		
Group A: p<	pns	pns	pns	0.01	pns	0.06	pns	0.02	0.001	0.001	0.01	0.001	0.01	0.001	0.03	0.001	pns	0.001
Group S: p<	pns	pns	pns	0.001	0.03	0.01	pns	0.01	0.001	0.001	0.001	0.001	0.001	0.001	0.001	0.001	0.001	0.01

CI = cardiac index; E = exercise; LVEDP = left ventricular end-diastolic pressure; LVEDVI = left ventricular end-diastolic volume index; LVEF = left ventricular ejection fraction; LVESVI = left ventricular end-systolic volume index; R = rest; SAP = systolic arterial pressure; ST ↓ = ST-segment depression; SVI = stroke volume index.

Table 16.3. Exercise Hemodynamic and Electrocardiographic Data Before and After Sublingual Nitroglycerin in Group A Patients

	Heart Rate (beats/min)		CI (l/min/m²)		SVI (ml/m²)		SAP (mm Hg)		DAP (mm Hg)		MAP (mm HG)		LVEDP (mm HG)		LVEDVI (ml/m²)		LVESVI (ml/m²)		LVEF (%)		ST ↓ (mm)	
Case	EC	EN	EC	EN	EC	EN	EC	EN	EC	EN	EC	EN	EC	EN	EC	EN	EC	EN	EC	EN	EC	EN
1	126	126	5.8	6.7	46	54	178	120	95	80	125	93	45	15	88	70	44	18	50	74	4.6	0.5
2	92	90	2.6	3.0	28	42	108	94	70	60	83	71	38	28	102	107	75	65	26	39	2.0	0.5
3	107	107	4.2	4.6	42	43	176	163	70	70	105	101	30	13	90	54	65	37	28	31	2.0	0.0
4	96	92	3.4	3.5	50	60	239	215	93	92	141	133	31	11	150	81	70	29	53	64	4.0	3.0
5	130	130	2.3	2.5	53	54	140	120	100	90	113	100	24	12	89	82	36	28	60	66	1.0	0.0
6	92	86	3.0	4.2	40	49	130	120	70	62	87	81	26	18	93	89	52	41	44	54	0.8	0.0
Mean	107	105	3.6	4.1	43	50	162	139	83	76	109	97	32	16	102	81	57	36	44	55	2.4	0.7
±	±	±	±	±	±	±	±	±	±	±	±	±	±	±	±	±	±	±	±	±	±	±
SD	17	19	1.3	1.5	9	7	46	43	14	14	22	21	8	6	24	19	15	16	14	17	1.6	1.2
p <	ns		ns		<0.01		<0.03		<0.03		<0.03		<0.005		ns		<0.008		<0.009		<0.01	

CI = cardiac index; DAP = diastolic arterial pressure; EC = exercise without nitroglycerin; EN = exercise following sublingual nitroglycerin; LVEDP = left ventricular end-diastolic pressure; LVEDVI = left ventricular end-diastolic volume index; LVEF = left ventricular ejection fraction; LVESI = left ventricular end-systolic volume index; MAP = mean arterial pressure; ns = not statistically significant; SAP = systolic arterial pressure; ST ↓ = ST-segment depression; SVI - stroke volume index.

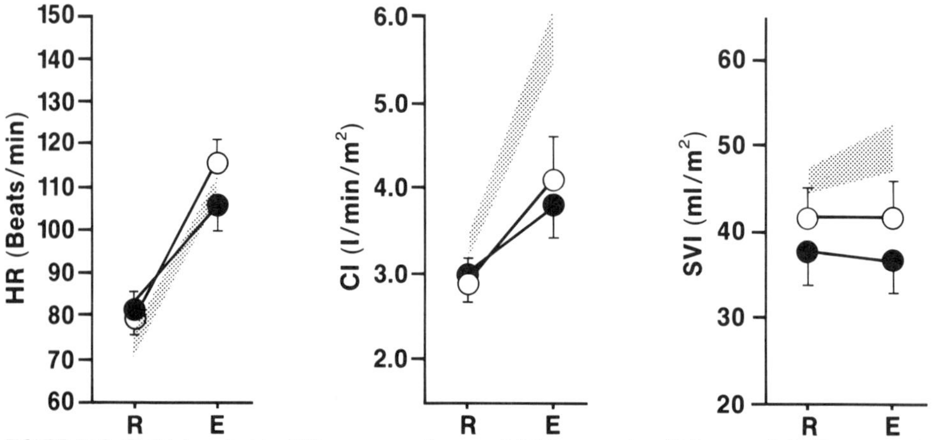

FIGURE 16.2. *Right,* heart rate (HR) response from rest (R) to exercise (E) is essentially the same in Group A patients (*open circles*), Group S patients (*closed circles*), and Group C (*stippled area*). *Center,* cardiac index (CI) is markedly higher in Group C than in either Group A or Group S patients. *Right,* stroke volume index (SVI) decreases in patients in both Groups A and S while increasing in Group C. Data are shown as the mean ± the standard error of the mean. The *stippled area* represents upper and lower limits of the standard error of the mean in Group C.

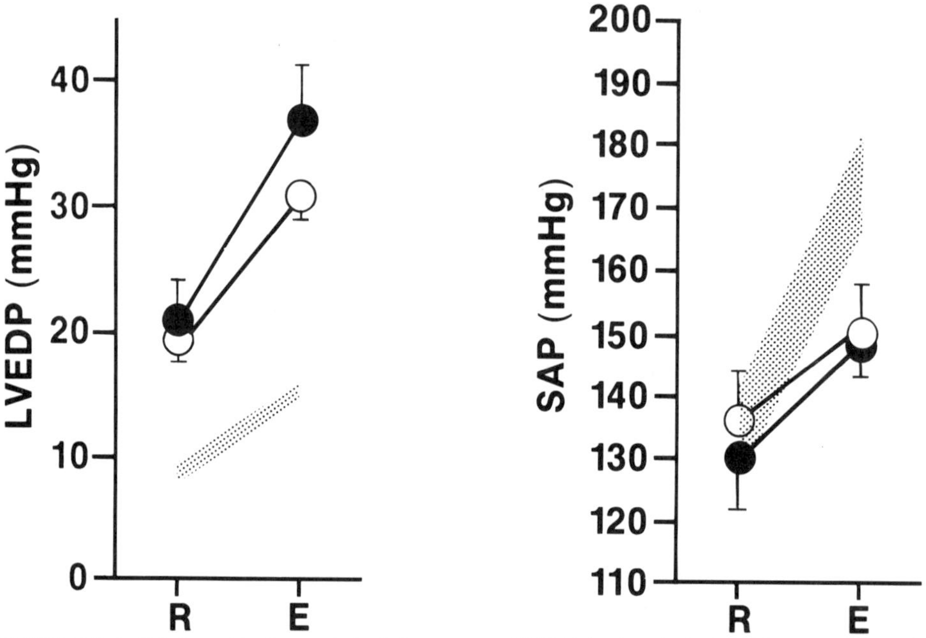

FIGURE 16.3. *Left,* left ventricular end-diastolic pressure (LVEDP) is elevated at rest (R) and increases markedly ($p < 0.02$) with exercise in Group A (*open circles*) and Group S patients (*closed circles*). Note the lower LVEDP at both rest and exercise in group C (*stippled area*). *Right,* at rest systolic aortic peak pressure (SAP) is essentially identical in all three groups, but with exercise Group C has a marked increase in SAP ($p < 0.02$ compared to Groups A or S). Data are shown as the mean ± the standard error of the mean. The *stippled area* represents upper and lower limits of the standard error of the mean in Group C.

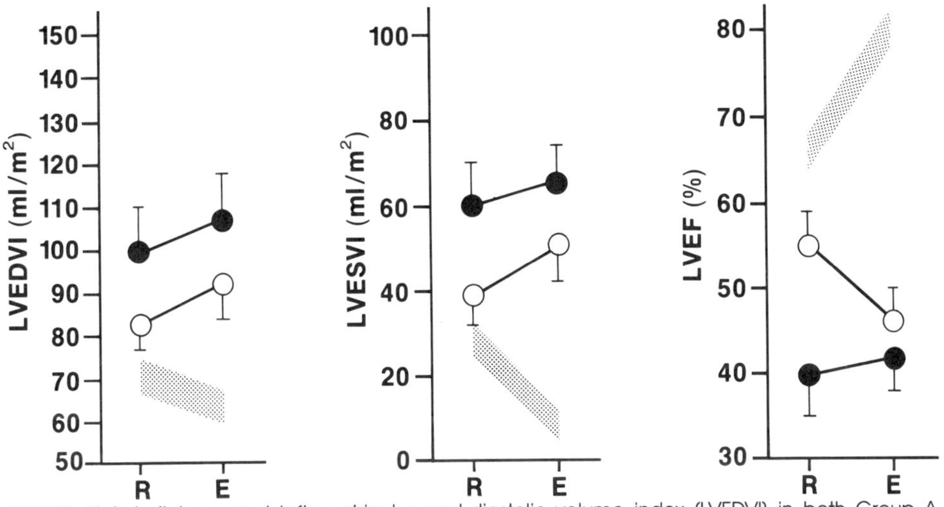

FIGURE 16.4. *Left,* increased left ventricular end-diastolic volume index (LVEDVI) in both Group A (*open circles*) and Group S (*closed circles*) patients from rest (R) to exercise (E) contrasts with decreased LVEDVI seen in Group C (*stippled area*). *Center,* both Group A and Group S patients show an increase in left ventricular end-systolic volume index (LVESVI), whereas Group C patients show a marked decrease in LVESVI. *Right,* left ventricular ejection fraction (LVEF) is greater in Group C. Group A subjects have higher LVEF at rest than do Group S patients, but they show a significant decrease in LVEF ($p < 0.01$) at exercise. Data shown are the mean ± the standard error of the mean. The *stippled area* represents upper and lower limits of the standard error of the mean in Group C.

without nitroglycerin in Group A, there was a concomitant decrease in LV end-diastolic pressure in all patients and a volume decrease in five of the six (Table 16.3).

Left Ventricular Frank-Starling Function Curve (Figures 16.6 and 16.7)

Left ventricular global systolic function was further assessed by plotting stroke volume index against LV end-diastolic pressure at rest and during exercise. These plots in both Groups A and S indicated no increase in stroke volume index with an increase in LV end-diastolic pressure during exercise. This global LV dysfunction was of similar magnitude in both Groups A and S and different from the relationship seen in Group C in which stroke volume increased with exercise. In the six Group A patients given sublingual nitroglycerin and re-exercised, a plot of LV stroke volume index versus end-diastolic pressure showed a decrease in LV filling pressure accompanied by an increase in stroke volume index.

DISCUSSION

This study obtained direct information regarding global and regional LV function during exercise in patients who sustained and survived out-of-hospital VF. Severe LV dysfunction was demonstrated during exercise associated with ST-segment depression without chest pain in patients in both Groups A and S. This dysfunction was characterized by increases in LV end-diastolic pressure, end-diastolic volume, and end-systolic volume without significant increases in stroke volume index and ejection fraction. Similar impaired myocardial performance was previously shown

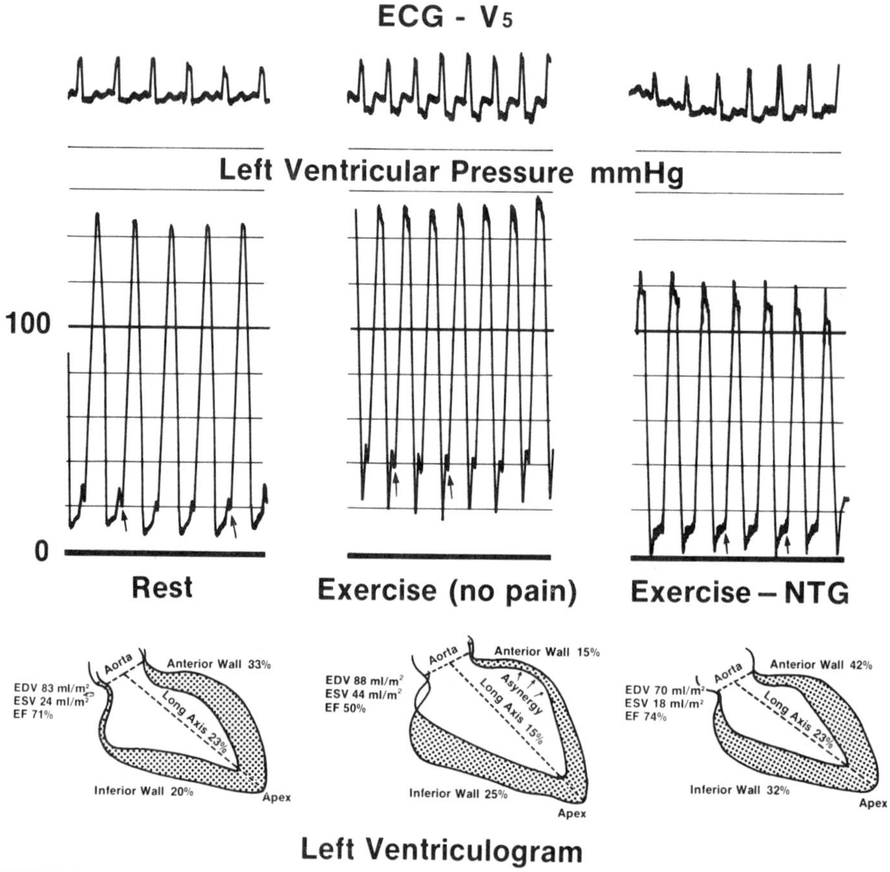

FIGURE 16.5. Simultaneous recording of chest lead V_5, left ventricular pressure, and ventriculogram during exercise, indicating ECG, hemodynamic, and left ventriculographic evidence of painless myocardial ischemia in a Group A patient with out-of-hospital ventricular fibrillation. Note the development of ST-segment depression, an increase in end-diastolic pressure (arrows), a decrease in ejection fraction (EF), and the development of anterolateral asynergy with exercise and reversal of this global and regional left ventricular dysfunction at exercise following 150 μg of sublingual nitroglycerin. EDV = end-diastolic volume; ESV = end-systolic volume.

during ischemia in isolated papillary muscle, intact experimental heart preparations,[15–18] and in man.[19–22] Our study also clearly demonstrates that during submaximal exercise, in the presence of ECG evidence of myocardial ischemia, regions of abnormal wall motion develop. These areas of reversible myocardial ischemia appear to correspond well to the distribution of significant coronary stenoses and are reversible with nitroglycerin. Such regional abnormalities are similar to those that occur during spontaneous angina[23] and during angina induced by atrial pacing,[21] exercise,[13,24] or both.[14]

The increase in LV end-diastolic volume with an increase in LV end-diastolic pressure during exercise-induced painless ischemia is an important finding of this study. Similar findings were reported in patients with spontaneous angina[23,25] or angina induced by atrial pacing[26] and by exercise.[13] Thus, an increase in LV end-diastolic and end-systolic volume with a concurrent rise in LV filling pressure seems to be an important hemodynamic feature of myocardial ischemia whether painless or not. This study further shows that for a given diastolic volume, LV end-diastolic

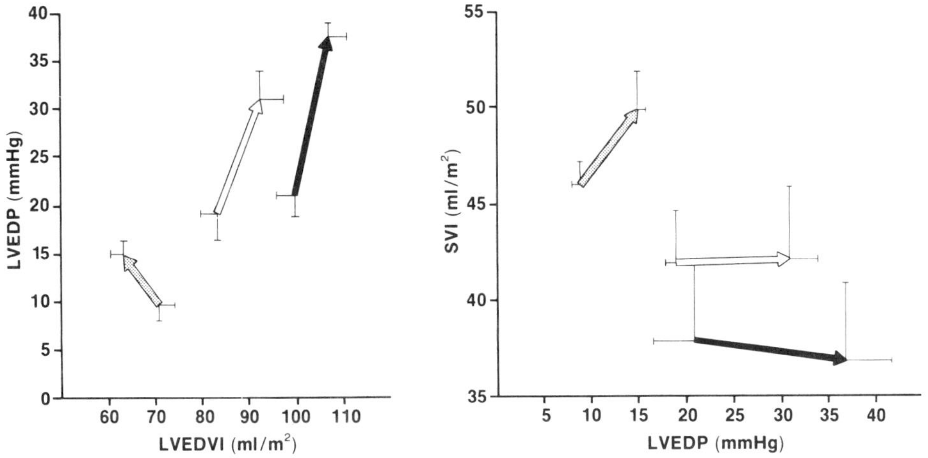

FIGURE 16.6. *Left,* changes in left ventricular pressure/volume relationship from rest to exercise. Note the decrease in left ventricular end-diastolic volume index (LVEDVI) associated with an increase in left ventricular end-diastolic pressure (LVEDP) in Group C (*stippled arrow*) compared to the increase in LVEDVI associated with a marked increase in LVEDP in both Group A (*open arrow*) and Group S (*closed arrow*). *Right,* changes in a modified Frank-Starling function curve. There is marked systolic dysfunction during exercise in Groups A and S as compared with Group C. SVI = stroke volume index.

pressure is higher during exercise-induced painless ischemia, which may indirectly indicate a change in diastolic properties of the left ventricle.[25,27]

The current study also clearly shows direct ECG and functional evidence for the reversal of exercise-induced painless myocardial ischemia by nitroglycerin. Previous investigations have demonstrated that nitroglycerin can improve LV function in patients with coronary artery disease at rest,[28,29] when given before exercise,[30] or when given during an episode of spontaneous angina.[23] The mechanisms involved in the reversal of the evidence of myocardial ischemia cannot be ascertained by this study, but an improvement in both LV systolic and diastolic function associated with a decrease in ST-segment depression was previously noted.[23] Current evidence sug-

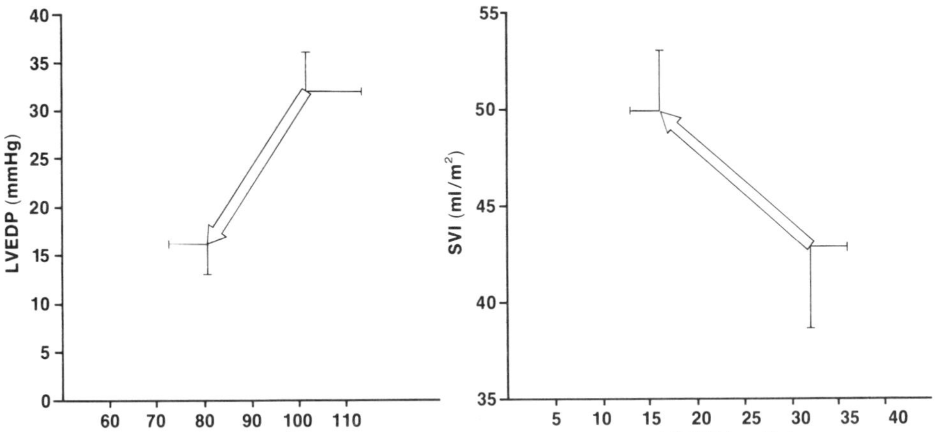

FIGURE 16.7. Effect of sublingual nitroglycerin on the diastolic pressure/volume relationship (*left*) and Frank-Starling curve (*right*) during exercise in six Group A patients. Data indicate an improvement in both following sublingual nitroglycerin. LVEDVI = left ventricular end-diastolic volume index; LVEDP = left ventricular end-diastolic pressure; SVI = stroke volume index.

gests that nitroglycerin, and nitrates in general, relieve myocardial ischemia by reducing both peripheral and coronary vasomotor tone.[31] These reductions are dose related, with smaller doses resulting in increased venous dilatation which reduces venous return and consequently LV end-diastolic pressure and volume.[32] Direct intracoronary nitroglycerin infusions will vasodilate epicardial coronary stenoses,[33] which will increase coronary flow and thus directly improve LV function. Sublingual nitroglycerin doses in the range used in our study increase peripheral arterial volume, resulting in a reduction of systolic pressures[34] which may indirectly improve LV systolic performance. Comparison of the results of exercise obtained before and after sublingual nitroglycerin in the current study suggests that the response to nitroglycerin in the presence of painless ischemia is typical and that asymptomatic survivors of sudden cardiac death benefit from favorable direct and indirect effects of nitroglycerin on the myocardial oxygen supply and demand relationship.

Under normal living conditions submaximal exercise without precipitation of angina may be frequently reached by patients who have sudden death. Thus, data from this study may be relevant to the normal life of these patients. The effects of the interaction between coronary arterial occlusion and exercise have been investigated to determine if myocardial ischemia facilitates the occurrence of malignant arrhythmia.[35,36] These experimental data show that VF is induced consistently by a trilogy of acute myocardial ischemia, coronary occlusion, and submaximal exercise. Extrapolation of these data to the clinical setting should be guarded. However, in a review, of 2,606 deaths in patients with cardiac symptoms, the majority of sudden cardiac deaths were exercise related.[37]

Prognosis with painless myocardial ischemia may be worse than that with overt angina pectoris, because it may remain unattended until a life-threatening cardiac event evolves. For example, myocardial infarction is known to occur without pain, and acute recurrent pulmonary edema is likely due to myocardial ischemia in patients with so-called asymptomatic severe coronary artery disease.[38] Recently the term "si lent" or "asymptomatic" has been used to describe this painless ischemia,[35–37,39] but as this study demonstrates, there is both ECG and ventriculographic evidence of ischemia. Painless myocardial ischemia might be a more descriptive term for this syndrome as it is neither silent nor asymptomatic. The current study also demonstrates that in addition to antiarrhythmics, victims of sudden death may benefit from relief of myocardial ischemia with therapeutic agents such as nitroglycerin.

SUMMARY AND CONCLUSIONS

Out-of-hospital ventricular fibrillation (VF) is the leading cause of sudden cardiac death. In 15 survivors of out-of-hospital VF, left ventricular (LV) function was assessed, both at rest and during submaximal exercise, to determine if painless myocardial ischemia is a significant factor in the pathogenesis of out-of-hospital VF. Patients were divided into two groups on the basis of a history of angina and/or myocardial infarction: Group A patients were asymptomatic ($n = 9$) and Group S patients were symptomatic ($n = 6$). The results of submaximal exercise in patients in Groups A and S were compared with those obtained in 13 patients undergoing an identical exercise protocol, but with no history of sudden death, coronary disease, LV dysfunction, or conduction abnormality (Group C). Groups A and S had significant ($\geq$70% diameter stenosis) coronary artery disease. At catheterization no patient developed angina during exercise, but 12 of the 15 survivors developed or had increased ST-segment depression (Group A, 1.9 $\pm$ 1.4 mm; Group S, 1.1 $\pm$ 1.2 mm) and 11 of the 15 developed abnormal wall motion. From rest to exercise, Group S patients had increased LV end-diastolic pressure (21 ± 9 to 37 ± 11 mm Hg; $p < 0.01$) and volume (100 ± 25 to 107 ± 26 ml/m^2; $p < 0.01$) with no significant change in LV ejection fraction (from 40 ± 13 to 42 ± 12%; p = ns). Group A patients had increased LV end-diastolic pressure (from 19 ± 4 to 31 ± 8 mm Hg; $p < 0.001$), but no significant change in end-diastolic volume (from 83 ± 13 to 92 ± 23 ml/m^2; p = ns) and ejection fraction (from 55 ± 13 to 46 ± 13%; p = ns). Both Groups A and S showed a response to exercise statistically different from that of Group C. In addition after 150 ± 50 μg of sublingual nitroglycerin, six Group A patients had a second identical submaximal exercise period. Hemodynamic, ventriculographic, and ECG evidence of exercise-induced myocardial ischemia was significantly decreased following nitroglycerin. Thus, survivors of out-of-hospital VF, either with or without a history of angina and/or myocardial infarction, do have exercise-inducible evidence of painless myocardial ischemia. This painless ischemia may have a preeminent role in the pathogenesis of out-of-hospital ventricular fibrillation.

REFERENCES

1. Littré E: *Oeuvres completes d'Hippocrates. Traduction avec le texte grec.* Paris, Basilliere, 1861, vol 5, p 601.
2. Myerburg RJ: Sudden cardiac death: Epidemiology, causes, and mechanisms. *Cardiology* 1987;74 (suppl 2):2–9.
3. Lown B: Sudden cardiac death: The major challenge confronting contemporary cardiology. *Am J Cardiol* 1979;43:313–328.
4. Kuller L, Lilienfeld A, Fisher R: Epidemiologic study of sudden and unexpected death due to arteriosclerotic heart disease. *Circulation* 1966;34:1056–1068.
5. Liberthson RR, Nagel EL, Hirschman JC, et al: Pathophysiologic observations in prehospital ventricular fibrillation and sudden cardiac death. *Circulation* 1974;49:790–798.
6. Shurtieff D: Some characteristics related to the incidence of cardiovascular disease and death: Framingham Study; 18 year follow up, in Kannel WB, Gordon T (eds): *The Framingham Study. An Epidemiologic Investigation of Cardiovascular Disease, section 30.* Publication No. (NIH) 74–599. Bethesda, Maryland, Department of Health, Education, and Welfare, Public Health, 1974, pp 1–40.
5. Axelrod PJ, Verrier RL, Lown B: Vulnerability to ventricular fibrillation during acute coronary arterial occlusion and release. *Am J Cardiol* 1975;36:776–782.
6. Kannel WB, Doyle JT, McNamara PM, et al: Precursors of sudden death. Factors related to the incidence of sudden death. *Circulation* 1975;51:606–613.
9. Doyle JT, Kannel WB, McNamara PM, et al: Factors related to suddenness of death from coronary disease: Combined Albany-Framingham studies. *Am J. Cardiol* 1976;37:1073–1078.
10. Weaver WD, Lorch GS, Alvarez HA, et al: Angiographic findings and prognostic indicators in patients resuscitated from sudden cardiac death. *Circulation* 1976;54:895–900.
11. Bruce RA, Hossack KF, DeRouen TA, et al: Enhanced risk assessment for primary coronary heart disease events by maximal exercise testing: 10 years experience of Seattle Heart Watch. *J Am Coll Cardiol* 1983;2:565–573.
12. Kasser IS, Kennedy JW: Measurement of left ventricular volume by single plane cine angiography. *Invest Radiol* 1969;4:83–90.
13. Sharma B, Raina S, Goodwin JF, Raphael MJ, Steiner R: Stress ventriculography in coronary heart disease. A comparative assessment of left ventricular function and wall motion during angina induced by exercise and atrial pacing, in Lichtlen PR (ed): *Coronary Angiography and Angina Pectoris.* Stuttgart, George Theime, 1976, pp 133–151.
14. Sharma B, Goodwin JF, Raphael MJ, et al: Left ventricular angiography on exercise: A new method of assessing left ventricular function in ischemic heart disease. *Br Heart J* 1976;38:59–70.

15. Tennant R, Wiggers CJ: The effect of coronary occlusion on myocardial contraction. *Am J Physiol* 1935;112:351–361.
16. Tyberg JV, Yeatman LA, Parmley WW, et al: Effect of hypoxia on mechanics of cardiac contraction. *Am J Physiol* 1970;218:1780–1788.
17. Sonnenblick EH, Kirk ES: Effect of hypoxia and ischemia on myocardial contraction. Alteration in the time course of force and ischemia-dependent inhomogeneity of contractility. *Cardiology* 1971;56:302–313.
18. Amsterdam EA: Function of the hypoxic myocardium: Experimental and clinical aspects. *Am J Cardiol* 1973;32:461–471.
19. Dwyer EM: Left ventricular pressure-volume alterations and regional disorders of contraction during myocardial ischemia induced by atrial pacing. *Circulation* 1970;42:1111–1122.
20. Sharma B, Taylor SH: Reversible left ventricular failure in angina pectoris. *Lancet* 1970;2:902–906.
21. Pasternac A, Haft JI, Kemp HG, et al: Abnormalities of ventricular motion induced by atrial pacing in coronary artery disease. *Circulation* 1972;45:1195–1205.
22. Parker JO, Ledwich JR, West RO, et al: Reversible cardiac failure during angina pectoris. Hemodynamic effects of atrial pacing in coronary artery disease. *Circulation* 1969;39:745–757.
23. Sharma B, Hodges M, Asinger RW, et al: Left ventricular function during spontaneous angina pectoris: Effect of sublingual nitroglycerin. *Am J Cardiol* 1980;46:34–41.
24. Sharma B, Taylor SH: Localization of left ventricular ischemia in angina pectoris by cine angiography during exercise. *Br Heart J* 1975;37:963–970.
25. Sharma B, Behrens TW, Erlein D, et al: Left ventricular diastolic properties and filling characteristics during spontaneous angina pectoris at rest. *Am J Cardiol* 1983;52:704–709.
26. McCans JL, Parker JO: Left ventricular pressure-volume relationship during myocardial ischemia in man. *Circulation* 1973;48:775–785.
27. Mann T, Goldberg S, Mudge GH Jr, et al: Factors contributing to altered left ventricular diastolic properties during angina pectoris. *Circulation* 1979;59:14–20.
28. Salel AF, Berman DS, DeNardo GL, et al: Radionuclide assessment of nitroglycerine influence on abnormal left ventricular sequential contraction in patients with coronary heart disease. Assesment by radio nuclide cineangiography in symptomatic and asymptomatic patients. *Circulation* 1976;53:975–82.
29. Helfant RH, Pine R, Meiser SG, et al: Nitroglycerin to unmask reversible asynergy. Correlation with post coronary bypass ventriculography. *Circulation* 1977;50:108–13.
30. Borer JS, Bacharach SL, Green MV, et al: Effect of nitroglycerin on exercise induced abnormalities of left ventricular regional function and ejection fraction in coronary artery disease. *Circulation* 1978;57:314–20.
31. McGregor M: Pathogenesis of angina pectoris and role of nitrates in relief of myocardial ischemia. *Am J Med* 1983;74(6B):21–27.
32. Thadani U: Current status of nitrates in angina pectoris. *Mod Con Cardiovasc Dis* 1987;56:49–54.
33. Brown B, Bolson E, Peterson RB, et al: The mechanisms of nitroglycerin action: Stenosis vasodilitation as a major component of the drug response *Circulation* 1981;64:1089–1097.
34. Fitchett D: The effect of nitroglycerin on forearm arterial compliance. *Clin Invest Med* 1982;5 (Supp 1):31.
35. Thompson PL, Lowen B: Coronary occlusion before, during and after strenuous exercise. *Cardiovasc Res* 1976;10:385–388.
36. Schang SJ Jr, Pepine CJ: Transient asymptomatic ST segments depression during daily activity. *Am J Cardiol* 1977;39:396–402.
37. Vuori I, Makarainen M, Jaaskellainen A: Sudden death and physical activity. *Cardiology* 1978;63:287–304.
38. Sharma B, Mikell F, Hodges M, et al: Left ventricular function during exercise and following nitroglycerin in patients with acute recurrent pulmonary edema of clinically undefined etiology (abstract). *Am J Cardiol* 1979;43:427.
39. Cecchi AC,DoVellini EV, Marchi F, et al: Silent myocardial ischemia during ambulatory electrocardiographic monitoring in patients with effort angina. *J Am Coll Cardiol* 1983;1:934–939.

CHAPTER 17

Relation of Amount and Distribution of Coronary Arterial Narrowing in Sudden Coronary Death to Previous Symptoms of Myocardial Ischemia

Carole A. Warnes, MD and William C. Roberts, MD

We studied at necropsy 70 victims of sudden coronary death (SCD) to determine the amount and distribution of cross-sectional area (CSA) luminal narrowing in each 5-mm segment of the four major coronary arteries, and compared the amount of narrowing both qualitatively and quantitatively in those with and without previous clinical evidence of myocardial ischemia.

PATIENT STUDIES AND METHODS

All patients fulfilled the following criteria: (1) Death was known to have occurred within 6 hours of the previously witnessed usual state of health. (2) Although the patient may have died in a hospital, he/she was not a hospitalized patient at the onset of symptoms suggestive of myocardial ischemia. (3) At necropsy, one or more of the four major (left main [LM], left anterior descending [LAD], left circumflex [LC], and right) coronary arteries was narrowed 76 to 100 percent in CSA. (4) Ventricular myocardial coagulation necrosis was absent at necropsy. (5) A cause of death, cardiac or noncardiac, other than coronary artery disease was absent. (6) Chronic congestive heart failure had never been present. (7) A cardiovascular operation had never been performed. Review of clinical and necropsy records in the Pathology Branch, National Heart, Lung, and Blood Institute, yielded 63 men and 7 women aged 22 to 81 years (mean 50) fulfilling these criteria (Figure 17.1). Of the 70 victims, 46 died outside the hospital. The other 24 had chest pain outside the hospital and had fatal cardiac arrest shortly after being brought to the hospital. The intact formalin-fixed heart in all 70 patients was submitted for detailed examination. The clinical information was obtained from the hospital where the patient had been hospitalized previously and/or from the patient's private physician, and often surviving family members were contacted for additional information.

The hearts were fixed in formalin for 24 hours or more. The four major coronary arteries were excised intact, X-rayed, and decalcified if necessary. Each artery was

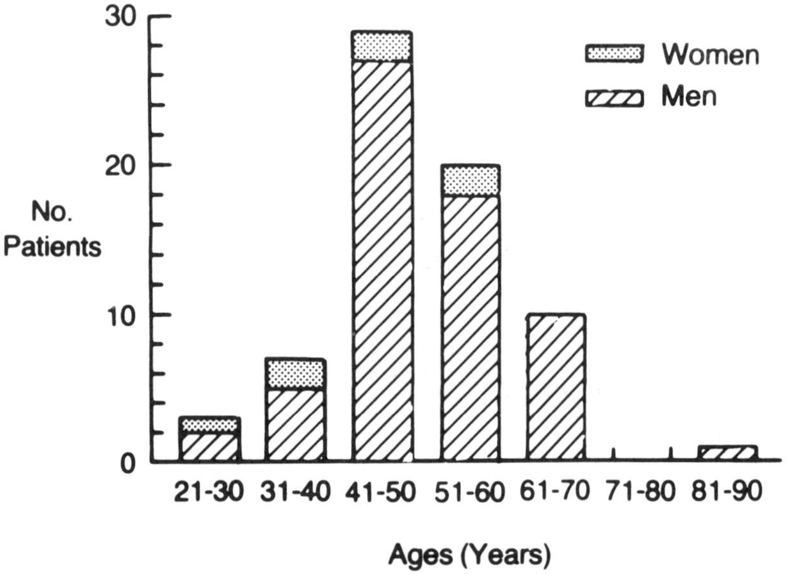

FIGURE 17.1. Age distribution in 70 patients with sudden coronary death.

then cut transversely into 5-mm segments and labeled sequentially, either from the aortic ostium or from its origin from the LM coronary artery. The segments were then dehydrated with alcohol and xylene and embedded in paraffin, and at least two histologic sections were cut from the paraffin block. Each histologic section was stained by the Movat technique.[1] The amount of luminal narrowing by atherosclerotic plaque was determined by visual inspection of these histologic sections when magnified 25 to 50 times. The percentage of CSA narrowing of each 5-mm segment was categorized into five groups: 0–25, 26–50, 51–75, 76–95, and 96–100. All sections were examined and the accuracy of the assessment of luminal narrowing was spot-checked by videoplanimetry. The agreement between these two techniques is approximately 95 percent.[2] A total of 3,484 5-mm segments from the 70 victims were examined (mean number of segments per patient was 50).

Chi square analysis was used to compare the amounts of coronary narrowing by quantitative means.

RESULTS

Qualitative Studies

Of the 70 patients, 11 (16%) had one major coronary artery narrowed 76 to 100 percent in CSA at some point, 19 (27%) had two arteries narrowed, 33 (47%) had three arteries narrowed, and 7 (10%) had four arteries narrowed. Of the 280 major epicardial coronary arteries in the 70 patients (four per patient), 176 (63%) were narrowed at some point 76 to 100 percent in CSA, a mean of 2.5 of 4.0 major coronary arteries per patient. Excluding the LM coronary artery, 167 (80%) of the other 210 major coronary arteries were narrowed 76 to 100 percent in CSA, an average of 2.4/3.0 coronary arteries per patient. Of the individual major coronary arteries, the LM was severely (76 to 100% in CSA) narrowed in 13 percent (9 of 70), the LAD in 86 percent (60 of 70), the LC in 74 percent, (52 of 70), and the right in 79 percent (55 of 70).

Comparison of the number of coronary arteries narrowed 76 to 100 percent CSA in the 39 previously asymptomatic patients to the 31 with previous acute myocardial infarction and/or angina pectoris disclosed the following (Figure 17.2): one major artery so narrowed in 8 (21%) versus 3 (10%) not significant (NS); two arteries in 11 (28%) versus 8 (26%) (NS); three arteries in 18 (46%) versus 15 (48%) (NS); and four arteries in 2 (5%) versus 5 (16%) (NS).

Comparison of the number of arteries narrowed 76 to 100 percent in CSA in the 39 patients without and the 31 with healed myocardial infarcts revealed the following (Figure 17.3): one major artery so narrowed in 9 (23%) versus 2 (7%) (NS); two arteries in 11 (28%) versus 8 (26%) (NS); three arteries in 13 (33%) versus 20 (64%) ($p < 0.02$); and four arteries in 6 (15%) versus 1 (3%) (NS).

Quantitative Studies

Analysis of the 3,484 5-mm coronary segments showed that 950 (27%) were narrowed 76 to 100 percent in CSA; 1,127 (32%), 51 to 75 percent; 689 (20%), 26 to 50 percent, and 718 (21%), 0 to 25 percent (Figure 17.4). The percentage of segments severely narrowed per patient, however, varied enormously, from 2 percent (1 of 50) to 88 percent (86 of 98). Sixteen patients had ≤10 percent of their 5-mm segments narrowed 76 to 100 percent in CSA; 15 patients had 11 to 20 percent of the segments so narrowed; 11 patients, 21 to 30 percent of the segments; 16 patients, 31 to 40 percent of the segments; 7 patients, 41 to 50 percent of the segments; 2 patients, 51 to 60 percent of the segments; 2 patients, 61 to 70 percent of the segments; and 1 patient had 81 to 90 percent of the segments so narrowed. The five categories of narrowing in each of the four major epicardial coronary arteries also

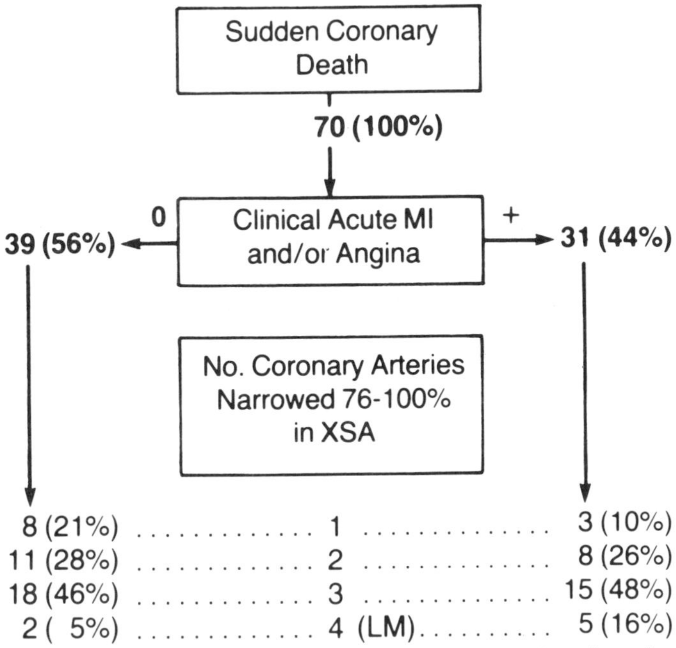

FIGURE 17.2. Qualitative comparison between the 39 previously asymptomatic patients and the 31 who experienced clinical acute myocardial infarction (MI) and/or angina pectoris before sudden coronary death. CSA = cross-sectional area; LM = left main coronary artery.

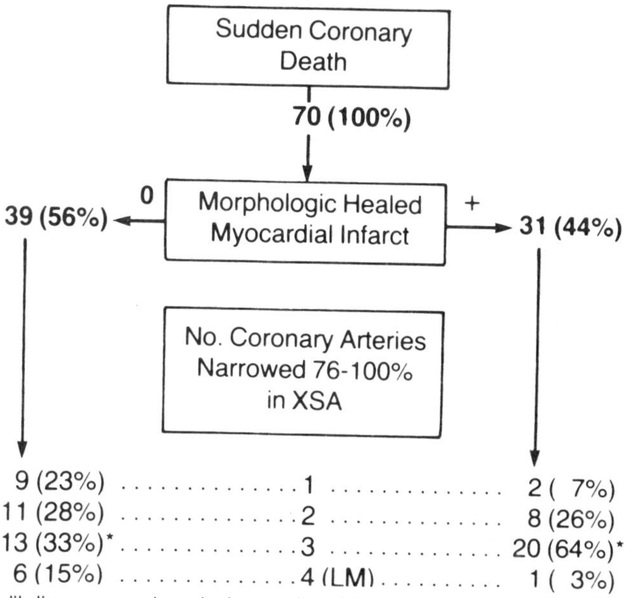

FIGURE 17.3. Qualitative comparison between the 39 patients who had no healed myocardial infarct at necropsy and the 31 who had a left ventricular scar. LM = left main coronary artery; XSA = cross-sectional area. *p < 0.02.

is shown in Figure 17.4. Comparison of the mean percentage of 5-mm segments narrowed 76 to 100 percent in CSA in the proximal and distal halves of the LAD, LC, and right coronary arteries disclosed a significantly higher percentage of severely narrowed segments proximally in the LAD and LC arteries. A similar distribution

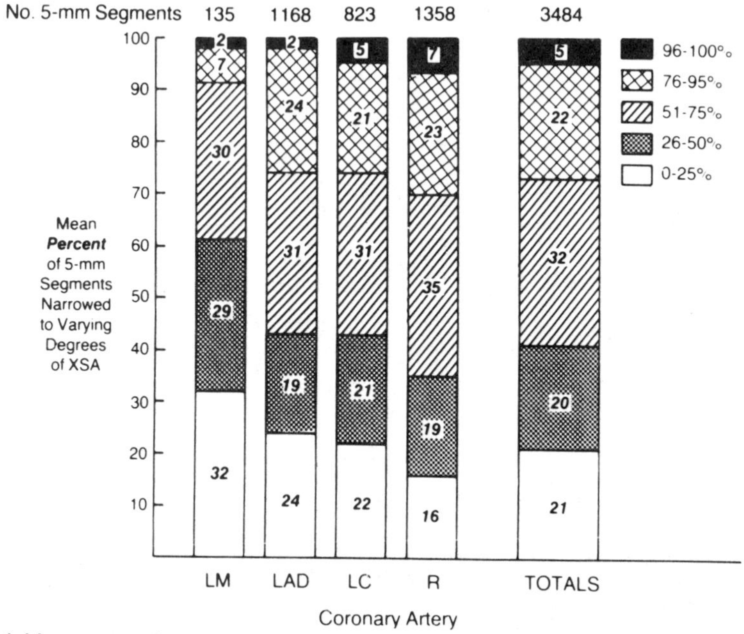

FIGURE 17.4. Mean percentages of 5-mm segments of the four major coronary arteries narrowed to varying degrees in cross-sectional area (CSA) in 70 patients with sudden coronary death. LAD = left anterior descending; LC = left circumflex; LM = left main; R = right.

of severe narrowing in the proximal and distal halves of these three arteries also was observed in patients with and without previous symptoms of myocardial ischemia and in patients with and without healed myocardial infarcts.

Among the 39 patients who had been asymptomatic, 502 (25%) of 1,991 5-mm segments were narrowed 76 to 100 percent in CSA compared to 448 (30%) of 1,493 5-mm segments in the 31 patients who had previously had clinical acute myocardial infarction or angina pectoris or both ($p < 0.005$) (Figure 17.5). Comparison of the mean percentages of segments in all five categories of CSA coronary narrowing between the previously asymptomatic and symptomatic groups disclosed significant differences in the category of minimal (0 to 25%) XSA narrowing (25% vs 15%, $p < 0.001$). Comparison of the amounts of narrowing in each of the four major coronary arteries disclosed a higher mean percentage of 5-mm segments narrowed 76 to 100 percent in CSA in symptomatic versus asymptomatic victims in the LM, LAD, and LC arteries but not in the right coronary artery, and a lower mean percentage of segments narrowed 0 to 25 percent in CSA in all four coronary arteries in the symptomatic group.

Comparison of the mean percentages of 5-mm segments in the five categories of narrowing between the 31 patients with and the 39 patients without left ventricular scars disclosed a higher mean percentage of segments narrowed 76 to 100 percent in the group with healed myocardial infarcts (33% vs 24%, $p < 0.001$) and a lower mean percentage of segments narrowed 0 to 25 percent (13% vs 26%, $p < 0.001$) than that of patients without healed myocardial infarcts (Figure 17.6). A higher mean percentage of 5-mm segments was minimally narrowed in those without healed infarcts and a higher mean percentage of segments was severely (76 to 100%) narrowed when a healed infarct was present. However, severe narrowing of the LM coronary artery occurred more frequently in those without healed infarcts.

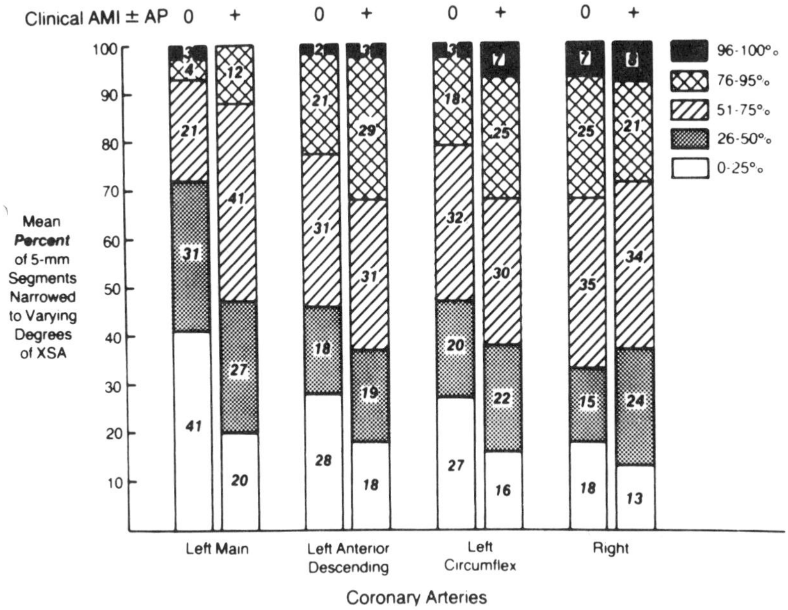

FIGURE 17.5. Mean percentages of 5-mm segments of the sum of the four major coronary arteries narrowed to varying degrees in cross-sectional area (CSA) in 70 patients with sudden coronary death. Comparison of 39 patients without and 31 patients with clinical acute myocardial infarcts and/or angina.

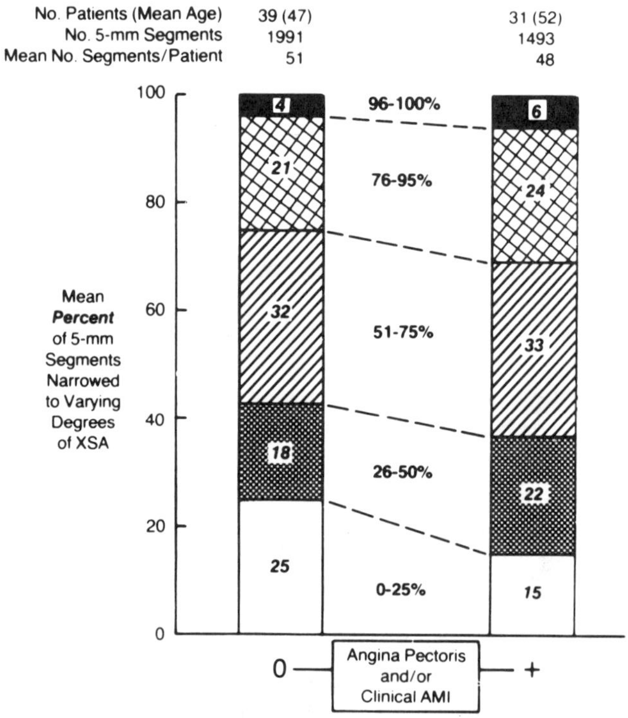

FIGURE 17.6. Mean percentages of 5-mm segments of the sum of the four major coronary arteries narrowed to varying degrees in cross-sectional area (CSA) in 70 patients with sudden coronary death: comparison of 39 patients without and 31 with a morphologic healed myocardial infarct (MI).

Of the 70 patients, 13 at necropsy had a thrombus in one coronary artery. In six patients, the thrombus consisted primarily of fibrin and erythrocytes, and in seven patients, nearly entirely of platelets. In all 13 patients, the thrombi were superimposed on atherosclerotic plaques that had already narrowed the lumina 26 to 50 percent (one patient), 51 to 75 percent (four patients), or 76 to 100 percent (eight patients) in CSA.

DISCUSSION

A major finding in our study was that sudden death victims had severe and extensive narrowing of the four major (LM, LAD, LC, and right) extramural coronary arteries by atherosclerotic plaque. Of the 70 patients, 59 (84%) had at least two major arteries narrowed to 76 to 100 percent in XSA and 11 (16%) had only one artery so narrowed by atherosclerotic plaque. Among the 59 patients with multivessel CAD, two arteries were severely (76 to 100% in CSA) narrowed in 19 patients (27%), three arteries in 33 patients (47%), and four arteries in 7 patients (10%). Of the four major coronary arteries per patient, 2.5 of 4 were severely narrowed. Of the 280 major coronary arteries in the 70 patients, 176 (63%) were narrowed severely, and of them the LAD was the most frequently (60 of 70 = 86%) narrowed artery. The 11 patients with one-vessel CAD (one artery narrowed 76 to 100% in CSA) were significantly younger than the 59 patients with multivessel CAD (mean age 41 vs 51 years). The severely narrowed artery in these 11 patients was the LAD in five, right in four, LC in one, and LM in one.

Qualitative studies describing, from gross inspection, the number of severely narrowed four major coronary arteries in nontraumatic sudden death victims have been performed by others.[3-7] Of the 720 necropsy subjects included in five studies, 499 (69%) had two or more major coronary arteries narrowed severely and 132 (18%) had only one coronary artery so narrowed. One difficulty in comparing any of these five previous necropsy studies with the present one is the varying criteria for inclusion of cases. To be included in our study, a patient had to have at least one of the four major coronary arteries narrowed 76 to 100 percent in CSA by atherosclerotic plaque. In the five previously reported studies, however, 89 (12%) of the 720 patients had none of the four coronary arteries narrowed to this extent; all apparently had at least one artery narrowed 51 to 75 percent in CSA. Another major problem in comparing our findings with those of previously reported studies concerns different temporal definitions of the term "sudden." We used a time period of 6 hours or less from the time of previously witnessed usual health to death, whereas Kuller and associates[3] and Friedman and colleagues[4] used a time period of less than 24 hours in their studies. The time frame used in the other three studies was not defined.[5-7] Our study also included only patients without histologic evidence of left ventricular myocardial coagulation necrosis, whereas 126 (18%) of the 720 patients included in the five previous studies cited had acute myocardial infarcts at necropsy.

Although four of the five previously reported studies mentioned the number and percentage of patients with previous clinical evidence of heart disease and with left ventricular scars at necropsy, none compared the amount of coronary narrowing in the groups with and without clinical evidence of myocardial ischemia or in the groups with and without left ventricular scars. We found the number of coronary arteries to be severely narrowed at some point (the qualitative approach) in patients with and without previous angina pectoris and/or myocardial infarction and in those with and without grossly visible left ventricular scars at necropsy to be roughly similar. Of our 70 patients, 31 (44%) had had clinical acute myocardial infarction (which healed), angina, or both and 39 did not. Comparison of those with and those without previous clinical evidence of myocardial ischemia disclosed similar percentages of total coronary arteries (four per patient) severely narrowed (84 of 124 [68%] vs 92 of 156 [59%]) and roughly similar percentages of two or more coronary arteries severely narrowed (28 of 31 [90%] vs 31 of 39 [79%]). Comparison of the 31 patients with and the 39 without left ventricular scars disclosed similar percentages of total coronary arteries severely narrowed (82 of 124 [66%] vs 94 of 156 [60%]) and similar percentages of two or more coronary arteries severely narrowed (29 of 31 [94%] vs 30 of 39 [77%]).

Cardiomegaly (heart weight >400 g) is frequently found at necropsy after sudden death from coronary artery disease. Of the 64 patients studied by Kuller and associates,[3] 37 (58%) had hearts weighing more than 450 g. Of the 208 victims studied by Baroldi and colleagues,[7] 157 (75%) had hearts weighing more than 400 g. In the 220 patients studied by Liberthson et al,[5] the mean heart weight for 190 men was 460 g, and for 30 women, 374 g. Only one of these necropsy studies[7] correlated the number of severely narrowed coronary arteries and heart weight. Comparison of our 35 patients with the 35 patients whose hearts weighed less than 450 g disclosed similar percentages of total coronary arteries severely narrowed (89 of 140 [64%] vs 87 of 140 [62%]) and similar percentages of two or more coronary arteries severely narrowed (30 of 35 [86%] vs 29 of 35 [83%]).

None of the previously reported five necropsy studies[3-7] provided quantitative information on the amount and distribution of coronary narrowing in sudden death victims. In our study of 70 patients, a total of 3,484 5-mm segments were examined; 27 percent of the segments were narrowed 76 to 100 percent in CSA, including 5 percent that were narrowed 96 to 100 percent. The 96 to 100 percent CSA narrowing is probably equivalent to angiographic total occlusion. Not a single 5-mm segment was entirely free of atherosclerotic plaque. A higher mean percentage of segments was severely narrowed in the proximal than in the distal halves of the three (LAD, LC, and right) major coronary arteries. A previous report from this laboratory,[8] which included 12 of the 70 patients in the present study, also emphasized the diffuse extent of atherosclerosis in sudden death victims. Although a control group was not included in the present study, a previous study[8] included 25 control subjects (mean age 49 years), and only 3 percent of the 5-mm segments of the four major coronary arteries were narrowed 76 to 100 percent in CSA by atherosclerotic plaque.

Of our 39 patients with no previous clinical evidence of myocardial ischemia (asymptomatic group), 25 percent of 5-mm segments were narrowed 76 to 100 percent in CSA compared with 30 percent in those who had had symptoms of ischemia (acute infarcts that healed and/or angina pectoris) ($p < 0.05$). The asymptomatic group also had a higher mean percentage of segments minimally narrowed (25% vs 15%, $p < 0.001$).

Similar differences were apparent in the quantitative comparisons between victims who had healed myocardial infarcts at necropsy and those who did not. More 5-mm segments were narrowed 76 to 100 percent in those with than in those without a left ventricular scar (33% vs 24%, $p < 0.001$); fewer 5-mm segments were minimally narrowed in those with than in those without healed infarcts (13% vs 26%, $p < 0.001$). Although a higher percentage of 5-mm segments from the sum of all four major coronary arteries were severely narrowed in patients with than in those without healed infarcts, analysis of the individual arteries disclosed that the LM coronary artery was different from the other three. In the 31 patients with healed infarcts, only 4 percent of the 57 5-mm segments of LM were severely narrowed; in contrast, in the 39 patients without healed infarcts, 12 percent of the 78 5-mm segments were severely narrowed.

Although our study patients as a group had severe and extensive coronary narrowing by atherosclerotic plaque, considerable variation in the percentage of 5-mm segments narrowed severely was observed. The range was 2 to 86 percent: 16 patients (23%) had less than 10 percent of their coronary segments narrowed 76 to 100 percent in CSA and 12 patients (17%) had more than 40 percent of their 5-mm segments severely narrowed. Thus, the extent of severe narrowing is difficult to predict in the individual patient, but it is predictable in groups of patients dying suddenly from coronary artery disease. The previously symptomatic patients clearly had more severe narrowing and less minimal narrowing than did the asymptomatic group, as did patients with healed myocardial infarcts.

REFERENCES

1. Movat HZ: Demonstration of all connective tissue elements in a single section. Pentachrome stains. *Arch Pathol* 1955;60:289–295.
2. Isner J, Wu M, Virmani R, Jones AA, Roberts WC: Comparison of degrees of coronary arterial luminal narrowing determined by visual inspection of histologic sections under magnification among three independent observers and comparison to that obtained by vid-

eoplanimetry. An analysis of 559 five-millimeter segments of 61 coronary arteries from eleven patients. *Lab Invest* 1980;42:566–570.
3. Kuller L, Cooper M, Perper J: Epidemiology of sudden death. *Arch Intern Med* 1972;129:714–719.
4. Friedman M, Manwaring JH, Rosenman RH, Donlon G, Ortega P, Grube SM: Instantaneous and sudden deaths. Clinical and pathological differentiation in coronary artery disease. *JAMA* 1973;225:1319–1328.
5. Liberthson RR, Nagel EL, Hirschman JC, Nussenfeld SR, Blackbourn BD, Davis JR: Pathophysiologic observations in prehospital ventricular fibrillation and sudden cardiac death. *Circulation* 1974;49:790–798.
6. Perper JA, Kuller LH, Cooper M: Arteriosclerosis of coronary arteries in sudden, unexpected deaths. *Circulation* 1975;51 and 52 (Suppl III):III-27–III-33.
7. Baroldi G, Falzi G, Mariani F. Sudden coronary death. A postmortem study in 208 selected cases compared to 97 "control" subjects. *Am Heart J* 1979;98:20–31.
8. Roberts WC, Jones AA: Quantitation of coronary arterial narrowing at necropsy in sudden coronary death. Analysis of 31 patients and comparison with 25 control subjects. *Am J Cardiol* 1979;44:39–45.

CHAPTER 18

Design of Studies to Critically Evaluate If Detection of Asymptomatic ST-Segment Deviation (Silent Ischemia) is of Medical or Public Health Importance

Salim Yusuf, MBBS, D Phil

In the last few years there has been growing interest in the phenomenon termed "silent ischemia." By this term investigators usually refer to "silent electrocardiographic abnormalities" (SEA) that are presumed to reflect underlying myocardial ischemia. This chapter will briefly review the literature to distinguish those aspects that are well supported by good data from those that are reasonable extrapolations. I shall then outline what further information is desirable and how studies to obtain this information can be designed.

OVERVIEW OF CURRENT WELL-ESTABLISHED FACTS AND REASONABLE EXTRAPOLATIONS

The following facts are reasonably well founded and established. Myocardial ischemia may or may not be associated with anginal pain.[2] In some patients, asymptomatic episodes of ischemia may be more frequent than episodes of angina, and the precipitating factors may be different (eg, the former tends to occur at relatively normal heart rates and the latter is usually associated with increased heart rate). At least one study has demonstrated a clear relation between both provoked and spontaneous ST-segment depression, whether painful or painless, and more sophisticated measures of reversible regional myocardial ischemia. Several studies have documented the close association between symptomatic and asymptomatic exercise-induced ST-segment abnormalities and other objective indexes of ischemia.

On the basis of these well-established facts, several reasonable extrapolations can be made. First, detecting spontaneous silent ECG abnormalities by ambulatory ECG monitoring is important because these abnormalities are associated with a high risk of myocardial infarction (MI) or cardiac death. These patients can only be identified by ambulatory monitoring. Treatment can then be focused specifically on these patients and unnecessary treatment avoided in others, thereby improving the prognosis of individuals and the community. If these tests truly did have a high degree of sensitivity, specificity, and adequate additional predictive value, we would have a remarkably cost-effective tool. This argument implies that we either have or are likely to have, in the foreseeable future, interventions that improve prognosis, prevent morbidity, and are specifically applicable only to these individuals and not to others. Moreover, because episodes of SEA are infrequent, prolonged monitoring may be necessary to detect all (or nearly all) these patients, without an appreciable loss of specificity.

Subsequent sections will examine: (1) the additional prognostic value of detecting SEA separately in normal individuals and subjects who have overt coronary artery disease (CAD); (2) whether the additional knowledge of the presence or absence of SEA favorably alters patient management or reduces costs; and (3) what the optimal duration of monitoring should be.

PROGNOSTIC VALUE OF DETECTING UNPROVOKED SILENT ELECTROCARDIOGRAPHIC ABNORMALITIES

The cornerstone of the evidence linking SEA to myocardial ischemia is the careful work by Deanfield et al.[1] These investigators studied the regional uptake of rubidium-82 in ischemic and nonischemic myocardium in 30 patients with severe angina and extensive coronary artery disease (CAD). During exercise, after cold pressor tests, and during unprovoked episodes of ECG abnormalities there was tomographic evidence of ischemia confined to segments that corresponded to the regions of ECG abnormalities. Moreover, tomographic evidence of ischemia was present whether or not angina occurred (eg, tomographic evidence of ischemia was present in 63 of 65 episodes associated with angina and during all 30 episodes of SEA). The patients in this study had angina an average of 6.5 years, had 18 attacks of angina per week, 26 of 30 had three-vessel disease or left main coronary artery disease, and two thirds had occlusion of at least one coronary artery. Based on this study we can be reasonably confident that in patients with clinically *severe* ischemia and extensive CAD, SEA are associated with other objective evidence of myocardial ischemia.

It is not clear, however, if the data obtained in such a select group can be extrapolated and applied to individuals with milder overt CAD or to apparently normal individuals. Until similar data are obtained in these populations, extreme caution should be used in assuming that all or a high proportion of individuals with detected SEA have ischemia and are consequently at high risk. Table 18.1 (adapted from Rozanski and Berman[2,3] 1987) summarizes the information from seven studies in normal individuals.[2–11] Electrocardiographic abnormalities, which might be called "ischemic," occurred in 48 of 367 individuals (13%). Twenty-eight percent of 74 individuals documented to have normal coronary arteries also demonstrated SEA. Although questions about the appropriateness of these "normal" subjects can be raised, an appreciable proportion of these SEA likely represent false-positive test results. These data lead to the obvious question about the specificity of SEA on ambulatory Holter monitoring in relation to reliable evidence of ischemia and the prediction of adverse clinical outcomes among individuals with little or no symptoms.

Limited data relating the prognostic significance of continuous ST-segment monitoring in patients with unstable angina are available in three relatively small studies[12–14] (Table 18.2). Two of these studies were retrospective analyses of data

Table 18.1. Frequency of ST-Segment Depression During Ambulatory Monitoring in Normal Subjects*

	Subjects (n)	Percentage
A. Catheterized Individuals		
Stern et al,[4] 1975	3/17	18
Crawford et al,[5] 1978	12/31	39
Quyyumi et al,[6] 1985	6/26	23
Subtotal	21/74	28
B. Volunteers		
Allen et al,[7] 1976	0/5	0
Armstrong et al,[8] 1982	15/50	30
Tanake and Goto,[9] 1983	0/18	0
Quyyumi et al,[10] 1983	10/120	8
Deanfield et al,[11] 1984	2/100	2
Subtotal	27/293	9

*Adapted from Rozanski and Berman[2] (1987).

collected primarily for other purposes, and the third was prospectively designed.[12,13] In the latter study,[14] clinical decisions were made by physicians unaware of the information on the Holter tapes, and the tapes were read without knowledge of the patients' clinical complications. These studies complement each other, and all consistently demonstrate a higher incidence of subsequent myocardial infarction or death (a four- to sevenfold higher risk) and more frequent surgery or angioplasty (two to four times) in those with ST-segment abnormalities. These data suggest that the presence of SEA is associated with a poorer prognosis and more aggressive patient management. It is not clear, however, whether SEA was an incremental prognostic factor that provided information not already available to the physicians (eg, a history of more frequent, prolonged, and severe chest pain at rest or information available from clinical examination or marked abnormalities on the resting ECG). Although coronary artery bypass graft (CABG) surgery and percutaneous transluminal coronary angioplasty (PTCA) were more frequent, the decisions in these studies were based on information that did not include SEA. Therefore, it is not clear if knowledge of

Table 18.2. Prognostic Importance of Continuous ST-Segment Monitoring in Patients with Unstable Angina

	MI or Deaths/ No. of Patients		CABG or PTCA/ No. of Patients	
Studies	ST-Segment Abnormal	ST-Segment Normal	ST-Segment Abnormal	ST-Segment Normal
Johnson et al,[12] 1982	3/21 (14%)	3/67 (5%)	9/21 (43%)	7/67 (10%)
Gottlieb et al,[13] 1986	6/37 (16%)	1/33 (3%)	10/37 (27%)	6/33 (18%)
Nademanee et al,[14] 1987	5/18 (28%)	1/29 (3%)	12/18 (67%)	3/29 (10%)
Total	14/76 (18.4%)	5/129 (3.9%)	22/76 (30%)	16/129 (12.4%)
Relative risk	4.7		2.4	

ABBREVIATIONS: CABG = coronary artery bypass grafts; MI = myocardial infarction; PTCA = percutaneous transluminal coronary angioplasty.

SEA will lead to further changes in the management of patients with unstable angina or if such changes will lead to improved patient prognosis.

Some studies have evaluated the prognostic importance of spontaneous SEA on Holter monitoring in unstable angina; however, there are no similar studies in patients with less severe angina or in normal individuals. However, there is substantial literature on the prognostic importance of ST-segment depression provoked by an exercise test in normal individuals and in those with angina or MI. Crawford et al[5] showed that in patients with stable angina pectoris, the sensitivity and specificity of ST-segment depression detected during an exercise test and during ambulatory monitoring are similar to those in detecting CAD. (In fact, in this study exercise tests were about 5 percent more sensitive and about 15 percent more specific.)[5] Others have demonstrated that Holter and standard ECG recordings obtained simultaneously during an exercise test detect similar degrees of ST-segment deviation equally reliably.[15] Therefore, given the lack of data relating SEA on Holter monitoring to prognosis, I shall turn to data from exercise tests to estimate the prognostic importance of SEA in asymptomatic individuals and in those following MI.

PROGNOSTIC VALUE OF EXERCISE-INDUCED ECG ABNORMALITIES IN NORMAL INDIVIDUALS AND THOSE WITH MYOCARDIAL INFARCTION

Table 18.3 summarizes the outcome in about 26,000 normal individuals with positive and negative exercise test results (ET) in 14 studies.[2,3,16,17] Overall, 221 of 2,950 (7.5%) with positive ET results had MI or died compared with 416 of 22,955 (1.8%) with normal ET results. Although these figures represent a 4.2-fold excess risk among those with positive ET results, twice as many events occurred in those with negative test results. Consequently, the sensitivity of the test is 37 percent, its specificity is 69 percent, and a positive test result has a predictive value of only 7.5 percent in this population. Similar data in patients after MI are presented in Table 18.4. Although an abnormal ET was associated with a 1.8-fold excess risk of MI and death, (74 of 396 [18.7%] with positive ET results and 125 of 1,193 [10.5%] with normal ET results), more events occurred in those with normal test results. These collective data indicate only a 37 percent sensitivity, a 77 percent specificity, and about a 19 percent predictive value for positive test results. Table 18.5 presents data separately

Table 18.3. Cardiac Events Among "Normal" Subjects Based on Exercise Test Results*

Studies	Exercise Test Results: Positive	Exercise Test Results: Negative	Risk Ratio	p Value
1. Rozanski & Berman,[2,3] 1987 (12 studies; follow-up 3 to 13 yr; all cardiac events)	151/1,034 (14.6%)	247/9,078 (2.7%)	5.4	0.001
2. MRFIT,[16] 1985 (Cardiac deaths; 7 yr)	49/1,601 (3.1%)	123/10,417 (1.2%)	2.6	0.001
3. LRC-CPPT,[17] 1988 (CHD deaths; 7.4 yrs)	21/315 (6.7%)	46/3,460 (1.3%)	5.1	0.001
Total	221/2,950 (7.5%)	416/22,955 (1.8%)	4.2	0.001

* Sensitivity = 37%; specificity = 89%; predictive value = 7.5%.

Table 18.4. Prognostic Significance of Exercise-Induced ST-Segment Depression Before Hospital Discharge After Myocardial Infarction*

Reference	No. of Cardiac Deaths or Reinfarction/No. of Patients (ST ≥ 0.1 mV) Yes	No	Ratio of Percentages	p Value
Kaku et al,[19] 1978	0/14	3/31	0.3	NS
Theroux et al,[26] 1979	16/64	2/146	19.7	<0.05
Smith et al,[24] 1979	6/20	2/42	7.3	<0.05
Sami et al,[23] 1979	6/18	8/67	3.6	NS
Starling et al,[22] 1980	10/42	12/88	2.0	NS
Srinivasan et al,[25] 1981	6/18	7/136	9.0	<0.05
Weld et al,[21] 1981	10/53	21/183	1.9	NS
Krone et al,[20] 1985	20/167	70/500	0.9	NS
Total	74/396	125/1193	1.8	<0.001

* Sensitivity = 37%; specificity = 77%; predictive value = 18.7%.

for MI and cardiac death and indicates interestingly that a positive ET result is strongly associated with a higher risk of cardiac death ($p < 0.0001$), whereas there is only a weak and marginally significant association with subsequent MI ($p < 0.05$).

These data, however, do not address whether a positive ET result confers additional prognostic information that is not available from other sources. Tibbits et al[27] in a study of patients after acute MI found that an ET did not provide incremental prognostic information when compared with simple clinical parameters and ejection fraction (Figure 18.1). In this study a positive ET result was not even a univariate predictor of outcome; therefore, lack of incremental prognostic significance of the ET is not necessarily surprising or informative. Therefore, similar analyses of existing and future studies could clarify the incremental prognostic importance of a positive ET result.

The information just presented casts doubt on the prognostic importance of the ET when applied to an individual subject and reflects the common dilemma shared by a number of classical risk factors (such as cholesterol, blood pressure, and smoking habits): "*Powerful risk factors are not common; common risk factors are not powerful.*" For example, a risk factor that predicts with a high degree of certainty the outcome in an individual patient (eg, cardiogenic shock in MI patients or individuals with very high LDL cholesterol above the 99.9 percentile) is usually not common enough to be of value in predicting outcome in a group of such patients as individuals. (Most patients with MI who die do not have antecedent cardiogenic shock, and most individuals who develop MI have "normal" cholesterol levels.) Conversely, a common risk factor (eg, cigarette smoking) has only a low predictive value in an individual (eg, three of four deaths among smokers are due to unrelated causes).

These considerations make it reasonable to expect the distribution of varying degrees of ECG abnormalities (a more sensitive analysis than simply dichotomizing ECG abnormalities into normal or abnormal tests) to follow the theoretic curves in Figure 18.2 with substantial overlap of the "risk factor" (in this case, the degree of ECG abnormality) without sharp separation in those who do and those who do not develop a cardiovascular event. Unlike the conventional risk factors known to have a *causal* relationship with coronary heart disease (CHD) so that modification of these is likely to decrease CHD, there does not appear to be any rationale in *confining*

Table 18.5. Prognostic Significance of a Positive Exercise Test in (A) Asymptomatic Individuals with Coronary Risk Factors (MRFIT + LRC-CPTT) and in (B) Postmyocardial Infarction Patients Before Hospital Discharge* (Summarized from the Eight Studies in Table 18.4)

		Exercise Test Results		Relative	
		Positive	Negative	Risk	p Value
A.					
Recurrent MI	MRFIT[16] (Usual care)	31/734 (4.2%)	183/5.471 (3.3%)	1.25	NS
	LRC[17]	28/265 (10.6%)	259/3.460 (7.5%)	1.2	NS
Cardiac deaths	MRFIT[16] (Usual care)	40/734 (5.4%)	90/5.471 (1.7%)	3.25	<0.01
	LRC[17]	21/265	46/3.460	5.7	<0.001
B.					
Recurrent MI		26/299 (8.7%)	67/880 (7.6%)	1.14	NS
Cardiac deaths		48/396 (12.1%)	58/1193 (4.9%)	2.47	<0.001
Overall		74/396 (18.7%)	125/1193 (10.5%)	1.8	<0.001

* Adapted from Moss et al,[26] 1987.

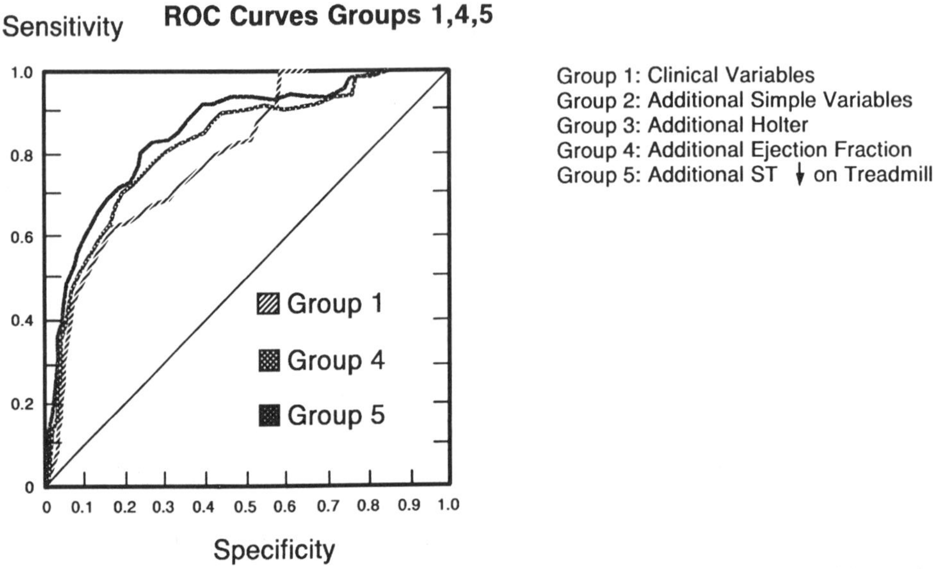

FIGURE 18.1. Sensitivity and specificity of the different variables in predicting one-year mortality acute myocardial infarction using receiver operator characteristic (ROC) curves. There is a significant increase in information by the addition of ejection fraction to the clinical variables. Note that ventricular arrhythmia recorded on a 24-hour Holter monitor did not provide additional information compared to clinical variables (not shown), nor did the results of ST-segment depression exercise testing (Group 5) when added to the clinical variables and ejection fraction. (From Tibbits et al[27] with the permission of the authors and the *American Journal of Cardiology*.)

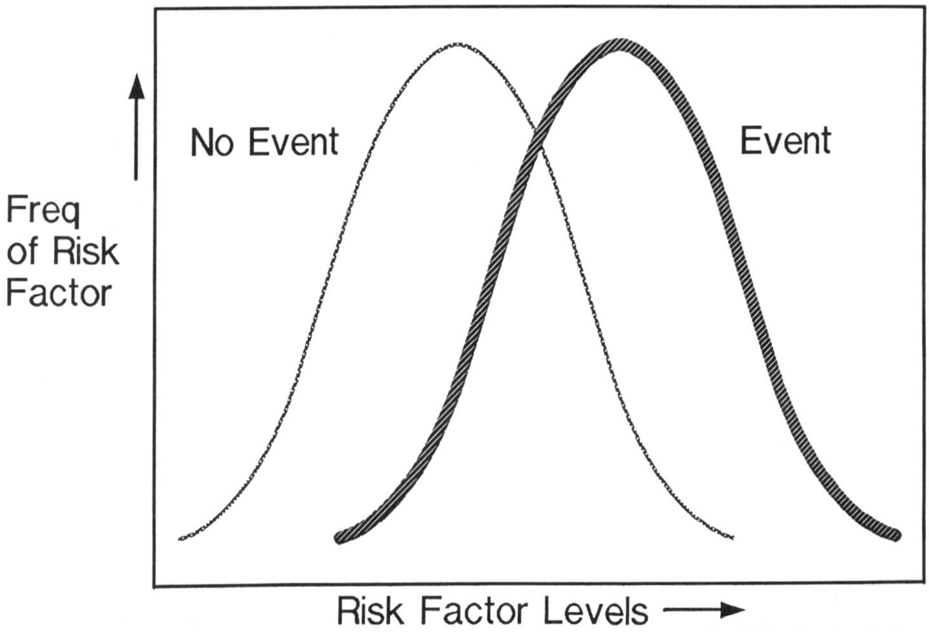

FIGURE 18.2. Theoretic demonstration of the frequency distribution of most risk factor levels (eg, cholesterol, blood pressure, and smoking) in individuals who suffer a particular event (MI, stroke, etc). Note the substantial overlap of the risk factors among those with and without an event. Consequently no particular "cut-point" can be used to precisely demarcate those who develop an event from those who do not. Extrapolating to SEA, it is therefore unlikely that ST-segment "abnormalities" will be highly predictive of those who will develop an adverse clinical outcome.

risk factor modification to those with a positive ET. Neither are there any current methods of preventing CHD specifically applicable only to such patients.

ISSUES IN ASSESSING THE OPTIMAL DURATION OF HOLTER RECORDINGS TO RELIABLY DETECT SEA

Because SEA is infrequent, it has been suggested that prolonged monitoring (eg, 72 hours) is required to detect nearly all patients with these ECG abnormalities. This suggestion is based on the study by Coy et al[28] who identified 11 asymptomatic individuals with ST-segment abnormality on ET and documented coronary artery disease. SEA was detected at the end of the first 24 hours of Holter recording in only about 65 percent of patients, by 48 hours in 75 percent, and by 72 hours in all patients (ie, increasing sensitivity with more prolonged recording). This study does not address whether increasing duration of recordings in "normal" individuals will lead to a progressive increase in the number of individuals who turn out to have "false-positive" results (ie, a decrease in specificity with an increase in the duration of recording). Table 18.2 suggests that a single 24-hour recording probably has about a 13 percent "false-positive rate," and it is possible that the number might be higher with more prolonged recordings.

This problem is illustrated by a study by Davis et al[29] who evaluated the prevalence, sensitivity, specificity, and predictive value of ventricular arrhythmia in relation to sudden death using different durations of recordings in patients after MI (Figure 18.3). With increasing duration of recording, the prevalence of arrhythmia and the sensitivity to predict sudden death increased. However, there was a concomitant decrease in specificity. Both the positive and negative predictive values were similar at 1, 2, 4, 6, 12, or 24 hours of recording. These data were confirmed by Coromilius et al (Personal Communication) using recordings from the Cardiac Arrhythmia Pilot Study. Therefore, in detecting SEA, careful evaluation of the optimal duration of recording requires that the sensitivity, specificity, and predictive value of different durations of recordings be compared in relatively unselected groups of normal subjects and those with CHD.

SUGGESTIONS FOR STUDY DESIGN TO EVALUATE THE INCREMENTAL PROGNOSTIC AND THERAPEUTIC IMPORTANCE OF DETECTING SILENT ECG ABNORMALITIES

Good General Methodology

Future studies should follow generally accepted principles that relate to careful and good scientific methods such as:

1. Formulation of questions or hypotheses in advance.
2. Prospective designs capable of addressing such questions or hypotheses.
3. Determining the adequate number of patients required for such studies.
4. Obtaining Holter tape recordings of optimal quality and duration. Because no such standards exist, it is reasonable to incorporate a convenient duration of recording such as 24 hours (unless a lot of resources are available) and then to assess the sensitivity, specificity, and predictive value of 1, 2, 4, 6, 12, or 24 hours of recording.

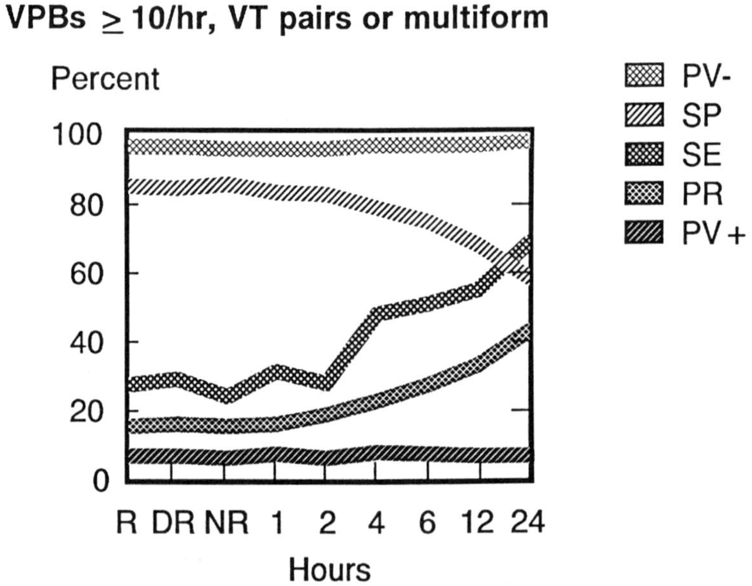

FIGURE 18.3. The positive and negative predictive values (PV+ and PV−), specificity (SP), sensitivity (SE), and prevalence (PR) of ventricular arrhythmia recorded on a Holter monitor during a random hour (R), daytime hour (DR), nighttime hour (NR), and during 1, 2, 4, 6, 12, and 24 consecutive hours in predicting sudden death. With increased duration of recording, the prevalence and sensitivity increase; however, specificity decreases, so that both the positive and negative predictive values are unchanged. Similar analyses of the duration of recording ST-segment deviation should be performed. It cannot be automatically assumed that longer duration of recording will be better. (From Davis et al[29] with the permission of the authors and the *American Heart Journal*.)

5. Unbiased analyses of the tape recordings in a uniform manner without knowledge of the patient's clinical status.
6. Unbiased ascertainment of clinical outcomes without knowledge of the results of the tape recordings. (This is only applicable in some designs, depending on the question. (Discussion will follow.)
7. Unbiased reporting of results, distinguishing the results of initially planned analysis from those that were data derived.

Suggested Design to Evaluate the Prognostic Significance of SEA on Ambulatory Monitoring in Apparently Healthy Individuals (Figure 18.4)

Individuals to be included are identified at random on the basis of screening from a population. Standard risk factors for CHD (eg, blood pressure, smoking history, cholesterol level, and fibrinogen) are then measured. Individuals are stratified into those with no, one, or several risk factors; ambulatory ECG recordings are obtained and analyzed for SEA. Several thousand individuals (5 or 10 thousand) are then followed for a sufficient period (about 10 years) so that several hundreds of events accrue. The independent and incremental contribution of SEA in predicting prognosis is then determined. This design can be modified to include exercise tests if the relative value of different methods of detecting SEA is to be compared. To be cost effective it might be appropriate to consider adding these tests to existing community studies.

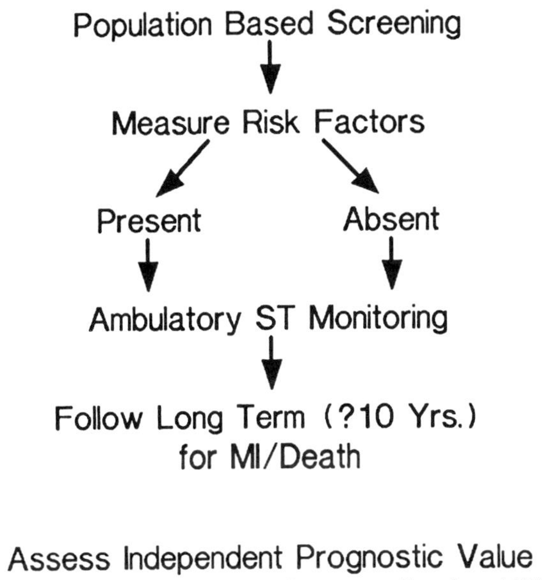

FIGURE 18.4. Suggested design for a study to assess the prognostic value of SEA in otherwise normal individuals.

Suggested Design to Assess the Prognostic and Therapeutic Importance of Detecting SEA in Patients with Clinical CAD (Figure 18.5)

The disease entity (stable angina, unstable angina, or MI) to be studied is initially defined. All consecutive patients with the particular disease are then enrolled. On the basis of available information (eg, clinical and other simple investigations) patients are stratified into two groups: one group in which the available information is thought to be adequate for patient management, and a second group in which the physician believes that additional information on SEA will be of value. Each stratum is then randomized into three groups: routine Holter monitoring, routine exercise

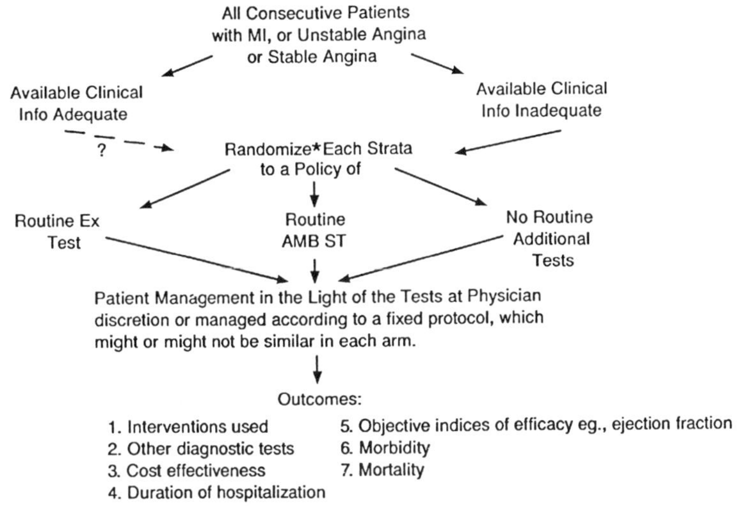

* Randomization could be further stratified by presence of ST segment deviation.

FIGURE 18.5. Suggested design to assess the prognostic and therapeutic importance of detecting asymptomatic ST-segment deviation in patients with classical COR ART disease.

test, and neither test performed routinely. (In some situations, such as unstable angina, it may not be possible to include a group randomized to ET.) Patients are then managed by the physicians to the best of their ability and judgment. The relation between SEA and clinical outcomes will be analyzed overall and separately in the initially defined strata. The outcomes of clinical interest in such a study could be more varied and could include more accurate prediction of prognosis, change in patient management in each stratum based on prior physician judgment (adequate or inadequate information from other sources), subsequent morbidity and mortality, or some objective measure of ventricular function. Additional outcomes could be the avoidance of other (and perhaps unnecessary) investigations, duration of hospital stay, cost effectiveness (balance of costs associated with the additional tests to detect SEA and costs associated with additional management versus costs saved by avoiding unnecessary investigations and treatment), and improvement in the quality of life of the patient (and physician!) due to reassurance. This design can be modified in a number of ways to take into account the prior training and level of expertise of the physician (more highly skilled clinicians might need fewer investigations) or the type of available hospital facilities (eg, ready access to the catheterization laboratory and cardiac surgery), which can all substantially influence how information on SEA is used. However, it is important in all analyses to evaluate the incremental contribution of knowledge about SEA in influencing outcomes. These designs can be modified to additionally evaluate the impact of a particular treatment (eg, CABG surgery) in patients with SEA. For example, patients with SEA are randomized to CABG surgery, PTCA, or medical treatment. A European collaborative group is conducting a similar study in post-MI patients with positive ET results. These patients are randomized to CABG surgery or medical treatment, and their long-term survival has been recorded since 1982. However, such studies, which include only patients with SEA, will be unable to distinguish whether intervention is effective only in those with SEA and without value in others or whether intervention is effective (or ineffective) in all patients irrespective of the presence or absence of SEA.

Because there are data to suggest that SEA has some prognostic value in patients with unstable angina, it would be useful to reanalyze the three completed studies to assess whether SEA provides incremental prognostic information in addition to other more readily available data. If this is the case, then it might be appropriate to conduct a study designed along the line of that just described in this group of patients. Such a study will probably require the randomization of about 2,500 patients into two groups (assuming a 10% incidence of MI or death, with 80% of these events occurring in those with ST-segment depression on a Holter monitor and this knowledge of SEA will lead to appropriate changes in management so that 30% of MIs or deaths will be prevented). However, this design may not be practicable for interventions that are already widely used in these patients (eg, PTCA or CABG surgery) and would be more suitable in evaluating new drugs, such as a new calcium antagonist.

Evaluating Whether an Intervention Should Specifically be Used Only in Patients with "Silent or "Overt" Ischemia (Figure 18.6)

Subjects are initially stratified according to the presence or absence of overt ischemia, SEA, a combination of both, or neither abnormality. (A particular study may have only two strata, the first two in patients with CAD and the last two in "normal"

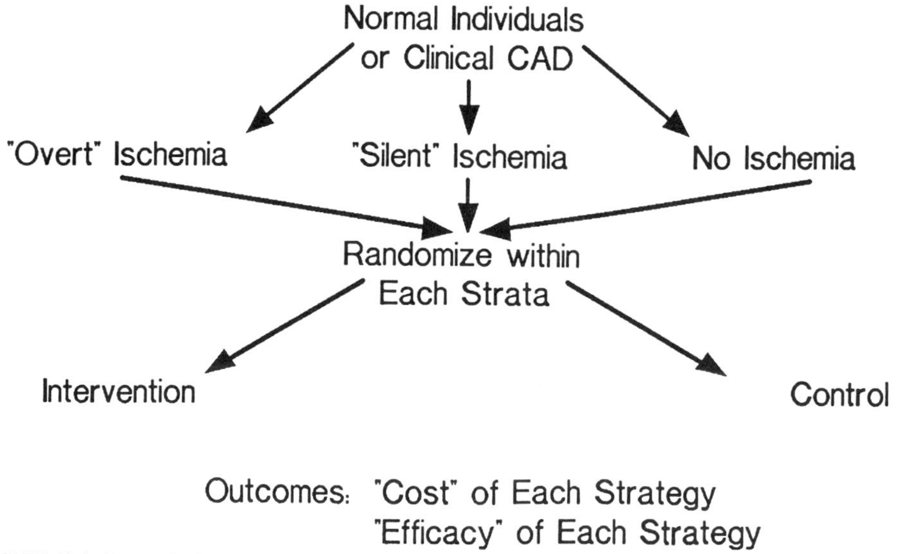

FIGURE 18.6. Suggested design for a study to assess whether an intervention should specifically be used in normal individuals or in those with "silent or "overt" ischemia.

individuals.) Each stratum is then randomized to an intervention or a control group. The outcome (cost and efficacy) of treatment is evaluated separately in each stratum. The two results are compared to assess whether the benefit observed in one stratum is significantly different from the benefit observed in the other. This is similar to the usual subgroup analyses in clinical trials, with the results being analyzed by statistical tests of interaction. An example of questions that might be addressed by such designs in patients with overt CAD involves a comparison of the value of an antiischemic agent that acts predominantly by increasing myocardial blood supply and another that is thought to act chiefly by decreasing myocardial oxygen demand. Such designs can also be used in asymptomatic subjects to compare the cost effectiveness of an expensive or inexpensive primary prevention strategy (intensive intervention in a few high-risk individuals versus mass low-cost strategy in all). The designs suggested in this section assume that the detection of SEA in normal individuals is of incremental prognostic value. Therefore, such studies are best conducted after this issue has been clarified by other studies described above.

CONCLUSIONS

Despite great interest in detecting SEA by Holter monitoring, there are few data to indicate its clinical usefulness or importance from a public health perspective. Unless large well-focused studies with appropriate designs are conducted, the true value of detecting SEA will not be known, and the field will continue, as present, to be dominated more by extrapolations and opinions than by facts.

REFERENCES

1. Deanfield JE, Shea M, Ribiero P, de Landsheere CM, Wilson RA, Horlock P, Selwyn AP: Transient ST-segment depression as a marker of myocardial ischemia during daily life. *Am J Cardiol* 1984;54:1195–1200.

2. Rozanski A, Berman DS: Silent myocardial ischemia: I Pathophysiology, frequency of occurrence and approaches toward detection. *Am Heart J* 1987;114:615–626.
3. Rozanski A, Berman DS: Silent myocardial ischemia: II Prognosis and implications for the clinical assessment of patients with coronary artery disease. *Am Heart J* 1987;114:627–638.
4. Stern S, Tzivoni D, Stern Z: Diagnostic accuracy of ambulatory ECG monitoring in ischemic heart disease. *Circulation* 1975;52:1045–1049.
5. Crawford NH, Mendoza CA, O'Rourke RA, White DH, Boucher CA, Gorwit J: Limitations of continuous ambulatory electrocardiogram monitoring for detecting coronary artery disease. *Ann Int Med* 1978;89:1–5.
6. Quyyumi AA, Mockus l, Wright C, Fox KM: Morphology of ambulatory ST-segment changes in patients with varying severity of coronary artery disease: Investigation of the frequency of nocturnal ischemia and coronary spasm. *Br Heart J* 1985;53:186–193.
7. Allen RD, Gettes LS, Phalan C, Avington ND: Painless ST-segment depression in patients with angina pectoris: Correlation with daily activities and cigarette smoking. *Chest* 1976;69:467–473.
8. Armstrong WF, Jordan JW, Morris SN, McHenry PL: Prevalence and magnitude of ST-segment and T wave abnormalities in normal men during continuous ambulatory electrocardiography. *Am J Cardiol* 1982;49:1636–1642.
9. Tanake T, Goto Y: Unstable angina pectoris—changes in the ST-segment during daily activities such as bathing, eating, defecating and urinating. *Jpn Circ J* 1983;47:451–458.
10. Quyyumi AA, Wright C, Fox K: Ambulatory electrocardiographic ST-segment changes in healthy volunteers. *Br Heart J* 1983;50:460–464.
11. Deanfield JE, Ribiero P, Oakley K, Krikler S, Selwyn AP: Analysis of ST-segment changes in normal subjects: Implications for ambulatory monitoring in angina pectoris: *Am J Cardiol* 1984;54:1321–1325.
12. Johnson SM, Mauritson DR, Winniford MD, Willerson JT, Firth BG, Cary JR, Hillis DL: Continuous electrocardiographic monitoring in patients with unstable angina pectoris: Identification of high risk subgroup with severe coronary disease, variant angina, and/or impaired early prognosis. *Am Heart J* 1982;103:4–12.
13. Gottlieb SO, Weisfeldt ML, Ouyang P, Mellits DE, Gerstenblith G: Silent ischemia as a marker for early unfavorable outcomes with unstable angina. *N Engl J Med* 1986;314:1214–1219.
14. Nademanee K, Intarachot V, Josephson MA, Rieders D, Mody Vaghaiwalla F, Singh BN: Prognostic significance of silent myocardial ischemia in patients with unstable angina. *J Am Coll Cardiol* 1987;10:1–9.
15. Tzivoni D, Gavish A, Benhorin J, Keren A, Stern S: Myocardial ischemia during daily activities and stress. *Am J Cardiol* 1986;58:47B–50B.
16. Rautaharji PM, Prineas RJ, Eifler WJ, Furberg CD, Neaton JD, Crow RS, Stamler J, Cutler JA: Prognostic value of exercise electrocardiogram in men at high risk of future coronary heart disease: Multiple Risk Factor Intervention Trial Experience. *J Am Coll Cardiol* 1986;8:1–10.
17. Lipid Research Clinic Program (LRCP): Coronary heart disease morbidity and mortality in hypercholesterolemic men predicted from an exercise test: The LRC coronary primary prevention trial. Submitted to *Circulation,* 1988.
18. Moss AJ, Bigger JT, Odoroff CL: Post infarct risk stratification. *Prog Cardiovasc Dis* 1987;29:389–412.
19. Kaku R, DeMaria AN, Salmon D, et al: Predischarge exercise testing following acute myocardial infarction: Value and limitatins. *Clin Res* 1978;26:242A.
20. Krone RJ, Gillespie JA, Weld, et al: Low level exercise testing after myocardial infarction: Usefulness in enhancing clinical risk stratification. *Circulation* 1985;71:80–89.
21. Weld FM, Chu KL, Bigger JT, et al: Risk stratification with low level exercise testing 2 weeks after acute myocardial infarction. *Circulation* 1981;64:306–314.
22. Starling MR, Crawford MH, Kennedy GT, et al: Exercise testing early after myocardial infarction: Predictive value for subsequent unstable angina and death. *Am J Cardiol* 1980;46:900–914.
23. Sami M, Kraemer H, DeBusk RF: The prognostic significance of serial exercise testing after myocardial infarction. *Circulation* 1979;60:1238–1246.

24. Smith JW, Dennis CA, Gassman A, et al: Exercise testing three weeks after myocardial infarction. *Chest* 1979;75:12–16.
25. Srinivasan M, Young A, Baker G, et al: The value of post cardiac infarction exercise stress testing: Identification of a group at high risk. *Med J Aust* 1981;1:466–467.
26. Theroux P, Waters DD, Halpern C, et al: Prognostic value of exercise testing soon after myocardial infarction. *N Engl J Med* 1979;301:341–345.
27. Tibbits PA, Evaul JE, Goldstein RE, Boccuzzi SJ, Therneau TM, Parker R, Wong D, and the Multicenter Post-infarction Research Group: Serial acquisition of data to predict one year mortality rate after acute myocardial infarction. *Am J Cardiol* 1987;60:451–455.
28. Coy KM, Imperi GA, Lambert CR, Pepine CJ: Silent myocardial ischemia during daily activities in asymptomatic men with positive exercise test responses. *Am J Cardiol* 1987;59:45–49.
29. Davis BR, Friedman LM, Lichstein E: Is 24 hours of ambulatory recording necessary for the post-infarction patient? *Am Heart J* 1988;115:83–91.

PART D

Therapeutic Implications

CHAPTER 19

Reproducibility of Ischemic Parameters

Relevance to the Choice of Therapeutic End Points

Koonlawee Nademanee MD

A myocardial ischemic episode can give rise to a series of unfavorable cardiac events: myocardial dysfunction,[1] ST-T wave changes on the electrocardiogram,[2] hemodynamic changes,[3–5] cardiac arrhythmias,[6] and angina.[5,6] These changes can readily be detected during exercise and daily activity and can be used as an indicator of myocardial ischemia.[7,8] Angina is the oldest and most frequently used parameter for representing myocardial ischemia. However, we now know that most myocardial ischemic episodes are not associated with angina.[9–11] Therefore, using angina frequency and nitroglycerin consumption as an index may not be truly representative of total ischemic episodes. ST-T wave changes during exercise tests are a relatively reliable indicator of provoked myocardial ischemia. Unfortunately, these ST-T wave changes may not correlate with myocardial ischemia which occurs spontaneously during daily activity. Although 24-hour ambulatory ECG monitoring in detecting ST-T wave changes during myocardial ischemia drew skepticism in the past, it has become an acceptable tool in detecting myocardial ischemic episodes.[12–14] Furthermore, ST-T wave changes detected on Holter monitoring have been accepted as an important indicator of spontaneous myocardial ischemia, even when not associated with angina.[15–17]

Debate as to which parameter is the most useful clinical marker of myocardial ischemia will perhaps continue. Nevertheless, evaluation of the efficacy of antiischemic treatment with these parameters in individual patients with coronary artery disease or in clinical trials of antiischemic agents could be problematic because of the variability of each parameter. For example, Figure 19.1 demonstrates variabilities in anginal frequency, nitroglycerin consumption, ischemic episodes on Holter monitoring (per week), and exercise duration on treadmill tests in a patient treated with placebo for 2 weeks. This patient had a substantial reduction in spontaneous ischemic episodes, anginal attacks, and nitroglycerin use during the first week of placebo A. However, the patient's exercise duration was less than baseline (from 6 to 5 minutes). Thus, placebo A mimicked an antianginal agent by improving the patient's subjective symptoms and spontaneous ischemia, but it did not improve exercise time on treadmill testing. After placebo B the anginal attacks recurred; however, the patient did not use nitroglycerin and had only one transient ischemic episode on Holter

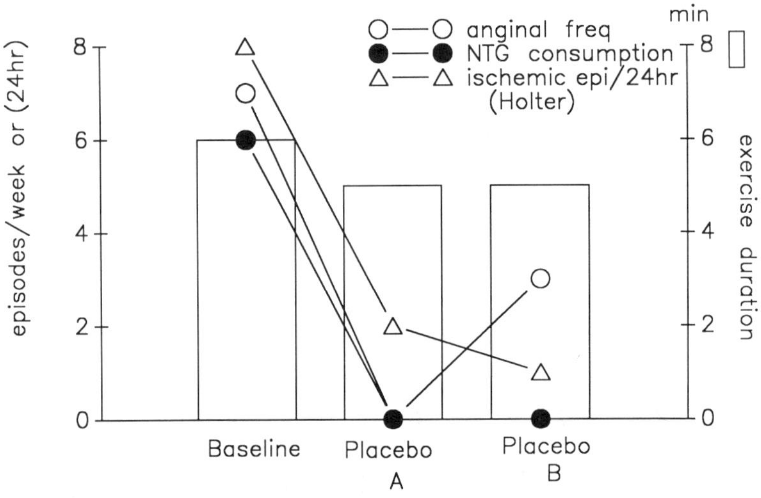

FIGURE 19.1. Example of the variability of ischemic parameters (exercise treadmill tests, Holter monitoring, and subjective symptoms) in a patient who underwent three treatment periods: baseline and two placebos.

monitoring compared to eight and two episodes during baseline and placebo A, respectively. Exercise duration did not change with placebo B. Clearly, this example illustrates the inherent variabilities of anginal symptoms, ischemic episodes detected on Holter monitoring, and exercise treadmill testing in provoked ischemia. Such variabilities will certainly confound the assessment of the efficacy of antiischemic treatment in this patient.

In addition, these findings raise the very important question as to which parameter is the most useful clinical marker of myocardial ischemia. Because of the lack of data on the relative variability among these parameters of myocardial ischemia, this study was performed to determine and compare the reproducibility and variability of ischemic parameters from various cardiac tests in patients with chronic stable angina. In this way the goal relevant to therapeutic end points and the guidelines for assessing efficacy of antianginal agents in both individuals and clinical trials can be defined rationally.

METHODS

Patient Population

We evaluated 65 male patients (mean age 59 years) with chronic stable angina, all of whom had unequivocal evidence of coronary artery disease. Forty-two had coronary artery stenoses detected by coronary angiography: 13 had one-vessel, 19 had two-vessel, and 10 had three-vessel coronary artery disease. Of the remaining 23 patients without prior coronary angiography, 11 had evidence of prior myocardial infarction by the presence of pathologic Q waves on the electrocardiogram and 12 had positive exercise treadmill tests for myocardial ischemia. All patients had had angina pectoris for at least 6 months before entry into the study.

Study Protocol

All patients were treated in a single-blind manner with placebo for three separate treatment periods, each lasting 1 week. All patients had a screening treadmill test showing a positive result for exercise-induced ischemia before the study. The first two consecutive placebo periods began after the patients had been withdrawn from antianginal treatment for at least five half-lives. All patients were then treated with either a calcium-channel blocker or nitrate for 2 to 3 weeks followed by the last placebo period for 1 week. Exercise treadmill tests and Holter monitoring were performed at the same time each day at the end of each placebo period. The patients were asked to maintain accurate diaries of their anginal attacks and nitroglycerin consumption. Because the third treatment period could be considered a "washout period" from previous antianginal therapy, we did not use this period in the analysis of anginal frequency or nitroglycerin consumption. The effects of previous antianginal agents may influence the anginal attacks on the first few days after treatment withdrawal, possibly by decreasing their frequency.

Holter Monitoring and Analysis

Twenty-four-hour Holter ECG recordings were obtained and analyzed by compact analog technique, whose details and validation have been described elsewhere.[9,17] It was found to be a highly reproducible technique for detecting the frequency and duration of myocardial ischemia when compared with real-time analysis of Holter recordings. ST-segment deviation was measured 0.08 seconds from the J junction. Episodes of ECG changes were considered to represent ischemia if they had at least 1 mm of ST-segment deviation from the baseline that lasted at least 30 seconds. ST-T wave changes associated with bundle branch block or changes in QRS complexes were excluded. All ischemic episodes were verified by real-time printouts of QRST complexes and overread blindly by a physician. In addition, a monthly quality assurance program was used with periodic full disclosure and recirculated known tapes, with adequate blinding into the analyst pool of tapes. In this context, the duplicate results were compared to determine their accuracy and repeatability. Our accuracy and precision of repeatability were more than 90 percent at any given time.

Exercise Treadmill Test

A modified Bruce exercise protocol was used in all patients. They all underwent a screening exercise test before the study and performed the exercise tests at the same time of day during each placebo period. The following parameters were systematically obtained for the analysis: (a) exercise duration, (b) the onset of 1-mm ST-segment depression, and (c) the onset of chest pain.

Criteria to stop exercise testing were:

1. Moderately severe (3+) chest pain (on a scale of 1 to 4, 4+ being the most severe)
2. Marked ST-T wave changes of 3 mm or more
3. Profound shortness of breath or fatigue.

Data and Statistical Analysis

Of the 65 patients evaluated in this study, 11 had to be excluded because of their need for antianginal treatment. Because of various contingent and social factors, not all of the remaining 54 patients completed all tests in all three placebo periods.

Summary statistics were generated for each parameter (Tables 1 and 2 presented later in sequence). The number of subjects includes those for whom at least two placebo replications were available. The number of observations is two to three times the number of subjects. The number of observations for anginal frequency and nitroglycerin consumption is exactly twice the number of subjects, because only the first two placebo periods were used for calculation to avoid carry over effects of antianginal treatment in the beginning of the last placebo period. We calculated the standard deviation and the mean over replications (each placebo period is one replication) for each subject and then averaged both the standard deviation and the mean over subjects. In addition, the coefficient of variation for each placebo period was calculated for each subject using the formula:

$$\text{Coefficient of Variation (CV)} = 100 \times \text{SD}/\text{Mean}$$

The coefficient of variation (CV) was averaged for all subjects, and this mean CV is presented in Table 19.2. The standard deviation among subjects within each placebo period was also calculated and averaged for these periods of placebo administration.

In all other calculations, log transformations were applied [x to log(x + 1)], because standard deviation tended to increase linearly with the means. An unbalanced, completely random component-of-variance analysis was performed on each log-transformed parameter, giving a component for within-subject variability and a component for among-subject variability.[18] The term "unbalanced" refers to the fact that subjects had varying numbers of placebo administrations (2 or 3) for the calculation. To adjust for the imbalance requires the following formulas:

$$V_w = \sum_{i=1}^{a} \sum_{j=1}^{n_i} \frac{(y_{ij} - \bar{y}_{i\cdot})^2}{(N - a)}$$

$$V_a = \frac{\sum_{i=1}^{a} \sum_{j=1}^{n_i} (\bar{y}_{i\cdot} - \bar{y}_{\cdot\cdot})^2 - (a - 1)V_w}{N - \sum_{i=1}^{a} \frac{n_i^2}{N}}$$

where V_w = within-subject variance component; V_a = among-subject variance component; y_{ij} = log value for the jth placebo administration for the ith subject; a = number of subjects; N = total number of observations; $\bar{y}_{i\cdot}$ = mean of n_i observations for the ith subject; and $\bar{y}.$ = mean overall N observations.

The last two columns of Table 19.2 present these variance components as the percentage of variation attributable to administration-to-administration differences and to subject-to-subject differences, using $V_w + V_a$ as total variation.

The number of subjects and the number of administrations per subject that are needed in a study for high (80%) statistical power of detecting differences of magnitude D, using p = 0.05, were determined. The formulas for k administrations are as follows:

1. Two-independent-samples protocol:

$$\text{number of subjects per group} = 1 + 15.7 \frac{\left(V_a + \frac{V_w}{k}\right)}{D^2}$$

2. Matched-pairs protocol:

$$\text{number of subjects} = 2 + 7.85\,\frac{\left(\frac{V_w}{k}\right)}{D^2}$$

Minimal sample sizes for the study designs and the various parameters used were determined to present the tradeoff between repeated measurements and the number of subjects and to give sample size estimates for planning studies. A significant level of 0.05 and a statistical power of 80 percent were used in all calculations. The calculation of variability of each parameter could be achieved by using an unbalanced, completely random components-of-variance analysis which circumvents the problem of missing data in each placebo period.

VARIABILITY OF ISCHEMIC PARAMETERS

The mean data of each parameter was averaged among subjects. The mean exercise duration, onset of chest pain on treadmill, and onset of 1-mm ST-segment depression were 434, 333, and 270 seconds, respectively. The mean number of ischemic episodes was 2.7 and the mean total duration of ischemia per 24 hours was 62 minutes. The mean anginal frequency and nitroglycerin consumption were 4.3 and 3.8 times per week, respectively.

To compare ischemic parameters or to examine parameters individually, various statistics expressing "variation" can be employed. Variance components can be used to determine the relative importance of factors (ie, treatments, subjects, and replications) and the minimal detectable changes in parameters both within subjects and among subject groups. The coefficient of variation expresses the expected deviations in a parameter relative to its mean value. A parameter with a smaller CV is more replicable and precise and is thus more sensitive in detecting differences between two measurements of a parameter (ie, that during placebo administration versus that during treatment). The exercise-induced ischemic parameters have a smaller CV than do the Holter or subjective parameters. The highest exercise-induced ischemic CV is 28 percent for the onset of 1-mm ST-segment depression, whereas the smallest CV for the Holter parameters, number of ischemic episodes per 24 hours, is 44 percent. Anginal frequency and nitroglycerin consumption have relatively larger CV, 56 percent and 55 percent, respectively. Thus, the exercise-induced ischemic parameters are the most sensitive in detecting changes in a subject whether due to the course of illness or to therapeutic treatment. Moreover, the number of ischemic episodes detected by Holter monitoring is more sensitive than are subjective symptoms in detecting an individual response to the therapeutic regimen. Surprisingly, the largest CV is found in the total duration of ischemic episodes per 24 hours, detected by Holter monitoring, which is indicative of the larger variability in this parameter compared with the others.

Similar findings are also found in the variability among subjects. The variability is much greater among subjects than within subjects. Our data show consistently that the variance components among subjects of each parameter are about twice as great as those within subjects. This is expected because the wide range in the severity of coronary artery disease among subjects will clearly give different degrees of severity and frequency of myocardial ischemia, whereas fewer variables will be involved in the development of myocardial ischemia in an individual.

It has long been known that anginal symptoms in patients with coronary artery disease could change in frequency and severity quite unpredictably.[19] Anginal syndrome is characterized by variability, exacerbations, and remissions,[20] which suggests that the occurrence of myocardial ischemia is subject to spontaneous variability that is naturally associated with factors involving the pathophysiology of myocardial ischemia. Interestingly, our findings indicate that transient myocardial ischemia detected by Holter monitoring has relatively the same magnitude of variability as does anginal frequency or nitroglycerin consumption, despite the fact that transient ischemic episodes were detected more frequently by Holter monitoring than by subjective symptoms. Thus, the variability of spontaneous ischemic parameters is most likely due to the inherent variability of precipitating factors of myocardial ischemia rather than to the tests themselves. Furthermore, it is now well accepted that transient myocardial ischemic episodes are probably caused by an intermittent reduction in blood supply.[4,21] This reduction is due to dynamic changes in the luminal stenosis of diseased coronary vessels from the increase in vasomobility in the area of normal smooth muscles opposing atherosclerotic plaques.[21]

The variability in ischemic parameters was more marked in spontaneous ischemic episodes than in exercise-induced ischemic episodes. Anginal frequency, nitroglycerin consumption, and ischemic episodes detected by Holter monitoring have a mean subject coefficient of variation ranging from 44 to 67 percent, and a percentage variation within subjects of 27 to 43 percent. In contrast, exercise duration, onset of chest pain, and 1-mm ST-segment depression had a mean subject coefficient of variation of 15 to 28 percent and a percentage variation within subjects of 20 to 33 percent. Thus, the exercise-induced ischemic parameters are more sensitive in detecting changes in a subject caused by either therapeutic treatment or progression of the disease. However, we should not extrapolate that the exercise treadmill test is necessarily the more useful parameter. In fact, spontaneous and exercise-induced ischemic parameters evaluate different aspects of the disease and therefore cannot be compared in this way. The former probably measures the threshold of myocardial ischemia which is caused by dynamic changes in the luminal stenosis of the diseased vessel. The latter measures the threshold of myocardial ischemia provoked by the increase in oxygen demand during exercise which exceeds the capabilities of the diseased vessel to provide enough blood for adequate perfusion.

MINIMAL INDIVIDUAL CHANGES IN EACH PARAMETER REQUIRED TO INDICATE SIGNIFICANT TREATMENT EFFECTS

To judge whether antianginal treatment in an individual patient is effective, account must be taken of the natural variability in these parameters. It cannot be assumed that the difference between the two measurements is the result of intervention or treatment. Using these variabilities in various ischemic parameters, one can determine the minimal detectable changes exceeding the boundary attributable to the variability of each individual parameter, so that the significant effects of any individual antiischemic effect can be determined. We found that the exercise-induced ischemic parameters require less percentage change for the significant change attributable to treatment (39% for exercise duration, 49% for onset of chest pain, and 67% for onset of 1-mm ST-segment depression), when compared with Holter parameters (72% for number of episodes per 24 hours and 95% for total duration of myocardial ischemia) and with anginal frequency (84%) and nitroglycerin consumption (77%).

In general, our data suggest that an improvement of approximately 3 minutes on exercise parameters or a reduction of at least two ischemic episodes detected by Holter monitoring or of four episodes of anginal attacks is required to obtain a significant antiischemic effect.

SAMPLE SIZE FOR A GIVEN PERCENTAGE OF CHANGE FOR EACH PARAMETER

Our data allow the rational design of clinical trials with respect to test frequency (number of replications), required percentage of change of each parameter, and sample size to reach the goal of the trials. In this context, we calculated sample sizes required for given percentages of change of different replications based on both a matched-pair protocol and two-independent-samples protocol. Figure 19.1 clearly shows that the increase in the number of replications results in a smaller sample size for a given percentage of change of each parameter. Hence, the higher the expected changes, the smaller the sample size needed for a given frequency of the test.

A two-independent-samples protocol needs a larger sample size than does a matched-pair protocol. However, the need could be minimized by increasing the number of test replications. In a matched-pair protocol, the increase in the number of replications results in a slight improvement in the sample size, but it may not warrant multiple measurements.

Comparing various parameters, exercise duration demands the smallest sample size to reach a goal set for the given expected percentage of change (p value = 0.05; 80% statistical power). Whereas the number of ischemic episodes on Holter monitoring is modest, the total duration of ischemia on Holter monitoring needs a much larger sample size for the same expected change. Anginal frequency and nitroglycerin consumption require a moderately large sample size between the two parameters from Holter monitoring.

In the past, many clinical trials for the evaluation of antianginal efficacy of investigational agents traditionally used exercise-induced ischemia, anginal frequency, and nitroglycerin consumption as the prime parameters. However, over the last 4 years Holter monitoring has gained popularity for detection of asymptomatic ischemic episodes by detecting silent ST-T wave changes which are now recognized as an important ischemic syndrome. Our study is the first to compare the variability of each parameter and to provide insights into the design of an antianginal study with respect to sample size and the number of measurements required for a given expected improvement in each parameter, which will indicate a significant drug effect. Clearly, our data follow the general principle that a matched-pairs protocol design (comparing baseline and treatment in the same patient) requires a much smaller sample size than does a two-independent-samples protocol. And the larger the expected percentage of change, the smaller the sample size needed. As shown in Table 19.4, an increase in the number of replications significantly reduces the sample size. However, increasing the number of replications beyond three in the matched-pairs protocol does not significantly reduce the sample size further. In fact, our data indicate that two replications are sufficient for all parameters in the matched-pairs protocol; for example, the sample sizes required for a 30% change (two replications) are 2, 3, 6, 7, 10, 14, and 35 subjects for total exercise duration, onset of chest pain during exercise, onset of 1-mm ST-segment depression during exercise, nitroglycerin consumption per week, anginal frequency per week, and total duration of myocardial ischemia per 24 hours, respectively.

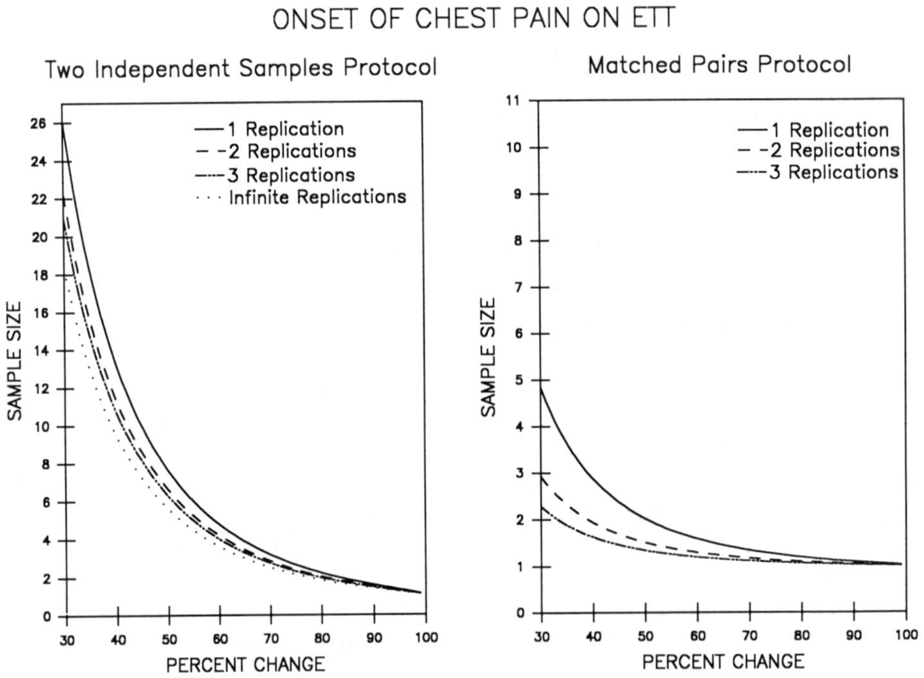

a

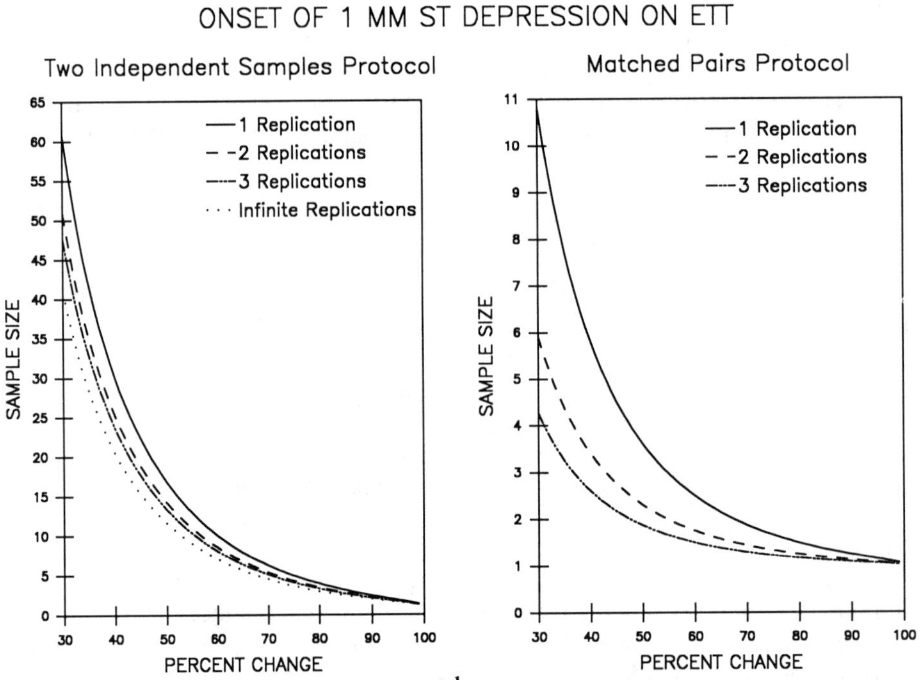

b

FIGURE 19.2. a-g: The relationship among sample sizes, expected percent changes, and number of replications of various ischemic parameters: onset of chest pain during exercise treadmill test (Figure 19.2a), onset of 1mm ST-depression during exercise (Figure 19.2b), total exercise duration (Figure 19.2c), total number and duration of 24 hours ischemic episodes on Holter monitoring (Figure 19.2d and 19.2e), anginal frequency (Figure 19.2f), and nitroglycerin consumption (Figure 19.2g). A comparison is made between the two independent samples protocol and matched pairs protocol.

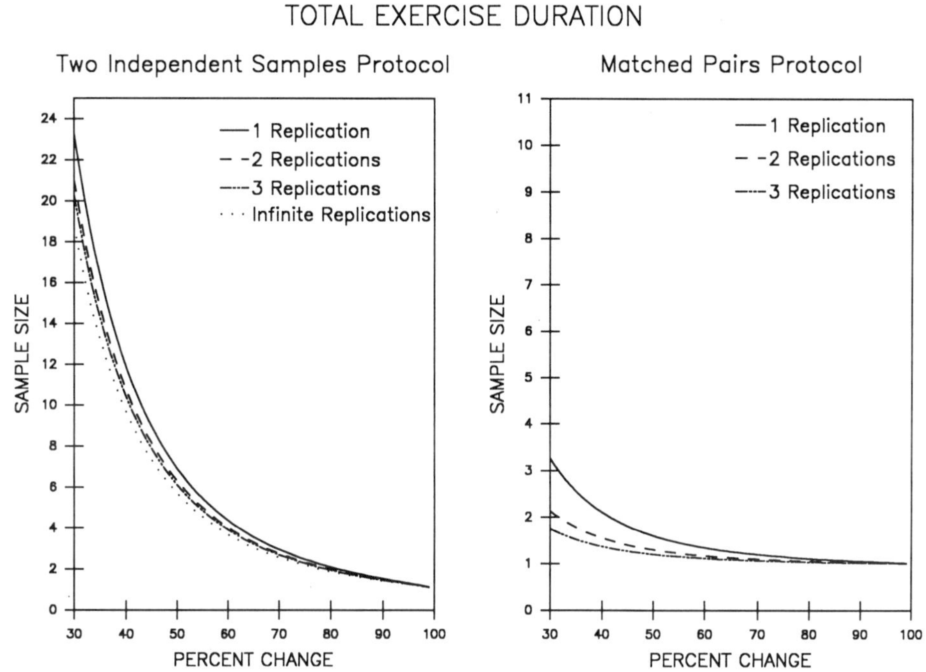

c

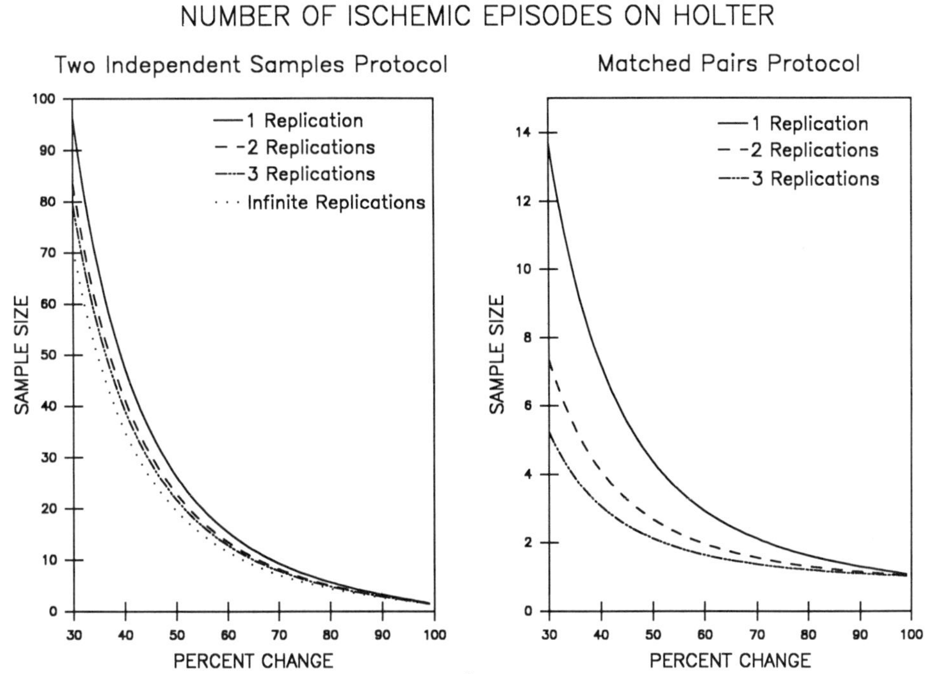

d

FIGURE 19.2. *(Continued)*

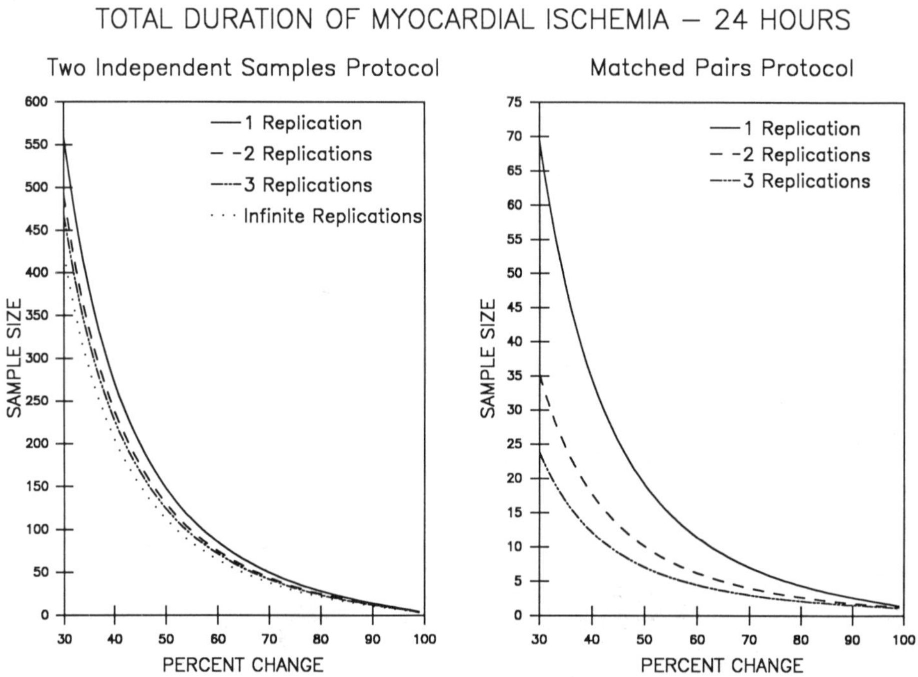

e

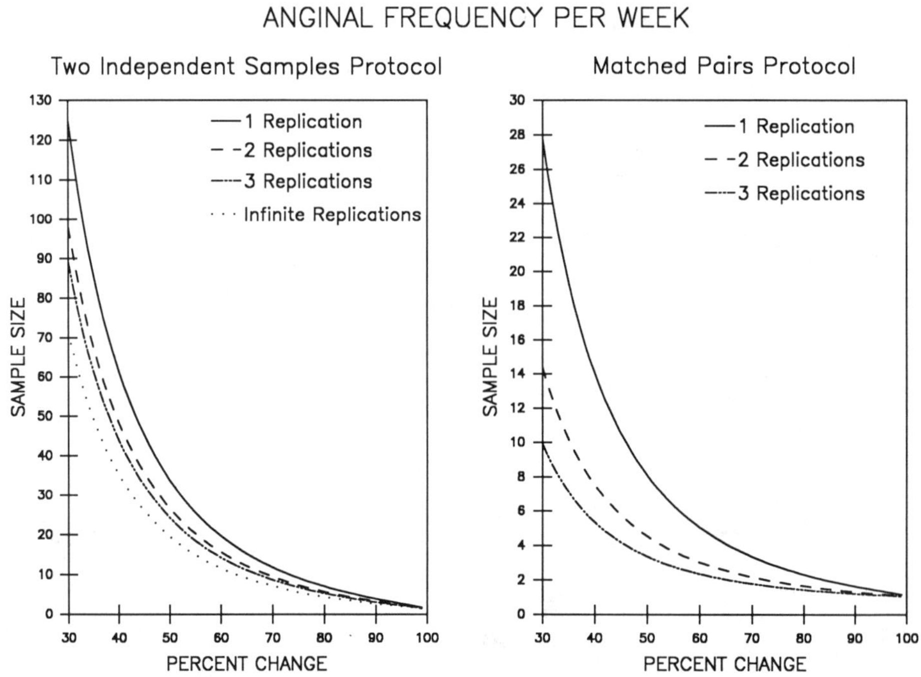

f

FIGURE 19.2. (*Continued*)

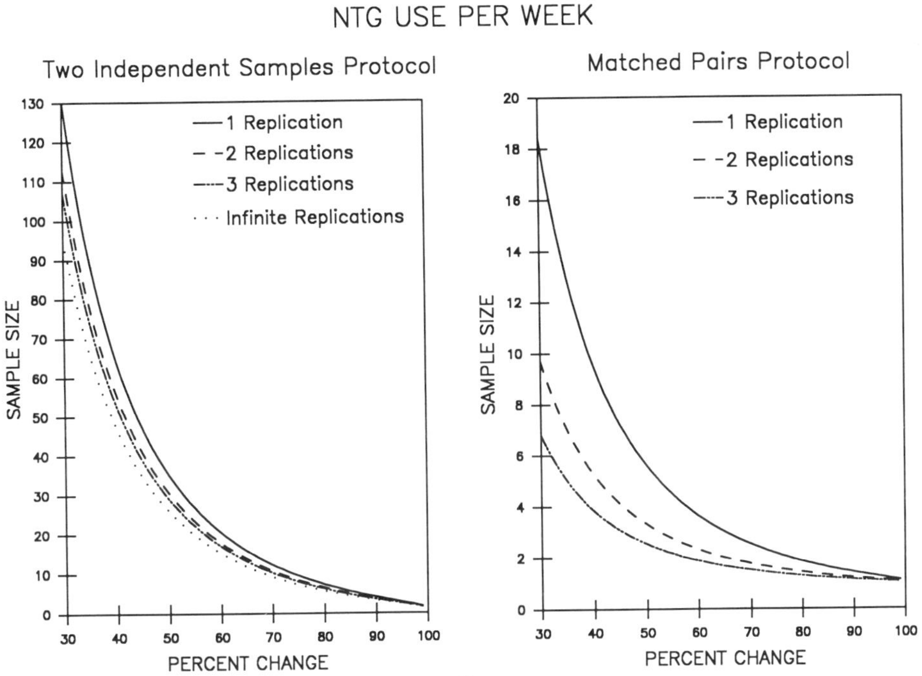

FIGURE 19.2. (*Continued*)

CLINICAL IMPLICATIONS AND LIMITATIONS OF THE STUDY

The findings of Morganroth et al[22] and Winkle[23] in the 1970s drew considerable attention to the variability of premature ventricular contractions detected on Holter monitoring and led to the criteria for determining the significant antiarrhythmic effects in suppressing ventricular arrhythmias. Similarly, our data can be used to determine the significant antianginal effects for individuals and for designing clincial trials. However, the present study cannot be used to infer which parameters are most useful in guiding antianginal treatment, nor does it imply that using the minimal detectable changes criteria in either parameter will prevent major cardiac ischemic events. Nevertheless, our study emphasizes that the variability of all parameters including exercise tests and Holter monitoring must be taken into account before any conclusions can be drawn on the efficacy of anginal treatment or intervention.

REFERENCES

1. Mitamura H, Ogawa HS, Yamajaki H, Handa S, Nakamura Y: Two-dimensional echocardiographic analysis of wall motion abnormalities during handgrip exercise in patients with coronary artery disease. *Am J Cardiol* 1981;48:1077.
2. Parodi O, Uthurralt N, Severi S, Bencivelli W, Michelassi C, L'Abbate A, Maseri A: Transient reduction of regional myocardial function during angina at rest with ST segment depression or normalization of negative T waves. *Circulation* 1981;63:1238.
3. Figueras J, Singh BN, Ganz W, Charuzi Y, Swan HJC: Mechanism of rest and nocturnal angina: Observations during continuous hemodynamic and electrocardiographic monitoring. *Circulation* 1979;59:955.
4. Chierchia S, Brunelli C, Simonetti I, Lazzari M, Maseri A: Sequence of events in angina at rest: Primary reduction in coronary flow. *Circulation* 1980;61:759.

5. Guazzi M, Polese A, Fiorentini C, Magrini F, Olivari MF, Bartorelli C: Left and right heart hemodynamics during spontaneous angina pectoris: Comparison between angina with ST segment depression and angina with ST segment elevation. *Br Heart J* 1975;37:401.
6. Maseri A: Pathogenetic mechanisms of angina pectoris: Expanding Views. *Br Heart J* 1980;43:648.
7. Borer J, Bacharach SL, Green MV, Kent KM, Epstein SE, Johnston GS: Real-time radionuclide cineangiography in the noninvasive evaluation of global and regional left ventricular function at rest and during exercise in patients with coronary artery disease. *N Engl J Med* 1977;296:839.
8. Deanfield JE, Maseri A, Selwyn AP, Ribesito P, Chierchia S, Krikler S: Myocardial ischemia during daily life in patients with angina: Its relation to symptoms and heart rate changes. *Lancet* 1983;2:753.
9. Nademanee K, Singh BN, Guerrero J, Hendrickson JA, Intarachot V, Baky S: Accurate rapid compact analog method for the quantification of frequency and duration of myocardial ischemia by semi-automated analysis of 24-hour Holter ECG recordings. *Am Heart J* 1982;103:802.
10. Schang SJ, Pepine CJ: Transient asymptomatic ST-segment depression during daily activity. *Am J Cardiol* 1977;39:396.
11. Deanfield JE, Shea M, Ribiero P, et al: Transient ST-segment depression as a marker of myocardial ischemia during daily life. *Am J Cardiol* 1984;54:1195.
12. Lambert CR, Imperi SA, Pepine CJ: Low-frequency requirements for recording ischemic ST-segment abnormalities in coronary artery disease. *Am J Cardiol* 1986;58:225.
13. Subramanian VB: Clinical and research applications of ambulatory Holter ST-segment and heart rate monitoring. *Am J Cardiol* 1986;58:11B.
14. Tzivoni D, Gavish A, Benhorin J, Keren A, Stern S: Myocardial ischemia during daily activities and stress. *Am J Cardiol* 1986;58:47B.
15. Singh BN, Nademanee K, Figueras J, Josephson MA: Hemodynamic and electrocardiographic correlates of symptomatic and silent myocardial ischemia: Pathophysiologic and therapeutic implications. *Am J Cardiol* 1986;58:3B.
16. Stern S, Tzivoni D: Early detection of silent ischemic heart disease by 24-hour electrocardiographic monitoring of active subjects. *Br Heart J* 1984;36:481.
17. Nademanee K, Intarachot V, Josephson MA, Rieders D, Vaghaiwalla FM, Singh BN: Prognostic significance of silent myocardial ischemia in patients with unstable angina. *J Am Coll Cardiol* 1987;10:1.
18. Searle SR: *Linear Models* New York; John Wiley & Sons, 1971, p 271.
19. Maseri A: The changing face of angina pectoris: Practical implication. *Lancet* 1983;1:746.
20. Kannel WB, Sorlie PD: Remission of clinical angina pectoris: The Framingham Study. *Am J Cardiol* 1978;42:119.
21. Brown BG, Bolson EL, Dodge HT: Dynamic mechanisms in human coronary stenosis. *Circulation* 1984;70:917.
22. Morganroth J, Michelson EL, Horowitz LN, Josephson ME, Pearlman AS, Dunkman WB: Limitations of routine long-term electrocardiographic monitoring to assess ventricular ectopic frequency. *Circulation* 1978;58:408.
23. Winkle RA: Antiarrhythmic drug effect mimicked by spontaneous variability of ventricular ectopy. *Circulation* 1978;57:1116.

CHAPTER 20

Nitroglycerin in the Myocardial Ischemic Syndromes

Focus on Silent Ischemia

William E. Shell, MD

Nitroglycerin has been used to treat angina pectoris for more than 100 years,[1] but its role remains controversial. Moreover, evaluation of the drug's effect in ischemia must take cognizance of the recent introduction of new delivery systems,[2] recognize the role of dynamic obstruction,[3] elucidate the incidence of silent events,[4–7] and delineate the potential tolerance effects to some of the pharmacologic actions of long-acting nitrates.[8,9] Moreover, it has been proposed that the therapy of myocardial ischemic syndromes should have as its goal the total elimination of ischemic events rather than the abolition of episodes of chest pain;[10] such a goal fosters the use of multiple therapies directed toward both the demand and the supply components of the ischemic process.

This discussion will focus on selected topics related to the use of nitroglycerin in acute reversible myocardial ischemia.

DEFINITION OF THE ISCHEMIC SYNDROMES: THREE FORMS OF ANGINA

Recently, we have begun to identify three forms of symptomatic ischemic syndromes: Heberden's, Prinzmetal's, and Maseri's angina. These forms, which can also be called demand angina, vasoconstrictive angina, and mixed angina, have independent prognostic and therapeutic implications. Silent ischemia occurs in patients with each of the three syndromes. The existence of three forms of the ischemic syndromes, each with symptomatic and asymptomatic events, implies variation in treatment strategies.

Ischemia results from an imbalance between the demand for oxygen and the supply. This imbalance can be initiated by either an increase in demand at fixed supply or a decrease in supply at fixed demand. Finally, the initiation of the event must be contrasted with its prolongation in which secondary increases in demand or secondary decreases in supply can occur. These underlying principles allow classification of the ischemic syndromes into three varieties. A brief comment about the salient features of these clinical entities will be made before critical discussion of the effects of nitrates on these syndromes.

Heberden's Angina

Stable exertional angina pectoris was described by Heberden[11] in 1772. The classic syndrome of exertional chest pain relieved by rest and nitroglycerin results from an increase in myocardial oxygen demand which outstrips flow through fixed coronary arterial obstruction. The laboratory model of Heberden's angina is ischemia evoked on an exercise treadmill.

Silent events have been described in Heberden's angina. It is well known that silent ST-segment depression frequently occurs during exercise testing in patients with established coronary arterial obstruction. In addition, silent ST-segment depression during "free" living exertion has been described using Holter monitoring. Cecchi et al,[12] for example, described silent ST-segment depression with exertion in patients with classic exertional angina documented by ambulatory monitoring; they found that the silent events induced by exertion were more frequent than the symptomatic events. These observations support an earlier report by Cocco et al[13] that also showed that silent ischemic events induced by exertion are more frequent than symptomatic events in patients with classic exertional angina.

Prinzmetal's Angina

Pure vasoconstrictive angina was described by Prinzmetal and colleagues[14] in 1959. The syndrome is associated with chest pain and ST-segment elevation. Usually the episodes are not provoked by an increase in myocardial oxygen demand. Vasoconstriction has been identified as the initiating event in Prinzmetal's angina. The laboratory model of vasoconstrictive angina is ergonovine-induced vasoconstriction. Silent Prinzmetal's angina has not been formally reported, but we recently observed a case.

Maseri's Angina

In the last several years, Maseri et al[15] introduced the concept of mixed angina. In this syndrome, events are precipitated by either an increase in myocardial oxygen demand or a spontaneous reduction in blood flow secondary to vasoconstriction. In patients with mixed ischemic syndromes, exercise-induced episodes of pain occur; they develop chest pain on the treadmill. In addition, spontaneous nonexercise-related events that are detectable by Holter monitoring occur; the spontaneous events are associated with chest pain, a decrease in thallium perfusion,[16] a decrease in myocardial perfusion indicated by Rubidium imaging,[17] a decrease in coronary sinus PO_2, and an increase in coronary sinus lactate production.[18]

The syndrome of spontaneous mixed angina is associated with chest pain and reversible ST-segment depression seen either on a standard electrocardiogram or by Holter monitoring. The symptoms occur at rest, with emotion, or with minimal activity. The poor correlation of symptoms with an increase in myocardial oxygen demand characterizes this syndrome. The spontaneous syndrome has also been called unstable angina, angina at rest, emotional angina, coronary insufficiency, or preinfarction angina,[19–22] depending on the particular characteristic of the syndrome under discussion. For this discussion, the term "spontaneous angina" has been selected to stress the lack of correlation of events with an increase in myocardial oxygen demand.

In Maseri's mixed angina, there is an admixture of exertional angina and vasoconstrictive spontaneous angina. The incidence of silent events in this syndrome is incompletely defined, but it appears to be quite significant. Biagini et al[23] documented 520 episodes of ST-segment changes in 11 patients fitting the profile of mixed angina, and only 12 percent of the episodes were symptomatic; the events occurred both with and without an increase in oxygen demand.

To plan therapeutic modalities for mixed angina, the mechanism of the spontaneous component must be appreciated and the treatment directed toward both the demand components and the spontaneous events. The conceptual framework for the pathogenesis of various forms of angina in relation to the role of dynamic stenosis has been presented at length by Brown and Smith elsewhere in this volume (see Chapter 2).

PHARMACOLOGIC CONSIDERATIONS

Nitroglycerin reduces many determinants of myocardial oxygen demand.[24] This reduction in demand is related to the peripheral effects of NTG; it is an important arteriolar dilator but a more potent venodilator. Thus, the drug decreases right and left atrial pressure, reduces arterial pressure, and reduces left ventricular end-diastolic pressure. The decrease in these filling pressures results in a substantial decrease in the demand for oxygen. The peripheral changes occur both at rest and after exercise. The peripheral effects of NTG, which are well documented, account for much of the acute effects of NTG on exercise-induced ischemia. It should also be emphasized that the decrease in ventricular filling pressure effected by NTG undoubtedly improves subendocardial coronary perfusion.

The peripheral hemodynamic effects of NTG rapidly attenuate.[25] At high-dose NTG, the reduction of filling pressures and the peripheral arteriolar dilatation return to baseline within 24 hours after the initial exposure. True tolerance does not develop, because these same subjects will respond to increases in NTG concentration. In physiologic concentrations, complete loss of response to an incremental dose of NTG has not been observed. The impact of the attenuation of peripheral vasodilatory and venodilatory responses on clinical use of NTG must be included in any dosing strategy for NTG.

NITROGLYCERIN AND THE CORONARY CIRCULATION

In terms of the net effects of NTG on the distribution of blood flow, the peripheral and central effects of the drug should be distinguished. Nitroglycerin is a potent dilator of epicardial coronary arteries and their stenotic segments.[26] In contrast, the calcium-channel blocking agents—nifedipine, verapamil, and diltiazem—are relatively weak dilators of epicardial coronary arteries.[26] These differences have been demonstrated in both animal models and human studies (see Chapter 2).

Nitroglycerin is a relatively weak dilator of coronary resistance vessels.[26] Dipyridamole and hydralazine are effective dilators of these resistance vessels.[26] The calcium-channel blockers have little effect at this level. Dilatation of the resistance vessels in the normal zones may account for the "coronary steal" phenomena seen with dipyridamole in some animal models.[26]

A number of physiologic stimuli and pharmacologic agents induce alpha-receptor-mediated vasoconstriction of coronary arteries.[26] Exercise, for example, is a potent stimulus for alpha-mediated vasoconstriction.[27–29] Nitroglycerin is a relatively weak inhibitor of alpha-mediated coronary vasoconstriction, whereas the calcium-channel blocking agents block the alpha-mediated coronary vasoconstriction.[26] These observations suggest that calcium-channel blocking agents may be more potent agents in the presence of exercise-induced ischemic events.

It is now well recognized that coronary stenoses can undergo vasodilatation (Chapter 2), particularly those with eccentric lesions and normally contracting smooth muscle segments.[26] Nitroglycerin dilates stenotic segments in approximately 70 percent of diseased coronary arteries, resulting in a substantial increase in luminal area. Importantly, resistance is related to the fourth power of the radius; a small change in the radius of a stenotic lesion will therefore result in a large reduction in resistance to flow.[26–28] Calcium-channel blocking agents are relatively weak direct dilators of stenotic lesions.[26] In the case of NTG, lesion dilatation must contribute importantly to the antiischemic action of the drug by promoting increased coronary blood flow.

ATTENUATION AND TOLERANCE IN THE ACTION OF NITROGLYCERIN

There is little available evidence concerning the development of attenuated responses of coronary artery vasodilatation secondary to NTG. Several studies failed to demonstrate a diminution of NTG in treating anginal symptoms. Recently, May et al,[30] using coronary sinus blood flow as an indirect guide to the state of coronary vasomotor tone, showed that after a 24-hour infusion of intravenous NTG, intracoronary NTG responses were attenuated by approximately 50 percent. It should be pointed out that the 24-hour infusions were of high dose and intravenous; despite such a high dose, the coronary arteries were still responsive to NTG, and the attenuation could be abolished by N-acetylcysteine. There are no data on the effects of continuous NTG on the attenuation of NTG-induced vasodilatation of stenotic segments. Moreover, the biologic implication of a 50 percent attenuation of coronary vasodilatory responses to high-dose NTG remains to be determined. Clearly, extensive evaluation of the effects of NTG on coronary vasodilator responses is still needed, particularly relative to NTG dose, route of administration, and nitrate-free periods.

ABOLITION OF SILENT ISCHEMIA

The existence of silent myocardial ischemia and its potential adverse prognostic implications may have substantial therapeutic impact. The existence of frequent silent ischemic events and the proposed mechanism raise a number of issues regarding therapy. First, all ischemia should be abolished, not only when symptomatic. Second, it must be recognized that ischemia, silent as well as symptomatic, can be induced both by an increase in myocardial oxygen demand secondary to an increase in heart rate, blood pressure, and contractility and by a reduction in blood flow induced by spontaneous vasoconstriction or thrombolytic occlusion. Ideally, therapy should be designed to decrease demand while maintaining blood flow.

Treatment of silent ischemia with the goal of eliminating all ischemic events is an evolving therapeutic concept that remains to be explored. For the present, it should be recognized that the assertion that all ischemic events should be eliminated is a hypothesis that is in need of critical testing. However, circumstantial evidence derived from observations concerning mechanical repair of coronary obstruction suggests that elimination of ischemia may alter morbidity and mortality. Percutaneous dilatation of the stenotic coronary artery can eliminate ischemia, both symptomatic and silent.[31] In addition, complete surgical revascularization procedures, particularly in unstable subsets, result in a reduced mortality rate.[32] It may be argued that the reduction in mortality induced by myocardial revascularization in certain subsets of patients with angina may stem from the elimination of ischemia, silent and symptomatic. There are advocates, therefore, of mechanical repair of coronary obstruction even in asymptomatic patients with silent ischemia;[33] this approach requires validation, although a randomized trial relative to this question has been proposed.[34]

Medical therapy of myocardial ischemia is complex, multifaceted, and nonstandardized in terms of end points or goals of treatment. Part of the difficulty stems from a failure (1) to quantify the total ischemic load, thereby ignoring the importance of silent ischemic episodes, and (2) to differentiate the treatment of demand from supply ischemia. In our own work related to initial attempts to explore the therapy of ischemia, we set two therapeutic goals: (1) total elimination of ischemia, and (2) specific treatment of both demand and vasoconstrictive components. We have concentrated on elimination of all ischemic events detected by Holter monitoring which include events occurring in real life both those induced by exercise and those occurring spontaneously. We have focused on prolonging exercise-induced ischemia assessed by exercise stress testing which has been the cornerstone of objectively judging efficacy.

A number of agents have the potential both to abolish spontaneous vasoconstrictive events and to reduce the determinants of myocardial oxygen demand. These agents include nitrates, beta-blocking agents, calcium-blocking agents, and antiplatelet drugs.

NITROGLYCERIN IN THE TREATMENT OF SPONTANEOUS SILENT ISCHEMIA

Our initial studies dealt with the use of transdermal NTG in silent myocardial ischemia.[35] There were several reasons for the choice of this agent in this setting. First, we wished specifically to explore vasoconstrictive events. Second, nitrates have a long history in the treatment of spontaneous anginal events, and silent ischemia is analogous to spontaneous angina. Transdermal NTG is known to provide nearly constant plasma levels, which may be necessary in patients with silent ischemia because they are not aware when they experience ischemic episodes. In addition, the nitrates have a known safety profile without the propensity to decrease myocardial contractility. They can be titrated to high doses if necessary to treat the silent events.

Previous Studies

Schang and Pepine[36] studied the effects of sublingual nitrates compared to placebo on the frequency of silent myocardial ischemic events. Five patients were treated with either hourly sublingual NTG or placebo during 10-hour peirods of ambulatory ECG monitoring. Asymptomatic episodes of ST-segment depression were significantly less frequent with nitrate therapy than with placebo (3.7 versus 0.6 episodes per monitoring period). This was the first item of data that silent myocardial ischemia was amenable to pharmacologic suppression.

Open-Label Trial

We recently completed an open-label trial to test the effects of transdermal NTG on the number, duration, and magnitude of ischemic events.[35] In eight patients with chronic stable angina, we performed 24-hour ambulatory monitoring using a calibrated system (DMI Instruments). From each tape a 24-hour full disclosure record was displayed on hard copy. From the hard copy printout, the onset and offset of each ST-segment event of either depression or elevation were identified. In addition, the maximum depth of either the depression or elevation was measured in millimeters. We then counted the number of events, measured the duration in total minutes, and estimated the magnitude of each event by multiplying the duration times the magnitude for each event—the so-called ischemia-magnitude integral. The baseline 24-hour tape was obtained in the presence of beta-blockade and sublingual NTG given for symptomatic episodes. The beta-blocking drugs were used to suppress demand angina by reducing rest and postexercise heart rate. Each patient had both symptomatic angina pectoris and silent ischemia on the regimen of beta-blockade and sublingual NTG.

We then titrated the dose of transdermal NTG in each patient beginning with 5 mg/24 hours (10 cm^2) and increasing the dose in 5 mg/24-hour increments. We increased the dose until the number of symptomatic events was abolished, and the 24-hour Holter recording was repeated. The mean dose was 10.4 mg/24 hours (range 5–20 mg or 10–40 cm^2).

All eight patients had a decrease in the number of symptomatic events. In addition, the total number of events fell from 5.8 to 0.8 per 24 hours ($p < 0.025$). As in other studies, 80 percent of the events were silent. This represents an 85 percent reduction in the total number of events per 24-hour period (Figure 20.1).

The duration of ischemic events also decreased from 95.8 min/24 hours to 17 min/24 hours ($p < 0.05$), representing an 82 percent reduction in the total duration of ischemia per 24 hours (Figure 20.2). It should be pointed out that there were no less than 2 weeks between the two sets of Holter recordings, and the possible effects of tolerance should have been evident if present. Long-term studies related to tolerance in silent ischemic events using ambulatory monitoring should be performed, but our data suggest that at least in this small cohort with both clinical and objective responses, tolerance was not observed.

Thus, in an open-label trial using a titration protocol, transdermal NTG in the presence of beta-blockade reduced the number, duration, and magnitude of ischemic events, both symptomatic and asymptomatic.

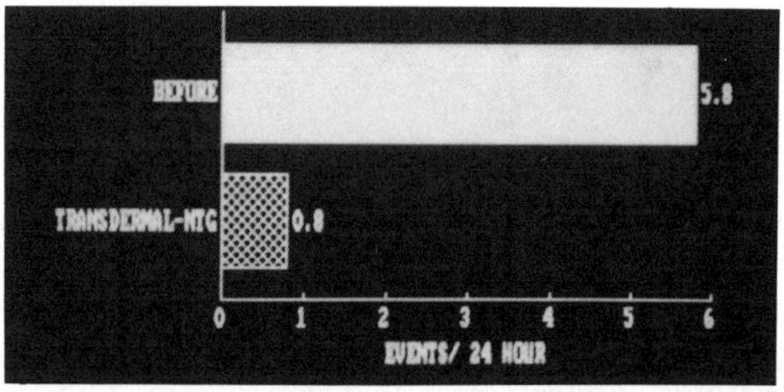

FIGURE 20.1. The effect of transdermal nitroglycerin (NTG) on the number of ischemic events. The number includes both the symptomatic and painless events. Painless episodes comprised about 80 percent of the total. Note the marked reduction in all episodes produced by transdermal NTG ($p < 0.025$).

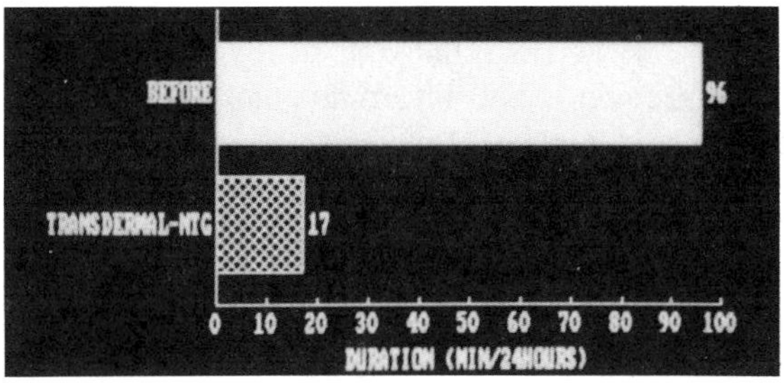

FIGURE 20.2. The decrease in the total ischemic load by transdermal nitroglycerin (NTG). The total ischemia time was 96 minutes per 24 hours before NTG and 17 minutes during NTG ($p < 0.05$).

Double-Blind Trial

We recently completed a crossover trial to confirm our initial results. The study design was a placebo-controlled, double-blind, double-dummy format with dose titration (Figure 20.3). The placebo washout period was 2 weeks, and the dose was changed every 2 weeks. Each patient received a 2-week placebo period, and the patients were then randomized to either placebo or active agent; there was no crossover and the patients were concomitantly given a beta-blocking agent. The Holter recordings were performed at fixed time intervals. In this study, in the active group at 20 mg/24 hours of transdermal NTG, total ischemic time fell from 143 ± 45 min/24 hours to 54 ± 28 (mean ± SE), $t = 1.8$, $p = 0.05$, and $n = 17$.

TREATMENT OF DEMAND ANGINA

The treatment of "pure" demand angina is more clearly defined, particularly because exercise stress testing is a useful and reasonably reproducible laboratory model. Calcium-blocking and beta-blocking agents appear to uniformly increase exercise treadmill time and reduce the frequency of exercise-induced angina.[33] Recently, Cohn et al[37] reported on a group of patients with silent ischemia induced on the treadmill; they treated eight patients with beta-blockade and found the time to ST-segment depression and maximum ST-segment depression was prolonged; also, the patients showed an improvement in the exercise ejection fraction determined by radionuclide ventriculography. These data suggest that beta-blockade can prolong exercise time, thereby reducing the frequency of exercise-induced silent ischemia.

The long-acting nitrates decrease the frequency of symptomatic angina[38] and at least acutely prolong exercise treadmill time at high doses.[8,9,39] When continuous transdermal NTG is applied, prolongation of exercise tolerance has been reported in

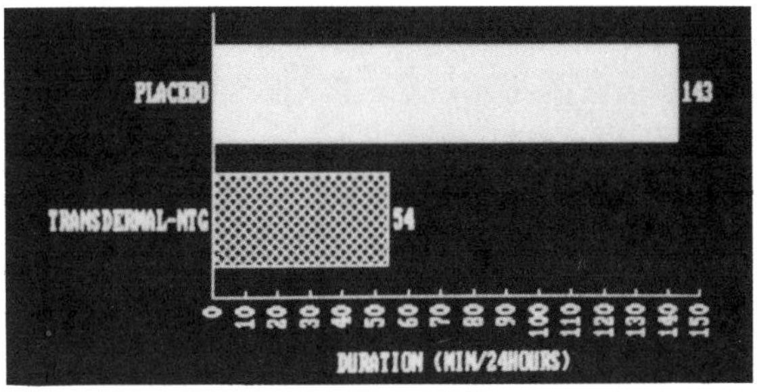

FIGURE 20.3. The effect of transdermal nitroglycerin (NTG) on the duration of ischemic events in a double-blind placebo-controlled trial. A significant reduction ($p < 0.05$) was effected by transdermal NTG (see text).

some studies[38–43] and attenuation in others.[8,9] In the largest study (n = 52) reported by Muiesan et al,[44] there was a small but statistically significant increase in exercise tolerance; the patients seemed to fall into three subsets: no attenuation, modest attenuation, and rapid-complete attenuation. Interestingly, the decrease in the reported chest pain incidents occurred even in patients experiencing marked attenuation of the exercise effects, suggesting that exercise tests may be a poor predictor of clinical and Holter-determined ischemic events.

The attenuation of exercise responses appears to be ameliorated by a nitrate-free period.[45] The duration of the nitrate-free period is uncertain, but approximately 8 hours appears to be sufficient.[46]

Despite the reported frequency of attenuated exercise responses, there are no reports of attenuation of either diary-reported chest pain or Holter-measured ischemic events. On the contrary, several large clinical studies using diary-defined chest pain show no hint of attenuation to transdermal NTG.[47] These observations also suggest that exercise testing may be a poor method to assess the clinical role of long-acting NTG.

CONCLUSIONS

Silent myocardial ischemia is a common manifestation of ischemic heart disease and occurs in all the ischemic syndromes. The current diagnostic standard for silent ischemia uses ambulatory ECG recordings. There is a paucity of data concerning the treatment of silent ischemic events. Our initial data suggest that transdermal NTG in the presence of beta-blockade and given in sufficient doses can reduce the number, duration, and magnitude of the ischemic events. These effects are consistent with the known physiologic effects of NTG on both the normal and stenotic epicardial coronary artery vasomotor tone. Therapy of ischemia should attempt to eliminate all ischemic events, and it appears reasonable to suggest that treatment should be designed to reduce myocardial oxygen demand and to prevent vasoconstriction or intraluminal thrombosis. Whether such an approach in the treatment of various ischemic syndromes based on the elimination of ischemia or a predefined degree of ischemia will necessarily lead to a reduction in morbid events remains uncertain. Controlled clinical trials will be needed to provide the rational basis for the use of Holter-documented ischemic episodes as an end point for gauging the efficacy of antiischemic therapy.

Acknowledgment: This work was supported in part by The Daniel E. Cohn Memorial Heart Fund.

REFERENCES

1. Murrell W: Nitroglycerin as a remedy for angina pectoris. *Lancet* 1879;1,113, 225, 284, 643–646.
2. Muller P, Imhof PR, Burkart F, Chu L-C, Geradin A: Human pharmacological studies of a new transdermal system containing nitroglycerin. *Eur J Pharmacol* 1982;22:473–480.
3. Maseri A: Role of coronary artery spasm in symptomatic and silent myocardial ischemia. *J Am Coll Cardiol* 1987;9:249–262.
4. Guazzi M, Fiorenti C, Polese A, Magrini F: Continuous electrocardiographic recordings in Prinzmetal's variant angina pectoris. A report of four cases. *Br Heart J* 1970;32:611–616.

5. Schang SJ, Pepine CJ: Transient asymptomatic ST-segment depression during daily activity. *Am J Cardiol* 1977;39:396–402.
6. Selwyn AP, Fox K, Eves M, et al: Myocardial ischemia in patients with frequent angina pectoris. *Br Med J* 1978;2:1594–1596.
7. Deanfield JE, Maseri A, Selwyn AP, et al: Myocardial ischemia during daily life in patients with stable angina: Its relation to symptoms and heart rate changes. *Lancet* 1983;2:753–758.
8. Reichek N, Priest C, Zimrin D, Chandler T, Sulton MSJ: Antianginal effects of nitroglycerin patches. *Am J Cardiol* 1984;54:1–7.
9. Parker JO, Fung H-L: Transdermal nitroglycerin in angina pectoris. *Am J Cardiol* 1984;54:471–477.
10. Pepine CJ, Hill JA: Management of the total ischemic burden in angina pectoris. *Am J Cardiol* 1987;59:7C–12C.
11. Heberden W: Some account of a disorder of the breast. *Med Trans Coll Physicians (London)* 1772;2:59.
12. Cecchi AC, Dovellini EV, Marchi F, et al: Silent myocardial ischemia during ambulatory electrocardiographic monitoring in patients with effort angina. *J Am Coll Cardiol* 1983;1:934–939.
13. Cocco G, Braun S, Strozzi C, et al: Asymptomatic myocardial ischemia in patients with stable and typical angina pectoris. *Clin Cardiol* 1982;5:403–408.
14. Prinzmetal M, Kennamer R, Merliss R, et al: Angina pectoris. 1. A variant form of angina pectoris. *Am J Med* 1959;27:375–388.
15. Maseri A, Severi S, De Nes M, et al: "Variant" angina: One aspect of a continuous spectrum of vasospastic myocardial ischemia. *Am J Cardiol* 1978;42:1019–1035.
16. Maseri A, Parodi O, Severi S, Pesola A: Transient transmural reduction of myocardial blood flow, demonstrated by thallium-201 scintigraphy, as a cause of variant angina. *Circulation* 1986;54:280–288.
17. Maseri A, Chierchia S, Davies G, Glazier J: Mechanisms of ischemic cardiac pain and silent myocardial ischemia. *Am J Med* 1985;79:7–11.
18. Chierchia S, Maseri A, Simonetti I, Brunelli C: Oxygen myocardial extraction in angina at rest. Evidence of a primary reduction of blood supply (abstract). *Circulation* 1977;55 & 56 (suppl III):37.
19. Fowler NO: Preinfarction angina. *Circulation* 1971;44:755–760.
20. Osler W: *The Principles and Practice of Medicine*. New York, Appleton, 1892.
21. White PD: Coronary insufficiency, angina pectoris. In: *Heart Disease*. New York, MacMillan, 1937.
22. Beamish RE, Storrie VM: Impending myocardial infarction: Recognition and management. *Circulation* 1960;21:1107–1110.
23. Biagini A, Mazzei MG, Carpeggiani C, et al: Vasospastic ischemic mechanism of frequent asymptomatic transient ST-T changes during continuous electrocardiographic monitoring in selected unstable angina patients. *Am Heart J* 1982;103:13–19.
24. Abrams J: Pharmacology of nitroglycerin and long-acting nitrates. *Am J Cardiol* 1985;56:12A–18A.
25. Roth A, Kulick D, Freidenberger L, Hong R, Rahimtoola SH, Elkayam U: Early tolerance to hemodynamic effects of high dose transdermal nitroglycerin in responders with severe chronic heart failure. *J Am Coll Cardiol* 1987;9:858–864.
26. Brown BG: Response of normal and diseased epicardial coronary arteries to vasoactive drugs: Quantitative arteriographic studies. *Am J Cardiol* 1985;56:23E–29E.
27. Epstein SE, Cannon RO, Talbot TL: Hemodynamic principles in the control of coronary blood flow. *Am J Cardiol* 1985;56:4E–10E.
28. Vatner SF: Regulation of coronary resistance vessels and large coronary arteries. *Am J Cardiol* 1985;56:16E–22E.
29. Berkenboom GM, Abramowicz M, Vandermoten P, Degre SG: Role of alpha-adrenergic coronary tone in exercise-induced angina pectoris. *Am J Cardiol* 1986;57:195–198.
30. May DC, Popma JJ, Black WH, Schaefer S, Lee HR, Levine BD, Hillis LD: In vivo induction and reversal of nitroglycerin tolerance in human coronary arteries. *N Engl J Med* 1987;317:805–809.
31. Josephson MA, Nademanee K, Intarachot V, Lewis H, Singh BN: Abolition of Holter-

detected silent myocardial ischemia after percutaneous transluminal coronary angioplasty. *J Am Coll Cardiol* 1987;10:499–503.

32. Bonow RO, Epstein SE: Indications for coronary artery bypass surgery in patients with chronic angina pectoris: Implications of the multicenter randomized trials. *Circulation* 1985;72(supplV):V–23.
33. FitzGibbon GM, Burton JR, Keon WJ: Aortocoronary bypass surgery in "asymptomatic" patients with coronary artery disease, in Rutishauser W, Roskamm H (eds): *Silent Myocardial Ischemia*. Berlin, Springer-Verlag; 1984, p 180.
34. Gottlieb SO, Weisfeldt ML, Ouyang P, Achuff SC, et al: Effect of the addition of propranolol to therapy with nifedipine for unstable angina pectoris: A randomized, double-blind, placebo controlled trial. *Circulation* 1986;73:331–337.
35. Shell WE: Mechanisms and therapy of silent myocardial ischemia and the effect of transdermal nitroglycerin. *Am J Cardiol* 1985;56:231–237.
36. Schang SJ, Pepine CJ: Transient asymptomatic ST-segment depression during daily activity. *Am J Cardiol* 1977;39:396–402.
37. Cohn PF, Brown EJ Jr, Swinford R, Atkins HL: Effect of beta blockade on silent regional left ventricular wall motion abnormalities. *Am J Cardiol* 1986;57:521–526.
38. Naafs MAB, de Boer AC, Koster RW, Klazen CW, Dunning AJ: Exercise capacity with transdermal nitroglycerin in patients with stable angina pectoris. *Eur Heart J* 1984;5:705–709.
39. Cerri B, Grasso F, Cefis M, Pollavini G: Comparative evaluation of the effect of two doses of nitroderm TTS on exercise-related parameters in patients with angina pectoris. *Eur Heart J* 1984;5:710–715.
40. Pucci P, Zambaldi G, Cerisano G, Roccanti P: Valutazione di un nuovo preparto de nitroglicerina percutanea nell-angina da sforsa. *G Ital Cardiol* 1983;13:167–171.
41. Thompson RH: The clinical use of transdermal delivery devices with nitroglycerin. *Angiology* 1983;34:23–31.
42. Martines C: Comparison of the prophylactic antianginal effect of two doses of nitroderm TTS in outpatients with stable angina pectoris. *Curr Ther Res* 1984;36:483–489.
43. Imhof PR, Georgopoulos AJ, Garnier G: Nitroderm TTS versus oral isosorbide dinitrate: A double-blind trial in patients with angina pectoris. *Acta Therapeutica* 1985;11:155–170.
44. Muiesan G, Agabiti-Rosei E, Muiesan L, Romanelli G, Pollavini P, et al: A multicenter trial of transdermal nitroglycerin in exercise-induced angina: Individual antianginal response after repeated administration. *Am Heart J* 1986;112:223–238.
45. Silber S, Krause KH, Theisen K: Nitrate-tolerance: Dependence on dosage intervals. *Circulation* 1984;70(suppl II):II–189.
46. Abrams J: Tolerance to organic nitrates. *Circulation* 1986;74:1181–1185.
47. Brody EL, Gold O, Rosenbach H: Transdermal NTG. *Cardiovasc Drugs & Therapy* 1987;1:218–221.

CHAPTER 21

Comparative Influence of Beta-Blocker and Calcium-Channel Blocker Therapy on Transient Myocardial Ischemia in Unstable and Vasospastic Angina

Michael H. Crawford, MD

Beta-blockers and calcium-channel blockers now have an established role in the treatment of various myocardial ischemic syndromes.[1,2] From the standpoint of mechanism, their role in chronic stable angina is reasonably well defined in terms of their property for decreasing cardiac work during exercise. Thus, both classes of drugs augment exercise duration on treadmill and the time to the development of a defined degree of ST-segment depression on the electrocardiogram. The precise mechanisms whereby these agents produce the salutary actions on myocardial oxygen consumption undoubtedly differ, although their net effects are quantitatively similar.

There is now emerging data to indicate that the pathophysiologic mechanisms of unstable angina and especially of Prinzmetal's angina differ from those of chronic stable angina[3] (see Chapter 2). Recent data have focused on thrombotic and vasospastic components in the pathogenesis of unstable angina (see Chapter 3), but compelling evidence has been adduced for focal vasospasm in the care of Prinzmetal's angina.[4] The purpose of this chapter is to examine the roles of calcium-channel blockers and beta-blockers in the control of ischemia in unstable and vasospastic angina in relation to the underlying pathophysiologic mechanism involved in these ischemic syndromes.

CLINICAL PRESENTATION AND PATHOPHYSIOLOGY OF UNSTABLE ANGINA

Unstable angina pectoris is a clinical diagnosis that encompasses a variety of situations characterized by the presence of episodes of myocardial ischemia that are unprovoked in the usual sense of being related to significant exertion and yet do not culminate immediately in acute transmural myocardial infarction. The mildest form of unstable angina is crescendo angina which is defined an as increase in the frequency and duration of angina attacks and provocation of these attacks by stimuli of increasingly lesser magnitude. If unchecked, crescendo angina may eventually result in angina decubitus (angina at rest) which can also appear without antecedent crescendo angina. Angina decubitus is completely unprovoked in the usual sense of being related to exertion or emotional stress and appears to be totally spontaneous. If unchecked, angina decubitus can lead to acute coronary insufficiency, a syndrome that can also occur de novo. Coronary insufficiency designates a situation in which chest pain and evidence of myocardial ischemia persist longer than the usual angina attack ($>$10 minutes), but it is not associated with electrocardiographic evidence of transmural myocardial infarction. Some physicians would permit mild elevations in serum creatine kinase in the coronary insufficiency syndrome ($\leq$2 times normal). Occasionally, it is difficult to distinguish between coronary insufficiency and non-transmural or non-Q wave myocardial infarction. The operational definition of the latter is chest pain lasting longer than 20 minutes, persistent electrocardiographic ST-T wave changes ($\geq$24 hours) without the development of significant Q waves and higher elevations in serum creatine kinase (greater than 2 times normal).[5]

Variant angina is also a form of unstable angina because it is spontaneous in nature and usually unprovoked by traditional exercise and stress. However, it may have a circadian rhythm, being more frequent in the early morning hours than in the late afternoon and evening,[6] although such a clear circadian periodicity in the case of total ischemic episodes was not found in a recent study.[7] It is characterized by unprovoked chest pain associated with ST-segment elevation on the electrocardiogram indicative of transmural myocardial ischemia. If these attacks do not remit spontaneously or if they are not aborted with medical therapy, then presumably transmural myocardial infarction could result. However, this appears to be an unusual complication of variant angina. Thus, prognostically variant angina is not as serious as the angina syndromes just discussed. Nevertheless, this is an incapacitating syndrome with the potential for disastrous consequences that need to be dealt with urgently as do the other unstable angina syndromes.

The clinical setting of the patient presenting with unstable angina is as varied as the unstable angina syndromes themselves. The setting may be new onset angina in a patient without a previous history of cardiac disease or symptoms of chest pain. It is not known whether the unstable angina will become stable, because stable angina by definition requires a certain passage of time. Thus, new onset angina may not always carry as serious a prognosis as do other forms of unstable angina. Unstable angina can also develop in a patient with chronic stable angina. In fact, this is one of the most common clinical settings for the presentation of unstable angina. Patients with angina pectoris in the recovery phase from acute myocardial infarction must also be considered as having unstable angina, because these patients are usually on restricted activity. Also, the presence of recurrent ischemia close to a major ischemic event is prognostically worrisome. In addition, angina that develops following percutaneous coronary angioplasty or coronary artery bypass graft surgery is especially worrisome and innately unstable, because again these patients are frequently on limited activities and should have an adequate blood supply to the myocardium if the procedure was successful. Recurrent ischemia suggests failure of the procedure and needs immediate attention.

The pathophysiology of unstable angina pectoris in the industrialized nations of the world is usually related to progression of preexisting atherosclerotic coronary artery lesions. Recent evidence suggests that plaque rupture is a frequent basis for the development of unstable ischemic syndromes.[8] Rupture of an atherosclerotic plaque releases factors into the blood stream that attract platelets and promote the generation of thrombosis.[9] If coronary blood flow is adequate, the resultant aggregates and thrombi may be washed downstream and cleared by the body's thrombolytic system without an untoward event. However, if the plaque is in an area of critical stenosis or if the patient's thrombolytic system is overwhelmed by the effects of cigarette smoking and other potentiators of thrombosis, sharp reductions in coronary blood flow may result, causing the syndrome of unstable angina. In addition, plaque rupture may precipitate coronary artery spasm which would further narrow the lumen and aggravate the process. The reaction to plaque rupture may include an increase in sympathetic nervous system activity which would increase heart rate and blood pressure and thereby raise myocardial oxygen demand which may further aggravate the process. Thus, there may be a combination of mechanisms, possibly initiated by plaque disruption with release of factors into the circulation, that can induce coronary artery spasm and thrombosis. The sympathetic reaction to these events may lead to an increase in myocardial oxygen demand which may lead to a vicious cycle of increased demand/reduced supply, which if not broken could progress to acute myocardial infarction.

The pathophysiology just described suggests that a mechanical approach to alleviating or bypassing the newly created critical obstruction of the coronary artery may be the best long-term management strategy. An early cooperative trial to compare immediate surgical therapy with medical therapy with beta-blockers demonstrated that acute symptomatic relief and prevention of complications could be achieved by either form of therapy equally well.[10] However, during long-term follow-up the crossover rate from the medical group into the surgical group was approximately one third. Thus, this study popularized the concept that medical therapy was valuable for aborting the acute attacks and "buying" time, but that eventually patients would need more definitive therapy of their coronary artery lesions, unless of course they had "pure" vasospastic angina.

PHARMACOLOGIC THERAPEUTIC STRATEGIES

In terms of pharmacologic approaches to reduce or abolish transient episodes of ischemia, perhaps a distinction should be made as to whether the patient has Prinzmetal's angina or unstable angina in which vasospastic component may not play a dominant role in the pathogenesis of individual episodes. In the former, long-term therapy with coronary vasodilators especially calcium-channel blockers,[11–13] is highly efficacious. Two studies deserve particular emphasis. The first, reported by Antman et al,[12] involved 127 patients in a multicenter study in which nifedipine in doses of 40 to 60 mg per day completely eliminated spontaneous pain episodes in 63 percent of cases, there being at least a 50 percent decrease in such attacks in 87 percent. In a subsequent multicenter, randomized, double-blind withdrawal study comparing nifedipine to placebo, the calcium antagonist was more effective than placebo.[14] It should be emphasized that in neither of these studies was Holter monitoring undertaken to evaluate the effects of nifedipine on painful or painless episodes of myocardial ischemia. In a smaller but a double-blind placebo-controlled study reported by Johnson et al,[13] verapamil, as in the case of nifedipine, markedly reduced the frequency of silent as well as the symptomatic episodes of ST-segment deviations documented on Holter recordings; however, the authors did not distinguish between silent and symptomatic episodes.

It should be emphasized that the effects of beta-blockers have not been systematically evaluated in variant angina. Anecdotal reports suggest that these agents may aggravate some cases of the syndrome. However, there has been only one study in which a beta-blocker (propranolol) increased the duration of vasotonic angina in patients with angiographically normal coronary arteries.[15] It is likely that this agent is applicable in only a minority of patients.

CONTROL OF ISCHEMIA IN UNSTABLE ANGINA

The current management strategy is to hospitalize patients with unstable angina and to begin treatment with one or usually more antianginal agents. If they continue to have pain at rest in the hospital, intravenous therapy with agents such as nitroglycerin or beta-blockers, or both, usually is begun. If multiple combination therapy does not control the syndrome, then mechanical therapy with intraaortic balloon pumping is instituted in appropriate patients who can be taken expeditiously to the cardiac catheterization laboratory for an assessment of coronary anatomy by angiography with the hope of performing either percutaneous transluminal coronary angioplasty or coronary artery bypass surgery emergently. Patients who respond well to medical treatment can undergo cardiac catheterization at a later, more convenient time. Consideration of their coronary anatomy will then dictate whether they will continue to be treated medically or whether mechanical therapy is recommended. It was in this general therapeutic framework that calcium blockers became available. Thus, in the beginning these agents were treated as add-on therapy in patients with unstable angina who failed on beta-blocker and nitrate treatment. More recently, comparative studies have been performed. It is becoming standard therapy to combine nitrate with a calcium antagonist and beta-blockers. The rest of this chapter will discuss the studies in which the effects of beta-blockers and calcium blockers were compared in the treatment of unstable and vasospastic angina.

ADD-ON THERAPY STUDIES

The earliest studies performed in patients with unstable angina using the calcium-channel blockers were studies in which a calcium-channel blocker was added to conventional therapy in patients unresponsive to the conventional therapeutic regimen. These studies introduce bias in that they select patients unresponsive in conventional therapy which was usually beta-blockers and nitrates. Thus, a high proportion of patients with a prominent vasospastic component to their angina pectoris could be anticipated. In fact, comparison of the electrocardiographic data in these studies suggests a higher than normal incidence of patients with ST-segment elevation observed during chest pain. Some large trials attempted to get around this bias by comparing multiple drug regimens, but unfortunately not all possible combinations of available drug therapy were tested. Nevertheless, these earlier studies provided some helpful insights into the use of calcium-channel blockers in the management of unstable angina, but none of the studies has addressed the issue of the effects of therapy on transient myocardial ischemia using Holter monitoring in controlled studies.

Several small studies or subgroups of larger studies have tested the addition of nifedipine therapy in patients whose condition was refractory to beta-blocker and nitrate treatment.[16–20] All these studies demonstrated symptomatic benefit from adding nifedipine therapy. The implication from these studies is that failure of beta-blocker and nitrate therapy identifies a group of patients with unstable angina in whom coronary artery spasm is playing an important role that can be controlled by the addition of a potent coronary vasodilator such as nifedipine. However, because the incidence of subsequent ischemic events is unchanged, the basic pathophysiology of worsening coronary obstruction must eventually lead to coronary thrombosis despite triple drug therapy. Again, in these studies and in the Holland Interuniversity nifedipine/metoprolol trial (HINT), the effects of beta blockade (metoprolol) and calcium antagonism (nifedipine), or their combination, on transient myocardial ischemic episodes were not critically evaluated. It must be emphasized that although the HINT trial was large, the trial treatment groups were small, and the effects on clinical outcome merely indicated trends without demonstrating unequivocal statistically significant differences. It was nevertheless noteworthy that of all the treatments studied in this trial, only the addition of nifedipine to previous maintenance treatment with a beta-blocker was clearly beneficial. The data suggest the importance of combining calcium-channel blockers and beta-blockers in the control of symptomatic myocardial ischemia in unstable angina. It would be of particular interest to determine the effects of calcium-channel blockers, beta-blockers, and their combination in the suppression of silent and symptomatic ischemia in unstable angina and to determine the effects on clinical outcome.

An interesting twist to the add-on therapy studies, in which the effects of therapy on Holter-detected ischemia were tested, was reported by Gottlieb and co-workers.[22] They studied patients who, while receiving nifedipine and nitrates, presented with unstable angina and compared the effects of adding propranolol therapy to placebo. They noted a beneficial effect of propranolol therapy on both symptomatic and asymptomatic episodes of myocardial ischemia. Furthermore, beta-blocker therapy was not detrimental in any patient in whom it was administered. This study also supports the value of beta-blockers in unstable angina and suggests that combination therapy (beta-blockade, calcium-channel blockers, and nitrates) may be the best approach in hospitalized patients.

Parodi and co-workers[23] reported on a small group of patients with unstable angina who were on chronic nitrate therapy and in whom the addition of a beta-blocker or verapamil or placebo was tested. They found that verapamil was superior to beta-blockers in these patients; however, it is noteworthy that in 8 of the 10 subjects ST-segment elevation was observed during episodes of pain. Also, some of the patients were responsive to propranolol therapy, and propranolol did not aggravate symptoms in any of the patients. This study also supports a role for calcium-channel blocker therapy in patients with a major vasospastic component to their unstable angina.

Finally, Theroux et al[24] investigated a group of patients on chronic isosorbide dinitrate therapy who developed unstable angina and were randomized to either propranolol therapy or the calcium-channel blocker diltiazem.[16] There was no difference in symptom relief between the two treatments or in any of the subsequent outcomes (Figure 21.1). Interestingly, these investigators excluded patients with ST-segment elevation, and they concluded that if patients with ST-segment elevation are eliminated, coronary artery spasm is not a major factor in the pathogenesis of unstable angina and therefore that calcium-channel blockers do not add significantly to the management of patients in whom spasm is unlikely. However, this study did not address the issue of a possible difference between the two classes of drugs in the treatment of silent myocardial ischemia.

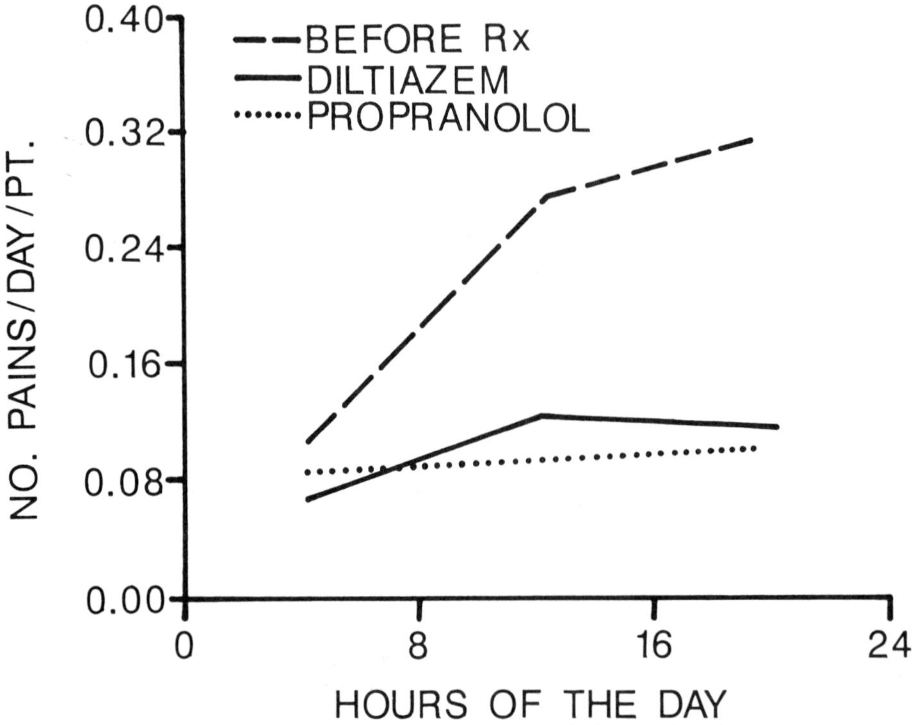

FIGURE 21.1. Effects of propranolol and diltiazem in pain-related episodes of ischemia in patients with unstable angina on nitrate therapy. The effects are compared to those of placebo. Silent ischemic episodes were not evaluated. Note that both calcium-channel blockers and beta-blockers have comparable potency in reducing pain. (From Theroux et al[24] with the permission of the authors and the *Journal of the American College of Cardiology*.)

COMPARISON STUDIES

With the exception of the Holland Interuniversity Study,[21] above, there have been few true comparison studies of beta-blockers and calcium blockers in the management of unstable and vasospastic angina. Even the available studies often contain subgroups in which true comparisons were not conducted. In most comparison studies, no placebo groups are included, because it would be dangerous to treat patients with unstable angina with nothing. This approach is understandable but leads to some concern regarding spontaneous changes in symptoms due to hospitalization alone. Although the study design in these trials was different from the additional therapy trials already mentioned, the results were not substantially different.

Andre-Fouet and colleagues[25] reported on a group of 70 patients with unstable angina, approximately one third of whom had ST-segment elevation observed with their episodes of chest pain, who were randomized to 49 hours of diltiazem therapy or propranolol. There was no overall difference between either therapy in the relief of symptoms; however, four patients with ST-segment elevation during their angina episodes were somewhat worse on propranolol therapy. The best criteria for selecting patients who would respond better to diltiazem were those found in the subgroup of patients who had rest angina only, irrespective of the nature of their ST-T wave changes. Again, this study supports the use of calcium-channel blockers for patients whose vasospasm is playing a prominent role in their unstable angina.

Muller and colleagues[20] reported on 126 patients with unstable angina who were randomly treated with propranolol plus isosorbide dinitrate or nifedipine in a blinded fashion. The comparison showed no difference in symptom relief or future ischemic events (Figure 21.2). Subgroup analysis of their trial revealed some interesting features. In the subgroup of 67 patients who had been on propranolol therapy before the trial, nifedipine was better than conventional therapy (Figure 21.3). However, the 59 patients who had not been on beta-blocker therapy before the trial achieved more rapid pain relief with beta-blocker therapy. Thus, they concluded that the overall lack of difference between the two treatment modalities was due to a counterbalancing effect of these two subgroups, and they suggested that if patients were already receiving beta-blockers, the addition of nifedipine was likely to be an effective treatment; however, if a patient had never been on beta-blocker therapy, then beta-blockers would be the first choice of therapy. The overall data clearly indicate the importance of combining beta-blockers and calcium-channel blockers.

Finally, Quyyumi and associates[26] reported on a small trial of nine patients with unstable angina in whom atenolol, nifedipine, and isosorbide mononitrate were compared in a triple crossover design. All three forms of therapy were beneficial, as shown in Figure 21.4. However, atenolol was best in decreasing exertion-related angina. Nifedipine and isosorbide mononitrate were best in controlling asymptomatic myocardial ischemic episodes, and all forms of therapy were equivalent in controlling nocturnal angina. Again, this trial points to a role for calcium blockers in patients likely to have a vasospastic component and the superiority of beta-blockers in

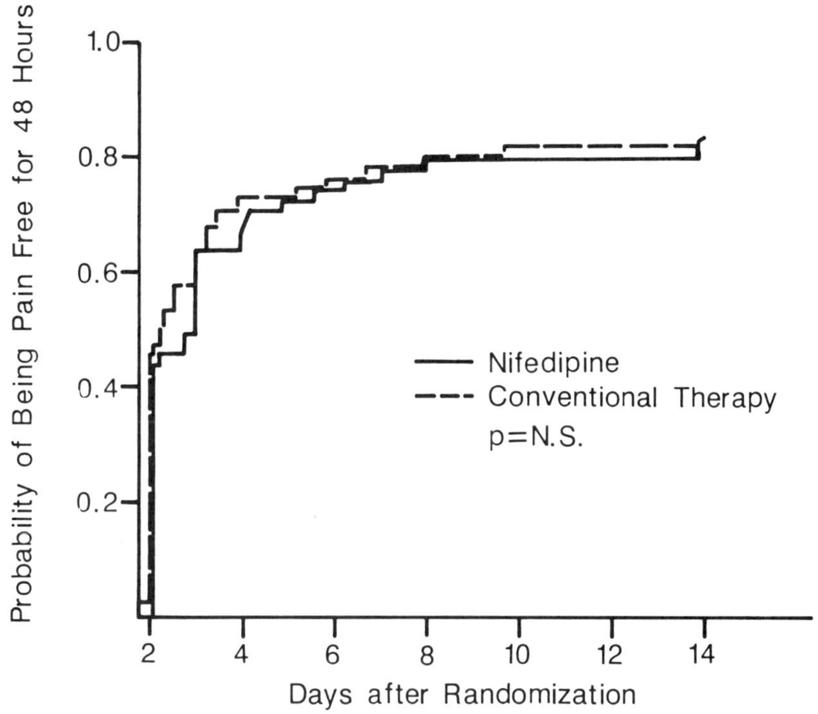

FIGURE 21.2. Probability of remaining pain free for ≥48 hours in all 126 patients with unstable angina randomly assigned to receive propranolol plus isosorbide dinitrate (conventional therapy) or nifedipine. Note there was no difference between the action of the calcium antagonist versus that of the combination of propranolol and isosorbide dinitrate. (From Muller et al[20] with permission of the authors and the American Heart Association.)

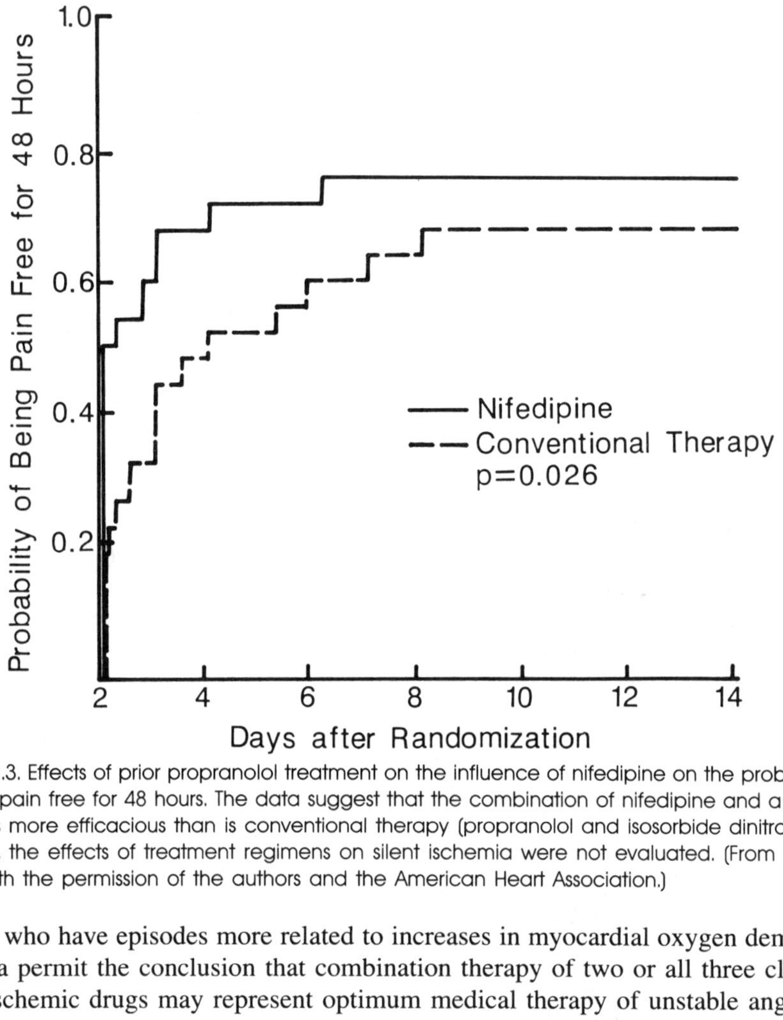

FIGURE 21.3. Effects of prior propranolol treatment on the influence of nifedipine on the probability of being pain free for 48 hours. The data suggest that the combination of nifedipine and a beta-blocker is more efficacious than is conventional therapy (propranolol and isosorbide dinitrate). In this study, the effects of treatment regimens on silent ischemia were not evaluated. (From Muller et al[20] with the permission of the authors and the American Heart Association.)

patients who have episodes more related to increases in myocardial oxygen demand. The data permit the conclusion that combination therapy of two or all three classes of antiischemic drugs may represent optimum medical therapy of unstable angina.

SUMMARY AND RECOMMENDATIONS

None of the trials conducted to date has been ideal, because not all therapies have been tested with the same study design and not all patients have been categorized and classified prospectively in a way that insures a lack of bias. Nevertheless, certain tentative conclusions can be derived from these studies which compare the influence of beta-blockers and calcium blockers in the treatment of transient myocardial ischemia in unstable and vasospastic angina. First, optimal therapy for unstable angina may be attained more readily with multiple drug therapy involving agents with coronary dilator actions and with a propensity for reducing oxygen demand. Second, monotherapy with individual agents may be effective or rarely deleterious in small subsets of patients, but the significance of the effects has not critically been determined nor have their effects on clinical outcome in the manner reported for aspirin involving controlled clinical trials of optimal protocol design and adequate sample size. Third, if a patient already on a beta-blocker develops unstable angina pectoris, the data suggest that the addition of nifedipine is likely to be efficacious in con-

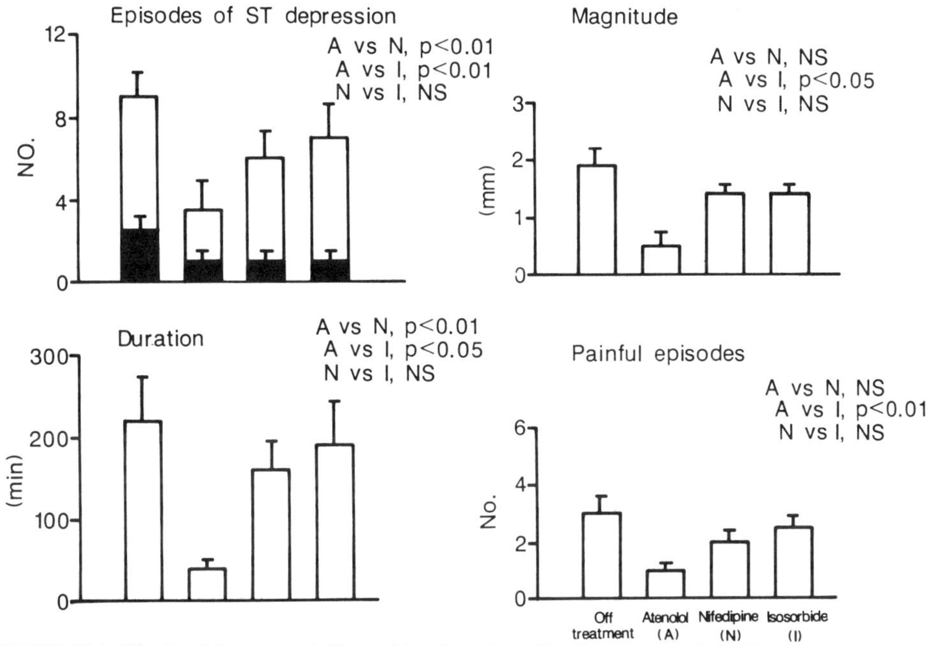

FIGURE 21.4. Effects of three modalities of treatment on the frequency of daytime and nocturnal (*shaded*) ischemic episodes (as assessed by ambulatory ECG monitoring), ST-segment depression, their duration and magnitude, and the frequency of painful episodes during the initial off-treatment period and during various treatment periods. Results represent means ± 1 SE. There was no significant difference between the action of nitrates and nifedipine, with atenolol being more effective. (From Quyyumi et al[26] with the permission of the authors and the *British Heart Journal*.)

trolling symptoms. Whether adding another calcium blocker would be equally efficacious is unclear from the reported studies, but there is no reason to believe that either verapamil or diltiazem would not be effective. Finally, if the patient is already receiving nitrate therapy, the studies would support adding either a beta-blocker or diltiazem; whether nifedipine or verapamil would be useful in this regard is unclear from the data currently available.

The comparative studies discussed did not always subclassify the patient in terms of other variables known to be important in the choice of one form of therapy over another. Also, some patient characteristics that might dictate one type of therapy over another were a cause for exclusion from some trials. Therefore, it is useful to address other specific indications for therapy with either beta-blockers or calcium blockers in patients with unstable angina.

In patients not receiving therapy who present with unstable angina there appear to be several potential indications for starting with beta-blocker therapy. One is increased heart rate not due to congestive heart failure. Because heart rate is an important determinant of myocardial oxygen demand, it seems important to bring this factor under control before considering other forms of treatment. Second, the presence of supraventricular or ventricular tachyarrhythmias are also an indication for considering beta-blocker therapy as first choice, because the use of beta-blockers alone or in combination with other antiarrhythmic agents is often efficacious in suppressing arrhythmias associated with myocardial ischemia, whereas calcium blockers are of less value in this regard. Third, hypertension could also be effectively managed by administration of a beta-blocker, which would also reduce myocardial oxygen demand and may control symptoms without having to resort to other forms of therapy. Obviously, calcium blockers can also decrease blood pressure as can a number of other agents, but considering the overall milieu of unstable angina, beta-blockers seem to be a good choice in this setting. Finally, it would appear from some of the data on patients with unstable angina that a strong history of exertional or demand-related angina in a patient whose angina had recently become unstable and who was not taking a beta-blocker would constitute an indication for trying beta-blocker therapy first.

There are also several situations in which a calcium blocker may be the best choice. First are patients who have contraindications to beta-blocker therapy, such as the presence of overt congestive heart failure or a history of bronchospastic disease. Second, patients who are likely to have coronary artery vasospasm as a major component of the pathophysiology of unstable angina apparently are best treated with a calcium blocker. These patients are those who had electrocardiographic ST-segment elevation associated with their episodes of pain. Also, patients with only rest pain that is unprovoked or spontaneous are more likely to have a coronary vasospastic mechanism and may respond best to calcium-channel blocker therapy. Finally, the patient with non-Q-wave myocardial infarction at this time would probably be best managed with diltiazem therapy, because it has been shown that this form of treatment can prevent recurrent ischemic events for up to 2 weeks following nontransmural myocardial infarction.[27]

The prognosis of patients with unstable and vasospastic angina is related to the underlying pathophysiology and, in the case of obstructive coronary artery disease, to the anatomy of the lesions. Those with minimal or no coronary occlusive disease who mainly have vasospasm are known to do well for long periods on medical management with calcium blockers and/or nitrates.[6] In fact, spontaneous remissions have been noted in these patients after the alleviation of certain stressful and emotional factors. Thus, these patients have an excellent prognosis. Those with occlusive coronary artery disease have a less favorable prognosis and should undergo cardiac catheterization as soon as feasible to identify the underlying anatomy. In appropriate patients, a mechanical solution to the coronary occlusive disease should be considered and carried out as soon as convenient. In patients in whom the anatomy of their coronary occlusive disease is not conducive to a mechanical solution, long-term medical therapy should be continued with periodic reevaluation of their status, because unstable angina is a highly variable syndrome with a diverse pathophysiology that may change in time and require adaptations of the therapeutic regimen along the lines indicated by the present discussion.

REFERENCES

1. Cruickshank JM, Prichard BNC: *Beta-Blockers in Clinical Practice*. Edinburgh, Churchill Livingstone, 1987 pp 505–576.
2. Singh BN, Ellrodt G, Nademanee K: Calcium antagonists: Cardiocirculatory effects and therapeutic applications, in Hurst JW (ed): *Clinical Essays of the Heart*. New York, McGraw-Hill Book Co., 1984; pp 65–97.
3. Maseri A: The role of coronary artery spasm in symptomatic and silent myocardial ischemia. *J Am Coll Cardiol* 1987;9:249–262.
4. Waters DD, Szlachcic J, Theroux P, Dauwe F, Mizgala H: Ergonovine testing to detect spontaneous remission of variant angina longterm. *Am J Cardiol* 1981;47:179–184.
5. Kingma JG, Denniss AR, Hearse DJ, et al: Limitation of infarct size for 24 hours by

combined treatment with allopurinol plus verapamil during acute myocardial infarction in the dog. *Circulation* 1987;75:V25–33.
6. Theroux P: A pathophysiologic basis for the clinical classification and management of unstable angina. *Circulation* 1987;75:V103–109.
7. Nademanee K, Intarachot V, Josephson MA, Singh BN: Circadian variation in occurrence of transient overt and silent myocardial ischemia in chronic stable angina and comparison with Prinzmetal angina in men. *Am J Cardiol* 1987;60:494–498.
8. Davies MJ, Thomas A: Thrombosis and acute coronary artery lesions in sudden cardiac ischemic death. *N Engl J Med* 1975;310:1137–1140.
9. Sherman CT, Litvak F, Grundfest W, et al: Coronary angioscopy in patients with unstable angina pectoris. *N Engl J Med* 1986;315:913–919.
10. Unstable Angina Pectoris Study Group: Unstable angina pectoris: National cooperative study group to compare surgical and medical therapy. II. In-hospital experience and initial follow-up results in patients with one-, two-, and three-vessel disease. *Am J Cardiol* 1978;42:839–848.
11. Schroeder JS, Lamb IH, Bristow MR, et al: Prevention of cardiovascular events in variant angina by long-term diltiazem therapy. *J Am Coll Cardiol* 1983;1:1507–1511.
12. Antman E, Muller JE, Goldberg S, et al: Nifedipine therapy for coronary artery spasm experience in 127 patients. *N Engl J Med* 1980;302:1269–1274.
13. Johnson SM, Mauritson DR, Willerson JT, Hillis LD: A controlled trial of verapamil for Prinzmetal's variant angina. *N Engl J Med* 1981;304:862–868.
14. Schick E: Randomized withdrawal from nifedipine—placebo controlled study in patients with coronary artery spasm. *Am Heart J* 1982;104:690–696.
15. Robertson RM, Wood AJJ, Vanghn WK, Robertson D: Exacerbation of vasotonic angina pectoris by propranolol. *Circulation* 1982;65:281–285.
16. Hugenholtz PG, Michels HR, Serruys PW, et al: Nifedipine in the treatment of unstable angina, coronary spasm and myocardial ischemia. *Am J Cardiol* 1981;47:163–173.
17. Moses JW, Wertheimer JH, Bodenheimer MM, et al: Efficacy of nifedipine in rest angina refractory to propranolol and nitrates in patients with obstructive coronary artery disease. *Ann Int Med* 1981;94:425–429.
18. Blaustein AS, Heller GV, Kolman RS: Adjunctive nifedipine therapy in high-risk, medically refractory, unstable angina. *Am J Cardiol* 1983;52:950–954.
19. Gerstenblith G, Ouyang P, Achuff SG, et al: Nifedipine in unstable angina. A double-blind randomized trial. *N Engl J Med* 1982;306:885–889.
20. Muller JE, Turi ZG, Pearle DL, et al: Nifedipine and conventional therapy for unstable angina pectoris: A randomized, double-blind comparison. *Circulation* 1984;69:728–739.
21. Report of the Holland Interuniversity Nifedipine/Metoprolol Trial (HINT) Research Group: Early treatment of unstable angina in the coronary care unit: A randomized, double blind, placebo controlled comparison of recurrent ischemia in patients treated with nifedipine or metoprolol or both. *Br Heart J* 1986;56:400–413.
22. Gottlieb SO, Weisfeldt ML, Ouyang P, et al: Effect of the addition of propranolol to therapy with nifedipine for unstable angina pectoris: A randomized, double-blind, placebo-controlled trial. *Circulation* 1986;73:331–337.
23. Parodi O, Simonetti I, Michelassi C, et al: Comparison of verapamil and propranolol therapy for angina pectoris at rest: A randomized, multiple-crossover, controlled trial in the coronary care unit. *Am J Cardiol* 1986;57:899–906.
24. Theroux P, Taeymans Y, Morissette D, et al: A randomized study comparing propranolol and diltiazem in the treatment of unstable angina. *J Am Coll Cardiol* 1985;5:717–722.
25. Andre-Fouet X, Usdin JP, Gayet CH, et al: Comparison of short-term efficacy of diltiazem and propranolol in unstable angina at rest. A randomized trial in 70 patients. *Eur Heart J* 1983;4:691–698.
26. Quyyumi AA, Crake T, Wright CM, et al: Medical treatment of patients with severe exertional and rest angina: Double blind comparison of beta blocker, calcium antagonist, and nitrate. *Br Heart J* 1987;57:505–511.
27. Gibson RS, Boden WE, Theroux P, et al: Diltiazem and reinfarction in patients with non-Q-wave myocardial infarction. Results of a double-blind, randomized, multicenter trial. *N Engl J Med* 1986;315:423–429.

CHAPTER 22

Treating the Complex Pathophysiology of Unstable Angina

Focus on Silent Ischemia and the Importance of Combination Therapy

Sidney O. Gottlieb, MD

Evolution of the pathophysiologic understanding of unstable angina involves a wider understanding of the importance of dynamic factors including inappropriate coronary vasoconstriction and platelet aggregation and thrombosis (see Chapter 3) superimposed upon atherosclerotic coronary artery disease.[1–7] Although progressive atherosclerotic obstruction is often present in patients with unstable angina,[8] events precipitating crescendo or resting symptoms may include disruption of an atherosclerotic plaque with subsequent platelet aggregation, which may lead to intermittent thrombotic occlusion of the vessel,[9] and vasoconstriction as a primary event or aggravated by vasoconstrictor mediators from aggregating platelets.[6,7] Attention has thus been directed to the relief of coronary vasoconstriction and platelet aggregation with coronary vasodilating agents such as nitrates and calcium antagonists, and antiplatelet and antithrombolytic drugs. This review will discuss the rationale for and results of clinical trials of combination medical therapy with nitrates, beta-blockers, and calcium antagonists in unstable angina, as well as the combined use of antiplatelet and antithrombotic strategies in an effort to reduce both symptomatic and silent ischemic events. The use of combination therapy presupposes a clear delineation of the mechanism of action and efficacy of individual agents.

BETA-BLOCKERS IN UNSTABLE ANGINA

Based largely on their documented efficacy in stable demand-related ischemia,[10,11] beta-blockers have been used for over 20 years in the management of patients with unstable angina; however, large controlled trials of their precise efficacy in preventing infarction or sudden death have not been reported. Although earlier reports suggested clinical benefit,[12,13] appreciation of the importance of coronary vasoconstriction in resting angina led to a theoretic concern that beta-blockers may potentiate myocardial ischemia in this setting by allowing for unopposed alpha-induced coronary vasoconstriction.[14,15] Reports of worsening ischemic symptoms with beta-blocker therapy including one small clinical placebo-controlled trial demonstrated prolongation of ischemic episodes by beta-blocker treatment detected by Holter monitoring in patients with vasospastic angina pectoris and little coronary artery disease.[16] Thus, reexamination of the role of beta-blockers in unstable angina was recently undertaken in a number of clinical trials addressing this issue.

Several studies compared the efficacy of beta-blockers and calcium antagonists in unstable angina. In the NAMIS Study,[17] a strategy of initial therapy with beta-blockers and nitrates was compared with nifedipine treatment. There was no significant difference between the effects of these two treatment regimens with regard to clinical outcomes, including frequency of recurrent angina. Of note, the subgroup in which nifedipine was added to prior ongoing beta-blocker therapy demonstrated the best clinical results. In another study, Theroux et al[18] examined monotherapy with diltiazem compared to propranolol in a double-blind randomized study. Although propranolol demonstrated no significant difference compared to placebo, diltiazem significantly reduced the number of symptomatic ischemic episodes. However, there was no significant difference in short-term prognosis between diltiazem and propranolol. Combination therapy was not studied. Parodi et al[19] compared the use of propranolol and verapamil to placebo in the control of symptomatic and silent ischemic episodes. In this crossover study involving prolonged periods of Holter monitoring in the coronary unit, propranolol was no better than placebo in reducing symptomatic and asymptomatic episodes of ischemia; however, verapamil significantly reduced or nearly eliminated all episodes. Thus, although beta-blockers may have variable clinical efficacy depending on the degree of underlying atherosclerotic coronary disease and the extent of superimposed vasopastic tendencies, clinical trials suggest that monotherapy with beta-blockers is not the ideal treatment for patients with resting symptoms in unstable angina.[16–20] However, it must be emphasized that it is entirely possible that in this study there may have been a preponderance of patients with vasospastic angina.

CALCIUM ANTAGONISTS IN UNSTABLE ANGINA

Early studies demonstrated the dramatic efficacy of certain calcium-antagonist drugs in reducing symptomatic and silent episodes in patients with vasospastic or Prinzmetal's angina. Nifedipine, diltiazem, and verapamil have demonstrated both short- and long-term efficacy in this setting.[20–22] More widespread application of these agents to the broad spectrum of patients with unstable angina has been studied, including the foregoing studies comparing calcium-blockers with beta-blockers and nitrates. In the HINT multicenter study,[23] therapy with nifedipine, metoprolol, and their combination was compared. In this trial, the only group to demonstrate statistically significant benefit of therapy was the combination group receiving both nifedipine and beta-blocker therapy. Thus, although calcium antagonists, when given alone, may have comparable efficacy to that of standard treatment, concern has been raised about monotherapy, and studies suggest that combination treatment with calcium antagonists and beta-blockers might be the most beneficial. There are theoretic reasons that suggest a combination might be the most effective regimen in reducing symptomatic as well as silent episodes of myocardial ischemia in this setting. This is relevant in clinical trials to examine the issue of suppression of silent ischemia relative to effects on the prognosis in unstable angina.

COMBINATION OF CALCIUM ANTAGONISTS AND BETA-BLOCKERS IN UNSTABLE ANGINA

In the Johns Hopkins Nifedipine Unstable Angina Trial,[24] the primary question addressed was the role of the addition of nifedipine to treatment with beta-blockers and nitrates. One hundred thirty-two patients were randomized to receive either nifedipine or placebo in addition to beta-blockers and nitrates after hospital admission to the coronary care unit. In this study, the addition of 80 mg of nifedipine per day resulted in a significant reduction in recurrent symptomatic events and thereby a reduction in the number of patients requiring bypass surgery for medically refractory angina. Although there was no significant difference between the groups with regard to survival or myocardial infarction rates in the overall population, the subgroup of patients with postinfarction angina did have a reduction in the number of deaths or reinfarctions with nifedipine treatment.[25]

In a subsequent follow-up study of combination therapy, the Johns Hopkins Propranolol Unstable Angina Study[26] randomized 81 patients with angina at rest to 160 mg of propranolol a day or placebo, added to the background therapy with nifedipine and nitrates. In this study, the addition of propranolol to nifedipine and nitrates significantly reduced the probability of recurrent rest angina and the number and duration of episodes of recurrent angina, and it also resulted in more than a 50 percent reduction in the number and duration of total episodes of ischemia on Holter monitoring (Figure 22.1). The resting heart rate was reduced in the propranolol group, but an important observation also was that the heart rate after the onset of ischemia increased significantly in the placebo group, but remained low and stable in the propranolol-treated group. Thus, although recurrent ischemic episodes are often asymptomatic, they may be associated with a reflex increase in heart rate, thus increasing in myocardial oxygen demands that may further aggravate ischemia. Beta-

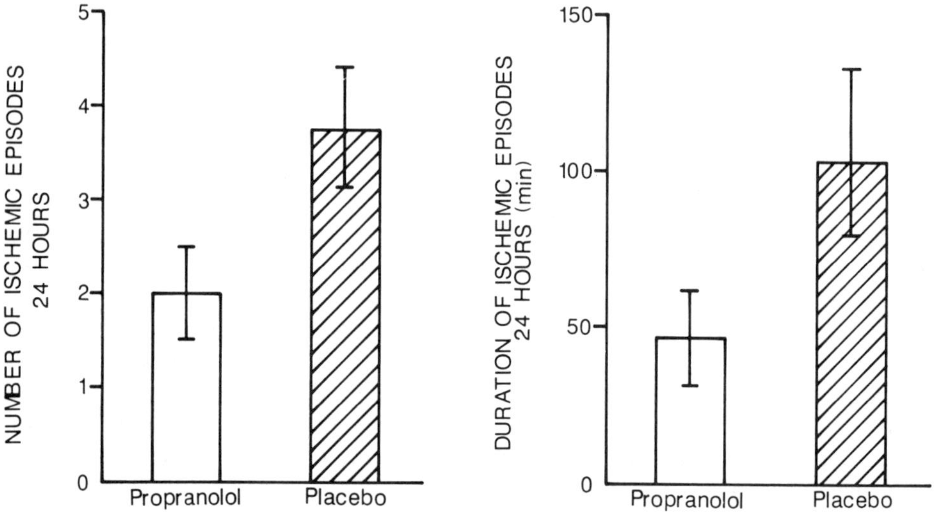

FIGURE 22.1. The number and duration of ischemic episodes per 24 hours as detected by continuous two-channel electrocardiographic monitoring during the first 2 days in patients with unstable angina treated with nifedipine (80 mg daily) and nitrates. Such patients were randomized in a double-blind protocol to propranolol (≥160 mg daily) and placebo. Note that the addition of propranolol to nifedipine and long-acting nitrates reduces the number ($p = 0.039$) and duration ($p = 0.036$) of ischemia when compared to the effects of placebo. (From Gottlieb et al[26] with the permission of the authors and the American Heart Association.)

blockers help both to reduce these ischemic episodes as well as to blunt the secondary increase in heart rate which may be detrimental. The effects of beta-blockade in this context are likely to lead to an attenuation of induced increases in heart rate, thereby shortening the overall duration of individual episodes of silent ischemia and preventing the attainment of the threshold perception of pain. Again, this emphasizes the significance of the combined effects of beta-blockers and the dihydropyridine types of calcium antagonists.

Other means whereby beta-blockers produce salutary effects in this setting should be considered. In addition to reducing myocardial oxygen demands, beta-blockers may reduce catecholamine-induced platelet aggregation;[27] they also allow for distribution of blood flow from the subepicardium to the subendocardium,[28] and may cause a rightward shift of the oxyhemoglobin dissociation curve, resulting in increased oxygen delivery to tissues.[29] Regardless of the mechanism or mechanisms responsible for this benefit, beta-blockers apparently have a synergistic benefit with calcium antagonists in reducing ischemic events.

Whereas the Johns Hopkins Unstable Angina Trials[24,26] examined the combination of nifedipine and propranolol, other calcium antagonists might be considered for this condition. Caution, however, is advised when considering the combination of verapamil and beta-blockers, because additive negative inotropic and atrioventricular conduction side effects may be noted with this combination. There appears to be less justification in combining verapamil with beta-blockers, particularly with prior impairment of left ventricular function or AV conduction. Diltiazem has been combined with beta-blockers in a number of instances, although the precipitation of severe bradycardia, heart block, or left ventricular dysfunction may be greater than that with nifedipine. Because nifedipine is the dihydropyridine prototype with more "pure" vasodilator properties, there is less risk of impairing left ventricular function or conduction when combined with beta-blockers. The role of the newer dihydropyridines in this setting has not been studied.

ANTIPLATELET AGENTS IN UNSTABLE ANGINA

Although symptomatic and silent ischemic episodes can be reduced by combining beta-blockers and calcium antagonists, there is little evidence to date that they significantly reduce the risk of death or myocardial infarction in this syndrome. Most reported studies were performed without the routine use of antiplatelet agents. Two large randomized trials demonstrated reduced death and infarction rates with aspirin in unstable angina. The first to be reported was the Multicenter Veterans Cooperative Trial[31] which demonstrated a 51 percent reduction in death or reinfarction in patients with unstable angina treated with 325 mg of aspirin per day. A subsequent Multicenter Canadian Trial[32] demonstrated that aspirin in a larger dose also resulted in a comparable 50 percent reduction in deaths or myocardial infarctions. Because side effects were extremely rare with the 325-mg dose in the VA study, it appears prudent to recommend this dosage to minimize gastrointestinal side effects. In the Canadian Multicenter Study,[32] the concomitant use of sulfinpyrazone was found to be of no clinical benefit. Thus, aspirin alone should be added to the combination of nitrates, beta-blockers, and calcium antagonists in unstable angina pectoris. It will be of particular interest to determine whether such a combination of agents will be synergistic in effect and whether such a potential action might be mediated through a reduction in silent ischemia.

ANTICOAGULANT AND THROMBOLYTIC THERAPY

Although heparin has been used by many clinicians in the in-hospital treatment of unstable angina, less information is available from clinical trials testing its efficacy. In one study, heparin was associated with a reduction in the progression to myocardial infarction.[33] In a more recent randomized trial, however, heparin demonstrated no significant clinical benefit.[34]

Thrombolytic therapy with streptokinase and tPA has been tested in subsets of patients with unstable angina. Vetrovec et al[35] demonstrated a resolution of intracoronary thrombus with intracoronary streptokinase. In a subset of patients with postinfarction angina, Shapiro et al[36] demonstrated the feasibility of intracoronary streptokinase therapy in restoring the patency of infarct-related vessels when thrombotic occlusion is present, and this was associated with a reduction in recurrent symptomatic episodes of angina. In a recent controlled trial, intravenous tPA reduced the incidence of thrombotic occlusion and recurrent symptomatic ischemic episodes compared to placebo.[37] In another recent study the benefit of tPA therapy was observed, but it appeared to be restricted to a subset with angiographically visible filling defects consistent with thrombus.[38] Thus, although thrombolytic therapy may be effective in certain subsets with significant degrees of thrombotic occlusion, its widespread use in the broad spectrum of patients with unstable angina is as yet undefined.

LIMITATIONS OF MEDICAL THERAPY: PROGNOSTIC SIGNIFICANCE OF PERSISTENT ISCHEMIA

Although combination medical therapy in most instances is sufficient to control symptoms, several studies demonstrated that a large percentage of patients continue to have persistent asymptomatic ischemia on Holter monitoring despite this clinically successful therapy.[39–41] The presence of persistent ischemia despite combination medical therapy has been associated with an increased incidence of adverse subsequent cardiac events, including death or myocardial infarction. Thus, reexamination of therapeutic goals in patients with unstable angina suggests that resolution of pain by itself may be an insufficient end point if objective evidence of recurrent ischemia is still present. Ongoing clinical trials will determine whether the therapy aimed at reducing silent ischemia will improve prognosis in patients with unstable angina. Until these results are available, it is reasonable to consider early revascularization in suitable candidates with coronary angioplasty or bypass surgery in the presence of ongoing silent ischemia despite maximally tolerated combination medical therapy.

REFERENCES

1. Maseri A, L'Abbate A, Baroldi G, et al: Coronary vasospasm as a possible cause of myocardial infarction. A conclusion derived from the study of preinfarction angina. *N Engl J Med* 1978;299:1271–1277.
2. Epstein SE, Palmieri ST: Mechanisms contributing to a precipitation of unstable angina and acute myocardial infarction: Implications regarding therapy. *Am J Cardiol* 1984;54:1245–1252.
3. Maseri A: Pathogenetic classification of unstable angina as a guideline to individual patient management and prognosis. *Am J Med* 1986;80(suppl 4C):48–55.
4. Gorlin R, Fuster V, Ambrose JA: Anatomic-physiologic links between acute coronary syndromes. (Editorial). *Circulation* 1986;74:6.

5. Ludmer PL, Selwyn AP, Shook TL, et al: Paradoxical vasoconstriction induced by acetylcholine in atherosclerotic coronary arteries. *N Engl J Med* 1986;315:1046–1051.
6. Fitzgerald DJ, Roy L, Catella F, Fitzgerald GA: Platelet activation in unstable coronary disease. *N Engl J Med* 1986;315:983.
7. Sherman T, Litvack F, Grundfest W, et al: Coronary angioscopy in patients with unstable angina pectoris. *N Engl J Med* 1986;315:913–919.
8. Moise A, Theroux P, Taeymans Y, et al: Unstable angina and progression of coronary atherosclerosis. *N Engl J Med* 1983;309:685.
9. Davies MJ, Thomas AC: Plaque fissuring—the cause of acute myocardial infarction, sudden ischaemic death, and crescendo angina. *Br Heart J* 1985;53:363–373.
10. Grant RHE, Keelan P, Kernohan RJ, Leonard JC, Nancekievill L, Sinclair K: Multicenter trial of propranolol in angina pectoris. *Am J Cardiol* 1966;18:361.
11. Alderman El, Daview RO, Crowley JJ, Lopes MG, Brooker JZ, Friedman JP, Graham AF, Matlof HJ, Harrison DC: Dose response effectiveness of propranolol for the treatment of angina pectoris. *Circulation* 1975;51:964.
12. Fischl SJ, Herman MV, Gorlin R: The intermediate coronary syndrome: Clinical, angiographic and therapeutic aspects. *N Engl J Med* 1973;288:1193.
13. Guazzi M, Fiorentini C, Polese A, Magrini F, Olivari MT: Treatment of spontaneous angina pectoris with beta blocking agents: A clinical, electrocardiographic and hemodynamic appraisal. *Br Heart J* 1975;37:1235.
14. Yasue H, Touyama M, Kato H, Tanaka S, Akiyama F: Prinzmetal's variant form of angina as a manifestation of alpha-adrenergic receptor-mediated coronary artery spasm: Documentation by coronary arteriography. *Am Heart J* 1976;91:148.
15. Kern MJ, Ganz P, Horowitz JD, Gaspar J, Barry WH, Lorell BN, Grossman W, Mudge GH: Potentiation of coronary vasoconstriction by beta-adrenergic blockade in patients with coronary artery disease. *Circulation* 1983;67:1178.
16. Robertson RM, Wood AJ, Vaughn WK, Robertson D: Exacerbation of vasotonic angina pectoris by propranolol. *Circulation* 1982;65:281.
17. Muller JE, Turi ZG, Pearle DL, Schneider JF, Serfas DH, Morrison J, Stone PH, Rude RE, Rosner B, Sobel BE, Tate C, Scheiner E, Roberts R, Hennekens CH, Braunwald E: Nifedipine and conventional therapy for unstable angina pectoris: A randomized, double-blind comparison. *Circulation* 1984;69:729.
18. Theroux P, Taeymans Y, Morissette D, Bosch X, Pelletier GB, Waters DD: A randomized study comparing propranolol and diltiazem in the treatment of unstable angina. *J Am Coll Cardiol* 1985;5:717.
19. Parodi O, Simonetti I, Michelassi C, Carpeggiania C, Biagini A, L'Abbate A, Maseri A: Comparison of verapamil and propranolol therapy for angina pectoris at rest: A randomized multiple-crossover, controlled trial in the coronary care unit. *Am J Cardiol* 1986;57:899–906.
20. Tilmant PY, LaBlanche JM, Thieuleux FA, Dupuis BA, Betrand ME: Detrimental effect of propranolol in patients with coronary arterial spasm countered by combination with diltiazem. *Am J Cardiol* 1983;52:230–233.
21. Pepine CJ, Feldman RL, Shittle J, Curry RC, Conti CR: Effect of diltiazem in patients with variant angina: A randomized double-blind trial. *Am Heart J* 1981;101:719–725.
22. Antman E, Muller J, Goldberg S, MacAlpin R, Rubenfire M, Tabatznik B, Liang CS, Heupler F, Achuff S, Reicheck N, Geltman E, Kerin NZ, Neff RK, Braunwald E: Nifedipine therapy for coronary artery spasm: Experience in 127 patients. *N Engl J Med* 1980;302:1269.
23. Holland Interuniversity Nifedipine/Metoprolol Trial (HINT) Research Group. Early treatment of unstable angina in the coronary care unit: A randomized, double-blind, placebo-controlled comparison of recurrent ischemia in patients treated with nifedipine or metoprolol or both. *Br Heart J* 1986;56:400.
24. Gerstenblith G, Ouyang P, Achuff SC, Bulkley BH, Becker LC, Mellits ED, Baughman KL, Weiss JL, Flaherty JT, Kallman CH, Llewellyn M, Weisfeldt M: Nifedipine in unstable angina—a double-blind, randomized trial. *N Engl J Med* 1982;306:885.
25. Ouyang P, Bulkley GH, Mellits ED, et al: A double-blind, randomized trial of nifedipine in post-infarction unstable angina. *Pract Cardiol* 1983;3:30–38.
26. Gottlieb SO, Weisfeldt ML, Ouyang P, et al: Effect of the addition of propranolol to

therapy with nifedipine for unstable angina pectoris: A randomized, double-blind, placebo-controlled trial. *Circulation* 1986;73:331–337.
27. Frishman WL, Weksler B, Christodoulou JP, Smithen C, Kilip T: Reversal of abnormal platelet aggregability and change in exercise tolerance in patients with angina pectoris following oral propranolol. *Circulation* 1974;50:887.
28. Buck JD, Hardman H, Warltier D, Gross G: Changes in ischemic blood flow distribution and dynamic severity of a coronary stenosis induced by beta blockade in the canine heart. *Circulation* 1981;64:708.
29. Schrumpf JD, Sheps DS, Wolfson S, Aronson AL, Cohen LS: Altered hemoglobin-oxygen affinity with long-term propranolol in patients with coronary artery disease. *Am J Cardiol* 1977;40:76.
30. Packer M, Meller J, Medina N, Yurchak M, Smith H, Holt J, Guerrero J, Todd GD, McAllister RG, JRl, Gorlin R: Hemodynamic consequences of combined beta-adrenergic and slow calcium channel blockade in man. *Circulation* 1982;65:660.
31. Lewis HD, Davis JW, Archibald DG, Steinke WE, Smitherman TC, Doherty JE, Schnaper HW, LeWinter MM, Linares E, Pouget JM, Sabharwal SC, Chester E, DeMots H: Protective effects of aspirin against myocardial infarction and death in men with unstable angina: Results of a Veteran's Administration Cooperative Study. *N Engl J Med* 1983;309:396.
32. Cairns JA, Gent M, Singer J, et al: Aspirin, sulfinpyrazone, or both in unstable angina: Results of a Canadian Multicenter Trial. *N Engl J Med* 1985;313:1368–1375.
33. Telford AM, Wilson C: Trial of heparin versus atenolol in prevention of myocardial infarction in intermediate coronary syndrome. *Lancet* 1981; I:1225–1228.
34. Zwerner PL, Gore JM, Corrao JM, Mahna CG, Goldberg RJ, Weiner B, Dalen JE: Heparin in the treatment of unstable angina: A randomized prospective trial (abstract). *Circulation* 1987;76(suppl IV):IV–108.
35. Vetrovec GW, Leinback RC, Gold HK, Cowley MJ: Intracoronary thrombolysis in syndromes of unstable ischemia: Angiographic and clinical results. *Am Heart J* 1982;104:946–952.
36. Shapiro EP, Brinker JA, Gottlieb SO, Guzman PA, Bulkley BH: Intracoronary thrombolysis 3 to 13 days after acute myocardial infarction for postinfarction angina pectoris. *Am J Cardiol* 1985;55:1453–1458.
37. Gold HK, Johns JA, Leinbach RC, Yasuda T, Grossbard E, Zusman R, Collen D: A randomized, blinded, placebo-controlled trial of recombinant human tissue-type plasminogen activator in patients with unstable angina pectoris. *Circulation* 1987;6:1192–1199.
38. Nicklas JM, Topol EJ, Kander N, Walton JA, Gorman L, Pitt B: Randomized, double-blind, placebo-controlled trial of rt-PA in unstable angina (abstract). *Circulation* 1987;76(suppl. IV):IV–180.
39. Gottlieb SO, Weisfeldt ML, Ouyang P, Mellits ED, Gerstenblith G: Silent ischemia as a marker for early unfavorable outcomes in patients with unstable angina. *N Engl J Med* 1986;314:1214–1219.
40. Nademanee K, Intarachot V, Singh PN, Josephson MA, Rieders D, Vaghaiwalla Mody F, Singh BN: Prognostic significance of silent myocardial ischemia in patients with unstable angina. *J Am Coll Cardiol* 1987;10:1–9.
41. Gottlieb SO, Weisfeldt ML, Ouyand P, Mellits ED, Gerstenblith G: Silent ischemia predicts infarction and death during 2 year follow-up of unstable angina. *J Am Coll Cardiol* 1987;10:756–760.

CHAPTER 23

Effect of Nifedipine on Silent Ischemia in Patients with Stable Angina and Those with Asymptomatic Coronary Artery Disease

Richard W. Nesto, MD, Kevin J. Kett, MD, and Lawrence S. Mc Auliffe, MD

It has been clearly established that the majority of ischemic episodes experienced by patients with documented coronary artery disease are painless or "silent."[1–5] Several studies using continuous ECG monitoring in hospitalized patients with unstable angina have shown that approximately 90 percent of episodes of ST-segment deviations occurred in the absence of chest pain.[6–8] In ambulatory patients with stable angina and a positive exercise tolerance test, approximately 75 percent of the episodes were also painless.[9–11] There is a growing appreciation of the fact that symptomatic and asymptomatic ischemia have similar prognostic significance and that the frequency and character of angina are insensitive indexes of the activity of coronary artery disease. Such a realization has raised issues regarding choices and end points of therapy.

There are clearly two objectives of therapy in this context: reduction of troublesome symptoms and prolongation of survival. At least in unstable angina, two studies[8,12] indicate that painless myocardial ischemia of a certain cumulative duration that persist after symptomatic episodes have been eliminated is associated with an enhanced incidence of adverse outcome: infarction, sudden death, or recrudescence of unstable angina requiring invasive intervention. The question has therefore arisen if elimination or a measurable reduction in silent ischemia by pharmacologic interventions in different subsets of patients with coronary artery disease might lead to a decrease in morbid coronary events associated with episodes of transient ischemia. To test such a hypothesis, a knowledge of the efficacy of various pharmacologic agents in reducing silent ischemia is essential to allow the rational choice of an agent. However, limited data are available in this regard. The purpose of this chapter is to describe two discrete studies[13,14] carried out to determine the efficacy of the dihydropyridine, nifedipine, in reducing episodes of transient myocardial episodes in patients with chronic stable angina[15] and in patients with asymptomatic coronary artery disease.[13]

NIFEDIPINE IN SILENT MYOCARDIAL ISCHEMIA IN ASYMPTOMATIC CORONARY DISEASE

Currently, there is very little data on the significance of silent myocardial ischemia detected by ambulatory ECG recordings in patients with asymptomatic coronary artery disease. However, a substantial body of data indicates that these patients who have unequivocally positive stress tests for ischemia electrocardiographically, have a markedly increased incidence of morbid coronary events despite the complete absence of pain during performance of the exercise treadmill test.[14]

Recently, Cohn and Lawson[13] reported on the effects of nifedipine in 15 male patients who had no history of angina or angina equivalents but who had angiographically documented coronary artery disease and a positive asymptomatic exercise stress test result. Twelve (42 to 72 years of age) of the 15 patients demonstrated more than one episode of ischemia on 48-hour ambulatory ECG monitoring. Three patients had prior Q-wave infarction, and one had non-Q-wave infarction. Six patients had triple-vessel coronary disease.

After the baseline Holter recordings in these 12 patients who had ischemic episodes, nifedipine, 10 or 20 mg three times daily (two patients had a larger dose) was given. After 2 to 3 days of treatment Holter recordings (48 hours) were repeated. During the initial or baseline recordings, 80 episodes of silent ischemia were identified (3 to 17 per patient). The total or cumulative duration was 1,487 minutes (range 14 to 699). There was a distinct circadian variation in the occurrence of the ischemic episodes, insofar as 40 percent of the episodes occurred between 6 AM and 12 noon. The effects of nifedipine on silent ischemia in the 12 patients are shown in Table 23.1.

The data indicate that 7 of the 12 patients in this study showed at least a 50 percent decrease in both the number and the duration of episodes, ischemia being eliminated in 2 patients. It was noteworthy that heart rate at the onset of ischemic episodes was not affected by nifedipine, neither was there a change in the circadian rhythmicity of the ischemic episodes.

NIFEDIPINE IN SILENT ISCHEMIA WITH CHRONIC STABLE ANGINA

There is limited experience in defining the effects of calcium antagonists on silent myocardial ischemia in patients with chronic stable angina. It is now widely appreciated that most episodes of ischemia in chronic stable angina (and in other ischemic

Table 23.1. Effects of Nifedipine on Silent Ischemia Documented on Holter Recordings in Patients with Asymptomatic Coronary Disease

	Before Treatment	With Nifedipine	p Value
Ischemic episodes	80	37	<0.01
Duration (min) of episodes	1,487	625	<0.05
Heart rate (bpm) at onset of episodes	87	88	NS
Episodes occurring between 6 AM and 12 noon	40	42	NS

syndromes) are silent. Preliminary data from uncontrolled studies[16–18] (which need to be extended and confirmed) indicate that, as in unstable angina, silent ischemia in chronic stable angina may be of prognostic significance.

Most asymptomatic episodes in chronic stable angina occur during activities associated with only mild increases in myocardial oxygen demand and well below the heart rate and blood pressure required to produce ischemia on exercise tolerance testing.[3,4] Variations in coronary blood flow, therefore, represent the major pathophysiologic mechanism accounting for the majority of ischemic events detected on ambulatory ST-segment monitoring. Agents that improve myocardial blood flow may therefore be of particular benefit in patients with asymptomatic ischemia. Of the three major classes of antianginal drugs (calcium-channel blockers, beta-blockers, and long-acting nitrates), calcium-channel antagonists may be ideally suited as treatment for silent ischemia, as they decrease coronary vascular resistance and improve coronary blood flow.[19]

To ascertain the effect of nifedipine on ischemia measured by exercise tolerance testing and ambulatory monitoring we performed a double-blind randomized crossover comparison of nifedipine versus placebo in 10 patients with documented coronary artery disease. The design of the protocol is shown in Figure 23.1. No patients were taking long-acting nitrates or calcium-channel blockers. Patients underwent a baseline exercise tolerance test and 48-hour Holter monitoring after which they were randomized to nifedipine therapy or placebo. Patients underwent a 1-week titration phase and then a 1-week efficacy phase. Repeat exercise tolerance test and 48-hour Holter monitoring were then carried out on the first limb of treatment, and then patients crossed over to the other limb of treatment with a similar 2-week period of drug monitoring. This was followed by another exercise tolerance test and 48-hour Holter monitoring. The mean dose of nifedipine attained was 20 mg four times daily.

The effect of nifedipine on the time to the development of 1-mm ST-segment depression compared to the baseline value ($p < 0.005$) and the value with the placebo ($p < 0.005$) is shown in Figure 23.2. A clearcut reduction induced by the drug is evident. Nifedipine also reduced systolic blood pressure at rest and during exercise compared with the values at baseline and those during placebo administration (Figure 23.3). On baseline 48-hour Holter monitoring, there were 5.5 episodes of silent isch-

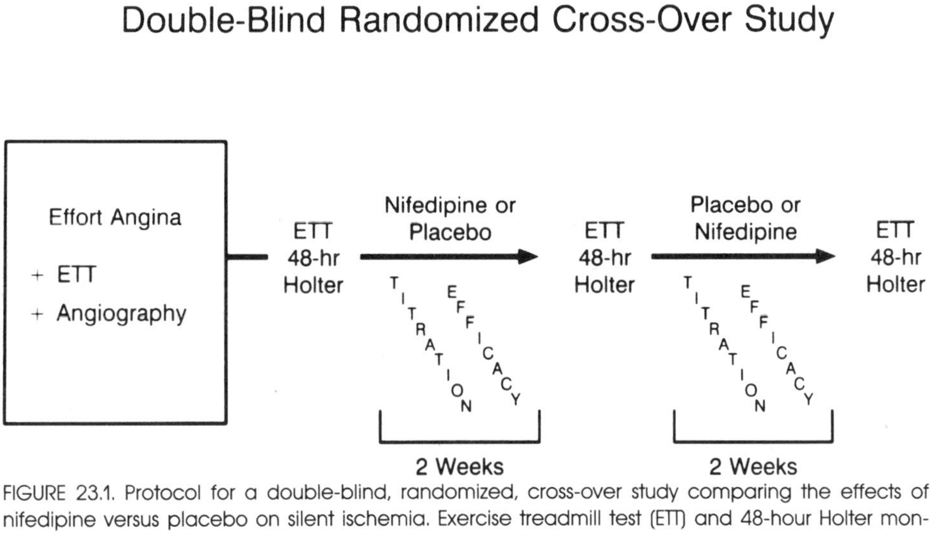

FIGURE 23.1. Protocol for a double-blind, randomized, cross-over study comparing the effects of nifedipine versus placebo on silent ischemia. Exercise treadmill test (ETT) and 48-hour Holter monitoring were conducted before randomization and at the end of each 2-week treatment period.

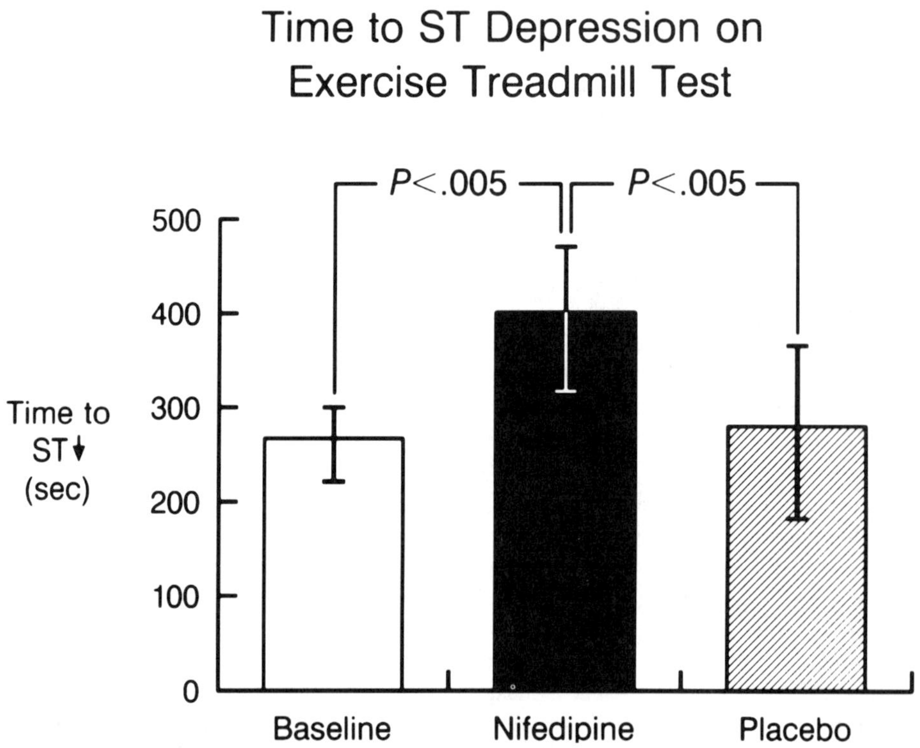

FIGURE 23.2. Time to ST-segment depression on exercise treadmill test (ETT). Nifedipine significantly increased time to ST-segment depression compared with baseline and with placebo.

emia (Figure 23.4) compared to 2.2 with nifedipine and 6.8 episodes with placebo (baseline vs nifedipine $p < 0.001$, nifedipine vs placebo $p < 0.02$). The total minutes of Holter monitor-detected ischemia was 97 at baseline compared to 35 minutes with nifedipine and 117 with placebo (baseline vs nifedipine $p < 0.01$, nifedipine vs placebo $p < 0.05$). The average duration of an ischemia event on Holter monitoring was reduced from 17.3 minutes at baseline to 10.7 minutes with nifedipine (Figure 23.5). Exercise capacity and time to ST-segment depression were also increased with nifedipine by virtue of a reduced double product at submaximal exercise. These results indicate that ischemia measured by exercise tolerance testing (increased myocardial demand) and Holter monitoring (presumably due to decreased coronary supply) is reduced by nifedipine. The salutary effect of nifedipine is probably multifactorial in ambulatory patients with coronary artery disease.

DISCUSSION

Until recently, the effectiveness of medical treatment in "stable" angina was based on reduction of chest pain. However, it is likely that despite a reduction in angina, patients may still experience episodes of asymptomatic ischemia that may bear on the subsequent clinical outcomes. In attempting to abolish a patient's "total ischemic activity," more aggressive treatment with larger doses of pharmacologic agents or their combinations may be necessary to significantly reduce or eliminate silent ischemia. Justification for this approach must be based on improving survival in these patients. As yet, no data exist to show the effect of treatment on survival in patients

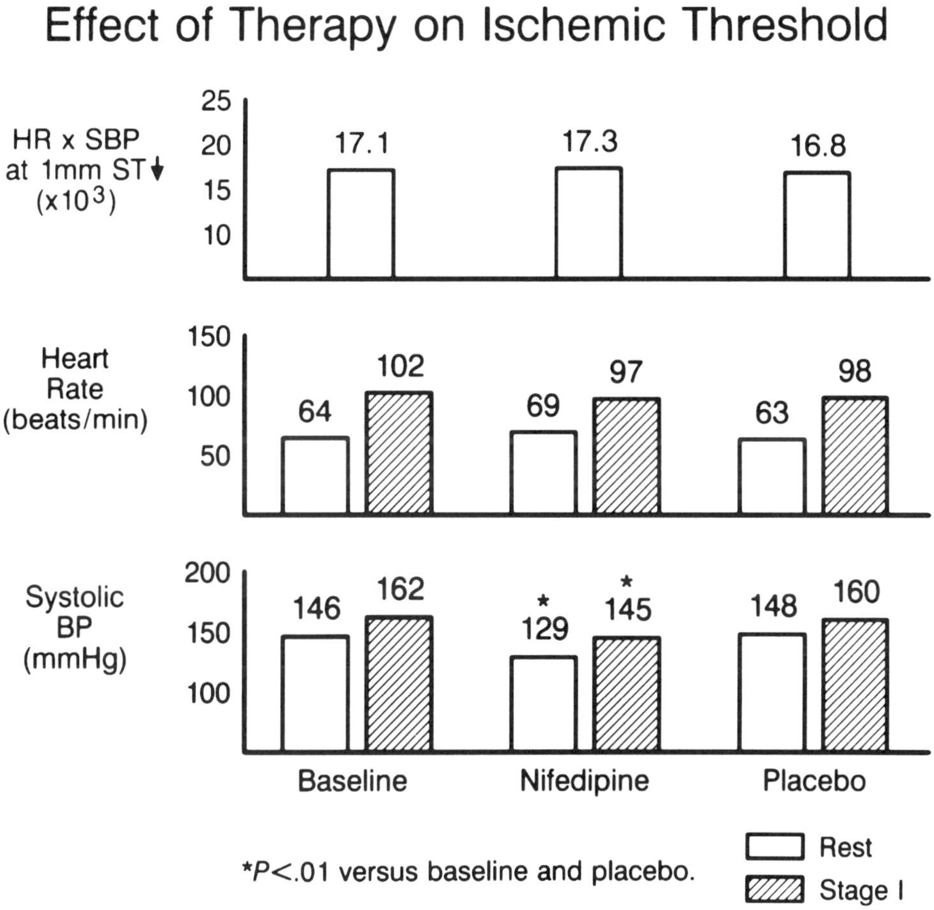

FIGURE 23.3. Effect of therapy on ischemic threshold. Nifedipine reduced systolic blood pressure (SBP) at rest and at exercise compared with baseline and with placebo. There were no significant differences in heart rate (HR) or double-product (HR × SBP).

in whom therapy has been specifically designed to reduce silent ischemia. It must be emphasized, however, that impact on survival in coronary artery disease by reduction or elimination of ischemia is as yet an unproven but tenable hypothesis.

The two studies cited herein, albeit small, demonstrate that nifedipine, a potent calcium antagonist, has the propensity to significantly reduce the frequency and duration of silent ischemia in two subsets of patients, namely, those with asymptomatic coronary artery disease with positive exercise treadmill test results and those with chronic stable angina. In this context, the data in patients with asymptomatic coronary artery disease are of particular interest in demonstrating an extremely high incidence of silent ischemia on 48-hour periods of Holter monitoring. Furthermore, the data showed that nifedipine reduced the number of silent episodes by 54 percent, the cumulative duration by 58 percent, while exerting no significant effect on the heart rate at the onset of the ischemic episode. In this limited study, the drug had no effect on the circadian distribution of myocardial ischemia, but a larger study will be required to confirm or negate these findings. However, the data clearly demonstrate the salutary effects of nifedipine on silent ischemia in patients with chronic stable angina as well as in those with asymptomatic coronary artery disease.

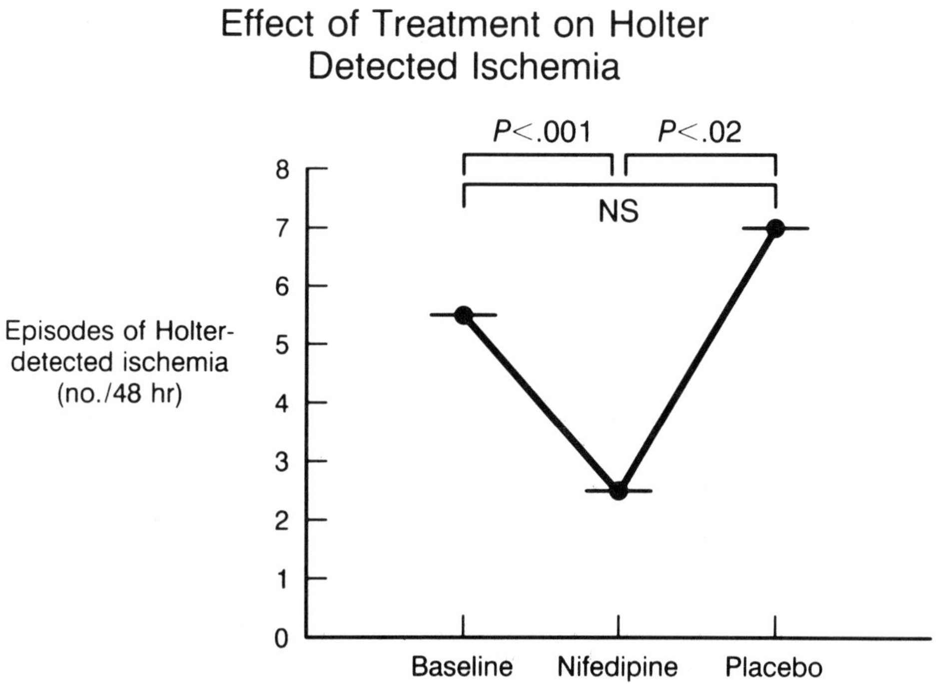

FIGURE 23.4. Effect of treatment on Holter-detected ischemia. Nifedipine reduced the number of ischemic episodes compared with baseline and placebo as detected by 48-hour Holter monitoring.

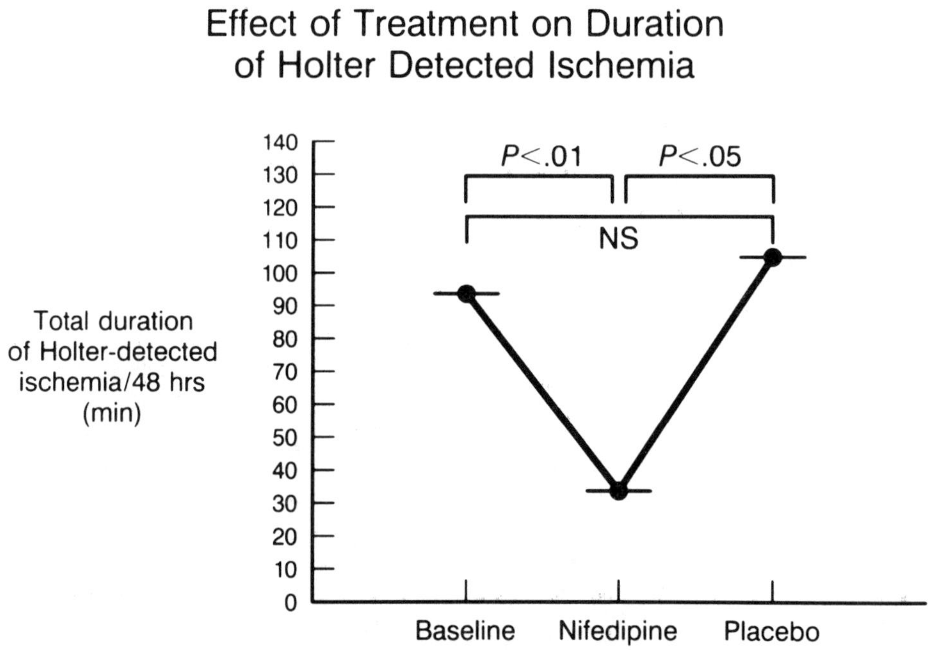

FIGURE 23.5. Effect of treatment on duration of Holter-detected ischemia. The total number of minutes of silent ischemia was significantly reduced by nifedipine compared with baseline and with placebo.

To date, there have been very few studies aimed directly at evaluating the use of nifedipine in silent ischemia in ambulatory patients. Oakley et al[20] studied six men with daily angina and strongly positive exercise test results. Each patient underwent four treatment periods of 1 week each: (1) glyceryl trinitrate alone, (2) propranolol 120 mg four times daily, (3) nifedipine 20 mg thrice daily, and (4) propranolol plus nifedipine in an unblinded, nonrandomized fashion. Twenty-four-hour ambulatory ST-segment monitoring was performed during each regimen. The combination of nifedipine and propranolol was significantly superior to either nifedipine or propranolol alone, although each of these three regimens was superior to the nitrate preparation in reducing the total number of episodes of ST-segment depression with or without pain. A similar study by Dargie et al[21] in 16 patients with stable angina and positive exercise test results evaluated nifedipine (30 and 60 mg/day), propranolol (240 and 480 mg/day), a combination of nifedipine and propranolol at two dosage levels (30 and 240 mg/day and 60 and 480 mg/day, respectively) against placebo in a single-blind randomized protocol. Fifty-nine percent of all episodes of ST-segment depression were painless. Both nifedipine and propranolol as monotherapies reduced silent ischemia with the greatest effect at the larger dose for each agent. The combination of nifedipine and propranolol produced a 95 percent reduction in silent episodes at the larger dosage regimen. Similar effects of treatment were noted in the frequency of angina, nitroglycerin consumption, and the area of ST-segment depression on exercise precordial ECG mapping. Monotherapy with propranolol reduced the rate-pressure product and decreased myocardial oxygen demand, accounting for its effectiveness. The beneficial effect of nifedipine in exercise-induced ischemia occurred without a significant change in rate-pressure product. In addition, the marked improvement in exercise-induced ischemia on combined therapy occurred without any further decrease in the double product. This observation, coupled with the observed dramatic reduction in Holter-detected ischemia with nifedipine either alone or in combination with the beta-blocker, suggests that an improvement in coronary blood supply is responsible for the benefit experienced with calcium-channel blocker therapy. In a single-blind, randomized parallel study[22] of 42 patients with stable angina undergoing Holter monitoring, 12 experienced silent ischemic episodes at rest. Nifedipine reduced or abolished silent ischemia in six of seven patients, whereas only one of five improved with pindolol treatment. These results also suggest that an agent that improves myocardial perfusion is effective therapy for silent ischemia.

CONCLUSIONS

The overall findings discussed herein provide the basis for the design of controlled clinical trials to determine the impact of elimination of silent ischemia on morbidity and mortality in coronary artery disease.

Enthusiasm for the treatment of silent ischemia stems from data indicating that asymptomatic ischemia detected by Holter monitoring in patients with stable angina may be associated with a poorer prognosis. Stern and Tzivoni[16] evaluated 80 patients with stable angina with ambulatory monitoring. Over a 1-year follow-up period, over 50 percent of the 37 patients with silent ischemia experienced clinical deterioration, whereas none of the 43 patients without silent ischemia experienced worsening. Rocco et al[17] followed 86 patients for a mean of 9 months after Holter monitoring. Cardiac death, infarction, or unstable angina occurred in 7 of 52 patients with silent ischemia, whereas no events occurred in the 34 patients without silent ischemia on ambulatory monitoring. DeWood and Rozanski[18] reported the 3-year follow-up of 59 patients who had undergone ECG monitoring. The occurrence of death, infarction, or worsening angina was fourfold higher in the 26 patients who manifested asymptomatic ischemia compared with the 33 patients without silent ischemia. These studies suggest that patients with spontaneous ischemia may have a different biology of disease that places them at high risk for morbid cardiac events.

It is also conceivable that more aggressive treatment of ischemia, whether symptomatic or silent, may also prevent myocardial "hibernation"[23] or persistent left ventricular dysfunction due to a "chronic" ischemic state in which left ventricular function is depressed in an adaptive fashion to match impaired coronary blood supply. Because an important determinant of survival in coronary artery disease is the status of left ventricular function,[24] it is conceivable that pharmacologic attempts to reduce silent ischemia in the ambulatory patient may improve prognosis by protecting the left ventricle from the consequences of ischemia. Long-term controlled studies involving adequate sample size will be required to demonstrate that treatment of silent ischemia in patients with stable angina may favorably alter morbidity and mortality in coronary artery disease.

REFERENCES

1. Deanfield JE, Selwyn AP, Chierchia S, Maseri A, Ribeiro P, Krikler S, Morgan MM: Myocardial ischemia during daily life in patients with stable angina: Its relation to symptoms and heart rate changes. *Lancet* 1983;1:753–758.
2. Cecchi AC, Dovellini EV, Marchi F, Pucci P, Santoro GM, Fazini PF: Silent myocardial ischemia during ambulatory electrocardiographic monitoring in patients with effort angina. *J Am Coll Cardiol* 1983;1:934–939.
3. Schang SJ, Pepine CJ: Transient asymptomatic ST-segment depression during daily activity. *Am J Cardiol* 1977;39:396–401.
4. Deanfield JE, Shea M, Ribiero P, et al: Transient ST-segment depression as a marker of myocardial ischemia during daily life. *Am J Cardiol* 1984;54:1195–1200.
5. Nesto RW, Phillips RT: Silent myocardial ischemia: Clinical characteristics, underlying mechanisms, and implications for treatment. *Am J Med* 1986;4:12–19.
6. Chierchia S, Lazzari M, Freedman B, Brunelli C, Maseri A: Impairment of myocardial perfusion and function during painless myocardial ischemia. *J Am Cardiol* 1983;1:924–930.
7. Biagini A, Mazzei MG, Carpeggiani C, Testa R, Antonelli R, Michaellasi C, L'Abbate A, Maseri A: Vasospastic ischemic mechanism of frequent asymptomatic transient ST-T changes during continuous electrocardiographic monitoring in selected unstable angina patients. *Am Heart J* 1982;103:13–20.
8. Nademanee K, Intarachot V, Josephson MA, Rieders D, Mody Vaghaiwalla F, Singh BN: Prognostic significance of silent myocardial ischemia in patients with unstable angina. *J Am Coll Cardiol* 1987;10:1–9.
9. von Armin T, Hofling B, Schreiber M: Characteristics of episodes of ST-elevation or ST-depression during ambulatory monitoring in patients subsequently undergoing angiography. *Br Heart J* 1985;54:484–488.
10. Cocco GX, Braun S, Strozzi C, Leishman B, Hons M, Chu D, Rochat N: Asymptomatic myocardial ischemia in patients with stable and typical angina pectoris. *Clin Cardiol* 1982;5:403–408.
11. Selwyn AP, Fox K, Eves M, Oakley D, Dargie H, Shillingford J: Myocardial ischemia in patients with frequent angina pectoris. *Br Med J* 1978;2:1594–1596.
12. Gottlieb SO, Weisfeldt ML, Ouyang P, Mellits ED, Gerstenblith G: Silent ischemia as a marker for early unfavorable outcomes in patients with unstable angina. *N Engl J Med* 1986;314:1214–1219.

13. Cohn PF, Lawson WE: Effect of nifedipine on out-of-hospital silent myocardial ischemia in asymptomatic men with coronary artery disease. *Am J Cardiol* 1988;61:908–910.
14. Erikssen J, Cohn PF, Thaulow E, Mowinckel P: Silent myocardial ischemia in middle aged men: Long term clinical course, in V. Arnim Th, Maseri A (eds): *Silent Ischemia*. New York, Springer-Verlag, 1987, pp 45–51.
15. Nesto RW, Kett KJ, McAuliffe LS: The use of nifedipine in the treatment of silent ischemia in patients with stable angina and in those with asymptomatic coronary artery disease. 1988; unpublished observations.
16. Stern S, Tzivoni D: Early detection of silent ischemia heart disease by 24-hour electrocardiographic monitoring of active subjects. *Br Heart J* 1985;54:484–488.
17. Rocco MB, Nabel EG, Campbell S, Goldham L, Barry J, Mead K, Selwyn P: Prognostic importance of myocardial ischemia detected by ambulatory monitoring in patients with coronary artery disease (abstr). *J Am Coll Cardiol* 1987;9:68A.
18. De Wood MB, Rozanski A: Long term prognosis of patients with and without silent ischemia (abstr). *Circulation* 1986; 94:II–59.
19. Singh BN, Hecht HS Nademanee K: Electrophysiologic and hemodynamic effects of slow-channel blocking drugs. *Prog Cardiovasc Dis* 1982;25:103–132.
20. Oakley GDG, Fox KM, Dargie HJ, Selwyn AP: Objective assessment of treatment in severe angina. *Br Med J* 1979;1:1540.
21. Dargie HJ, Lynch PC, Krikler DM, Harris L, Krikler S: Nifedipine and propranolol: A beneficial drug interaction. *Am J Med* 1981;71:676–682.
22. Cocco G, Strozzi C, Chu D, Amrein D, Castagnoli E: Therapeutic effects of pindolol and nifedipine in patients with stable angina pectoris and asymptomatic resting ischemia. *Eur J Cardiol* 1979;10:59–69.
23. Braunwald E, Rutherford JD: Reversible ischemic left ventricular dysfunction: Evidence for the "hibernating myocardium." *J Am Coll Cardiol* 1986;8:467–470.
24. Harris PH, Harrell FE, Lee Kl, Behar VS, Rosati RA: Survival in medically treated coronary artery disease. *Circulation* 1979;6:1259–1268.

CHAPTER 24

Calcium Antagonists and Beta-Blockers, Alone and in Combination, in the Suppression of Silent Myocardial Ischemia in Chronic Stable Angina

Bramah N. Singh, MD, D Phil and
Koonlawee Nademanee, MD

It has been recognized for some time that the overall spectrum of therapeutic activity of calcium antagonists is at least as wide as that of beta-blockers.[1] Beta-blockers and calcium antagonists are potent antianginal and antiischemic agents; both classes of compounds exert somewhat similar effects in supraventricular as well as ventricular tachyarrhythmias.[2,3] From experimental studies it also appears that calcium antagonists and beta-blockers exert a comparable degree of cardioprotective effects in terms of the magnitude of myocardial enzyme release and tissue histochemistry, structural and ultrastructural disorganization, gross anatomic infarct size, and the incidence of ventricular fibrillation after acute coronary artery ligation.[4] Both classes of agents have been shown to ameliorate symptomatic myocardial ischemia in patients with chronic stable angina, producing an increase in exercise capacity and increasing the time to the development of ischemic ST-segment depression during treadmill stress tests. In this respect the overall effects of the two compounds have been additive.[5]

In recent years, over two thirds of the episodes of ischemia in patients with chronic stable angina were found to be silent.[6–8] However, the effects of calcium-channel blockers and beta-antagonists on silent myocardial ischemia in chronic stable angina are not well defined. The issue has become of practical importance with the recent demonstration in unstable angina that persistent silent ischemia after the symptomatic episodes are eliminated by medical therapy is of prognostic significance.[9,10]

The purpose of this chapter is threefold. The first is to discuss the pharmacologic similarities and differences between beta-blockers and calcium antagonists. The second objective is to review preliminary evidence from the literature that beta-blockers and calcium-channel blockers exert a suppressant effect on silent ischemia documented by ambulatory ECG recordings in patients with chronic stable angina. Finally, we present our data from a controlled double-blind study in which the comparative efficacy of nicardipine and propranolol, when given alone or in combination, to suppress silent ischemia in chronic stable angina is determined.

PHARMACOLOGIC CONSIDERATIONS

With beta-adrenergic blocking drugs, the bulk of the pharmacologic effects can ultimately be attributed to the ability of these compounds to competitively antagonize beta-adrenoceptors. Structurally, these compounds are reasonably homogeneous: minor structural differences have produced compounds of variable beta-blocking potencies, varied pharmacokinetics, and associated features such as intrinsic sympathomimetic activity, cardioselectivity, and membrane-depressant propensities. However, although these features may influence the overall side effect profile of an individual agent, they have little or no effect on their therapeutic efficacy, which results essentially from blockade of beta-adrenoceptors. In contrast, calcium antagonists constitute a structurally heterogeneous group of compounds[11] that share two significant properties: (1) the ability to block the slow-calcium channel in cardiac muscle, and (2) the ability to inhibit transmembrane fluxes of calcium in smooth muscle especially in the coronary and peripheral circulations.[11]

Because of their often striking structural differences, individual calcium compounds may exhibit other pharmacologic actions (eg, verapamil and diltiazem have noncompetitive sympatholytic actions) which may lead to a complex interplay with their intrinsic properties demonstrable in isolated tissues and the reflex changes they may produce as a result of sympathetic activation due to peripheral vasodilatation.[11] Because of the reflex effects and the varying potencies of different calcium antagonists to induce peripheral vasodilatation, the in vitro and in vivo actions of calcium antagonists may differ markedly. This is particularly striking in the case of atrioventricular (AV) nodal conduction and refractoriness. For example, as with beta-blockers, calcium antagonists such as verapamil, diltiazem, tiapamil, or gallopamil predictably lengthen AV conduction and refractoriness both in vivo as well as in vitro. By contrast, the dihydropyridines (eg, nifedipine and nicardipine) are potent depressants of AV nodal conduction in isolated hearts, but this effect is nullified or even reversed by their reflex effects.[11] However, it must be emphasized that whereas calcium antagonists alter AV nodal conduction by blocking the slow-channel potentials in this structure, beta-blockers produce their negative dromotropic effects by altering the sympathetic impulse traffic in the AV node. Thus, the AV nodal effects of the two classes of compounds are likely to summate if they have similar effects individually (eg, propranolol versus verapamil or diltiazem); in the case of the dihydropyridines, concomitant beta-blockade is likely to convert a potentially facilitatory action on the AV node to a depressant one. These electrophysiologic features of the various compounds are of therapeutic significance in the choice of an agent or combination of agents for the control of ischemic syndromes in patients who may have preexisting conduction system disease. However, from the standpoint of controlling ischemia, the comparative cardiocirculatory effects of calcium antagonists and beta-antagonists are the most relevant pharmacologic effects.

It is now well established that most beta-antagonists, when administered intravenously or orally, depress heart rate, cardiac output, and indexes of ventricular contractility and increase the filling pressures of the ventricle. Thus, the major mechanism of their antiischemic action is a reduction in oxygen demand. These drugs may also reduce coronary blood flow commensurate with the reduction in myocardial oxygen demand. From studies utilizing quantitative angiography, it is also known that beta-blockers may produce coronary vasoconstriction, an effect that may aggravate the tendency to coronary vasospasm especially in Prinzmetal's angina in patients with normal coronary vessels. For this reason, beta-blockers are unlikely to eliminate episodes of ischemia that are triggered by coronary vasospasm. Conversely, in patients whose episodes of ischemia are triggered by vasospasm in the setting of advanced coronary artery disease, the increases in heart rate and blood pressure in response to ischemia are likely to augment the overall duration of ischemia. Beta-blockers are likely to curtail the duration of these ischemic episodes[12] and perhaps prevent them from reaching the threshold of pain perception. In contrast to the action of beta-blockers, the most striking hemodynamic effects of calcium antagonists consist of a predictable and consistent reduction in systemic vascular resistance accompanied by either no change or an increase in cardiac output.[11] Furthermore, unlike beta-blockers, calcium antagonists reduce coronary vascular resistance with a tendency for the coronary sinus flow to increase. Furthermore, these agents have the propensity to dilate resistance as well as capacitance vessels in the coronary circulation;[13,14] although this effect is modest in extent, lesion dilatation even of such a degree is of hemodynamic significance.[15] It may be an important component of the antiischemic actions of calcium-channel blockers.

The differing pharmacologic effects of beta-blockers and calcium-channel blockers therefore provide a rational basis for their combined therapy in the amelioration of transient myocardial ischemia. This issue is examined in the remainder of this chapter, with particular focus on silent episodes of ischemia documented by ambulatory ECG recordings in patients with chronic stable angina.

BETA-BLOCKERS AND SILENT MYOCARDIAL ISCHEMIA

At present there appears to be only limited data on this subject. A recent study,[16] however, has documented that beta-blockade does exert a salutary effect on silent myocardial ischemia in patients with chronic stable angina. Imperi et al[16] studied the effects of titrated doses of metoprolol (50 to 200 mg twice daily) in patients with positive ECG evidence of aysmptomatic ischemia but angiographically confirmed coronary artery disease. The frequency and duration of silent myocardial ischemia were quantified over 72 hours of Holter monitoring in each patient at baseline and after steady-state therapy at each dose of the beta-blocker. The effects on silent myocardial ischemia relative to dose are shown in Figure 24.1. A significant reduction was achieved at each dose level with a clearcut dose-response effect.

Other associated features of beta-blocker action were apparent. For example, the well-known circadian pattern of ischemia distribution[17,18] over 24 hours was markedly attenuated by metoprolol (Figure 24.2). It is tempting to speculate that blunting the circadian pattern of silent ischemia in patients with coronary artery disease may be one mechanism to reduce sudden death and reinfarction in the survivors of acute myocardial infarction given prophylactic beta-blockade. In the study reported by Imperi et al,[16] metoprolol also reduced the total ischemic time per 24 hours; it attenuated the heart rate at the onset of ischemia while reducing the increases in heart rate associated with individual episodes, the durations of which were also shortened. The effects of other beta-blockers are currently unknown, but the relative potencies of

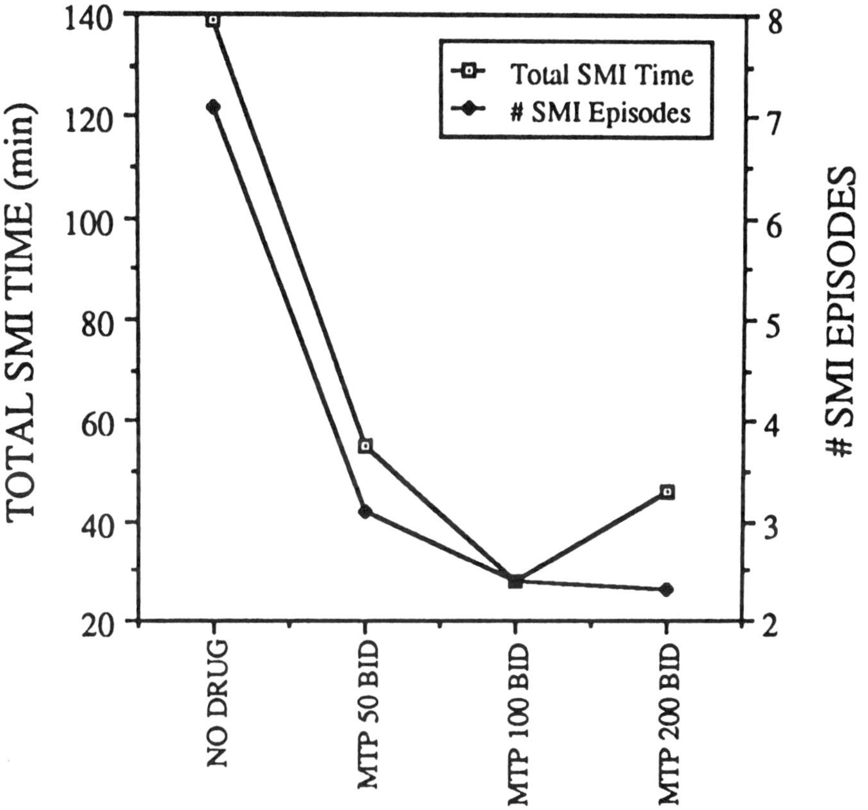

FIGURE 24.1. Effects of metoprolol on silent myocardial ischemia relative to dose in patients with coronary artery disease. Note a general dose-dependent reduction in the frequency of silent ischemia (#SMI episodes) as seven of nine patients showed dose-dependent reduction in the total time of silent myocardial ischemia with metoprolol (MTP). (From Imperi et al [16] with the permission of the authors and the *American Journal of Cardiology*.)

individual agents require critical appraisal by controlled clinical trials in appropriate subsets of patients.

CALCIUM-CHANNEL BLOCKERS AND SILENT ISCHEMIA IN CHRONIC STABLE ANGINA

Again, as with beta-blockers, limited data are available in chronic stable angina. Most of the reported data deal with the effects of calcium-channel blockers in vasospastic angina. In this case, the effects of all calcium-channel blockers in silent as well as symptomatic ischemia appear comparable, reflecting their somewhat similar coronary vasodilator propensity. The effects in chronic stable angina undoubtedly stem from a much more complex action of different classes of these agents in relation to the possibly equally complex mechanisms underlying different episodes of transient ischemia in this setting.

As emphasized, little systematic data are available on the effects of calcium-channel blockers on silent myocardial episodes in chronic stable angina. The earliest observations dealt with the effects of bepridil, a calcium antagonist with a complex pharmacologic profile.[19] When 300 mg/day of the compound were given to patients

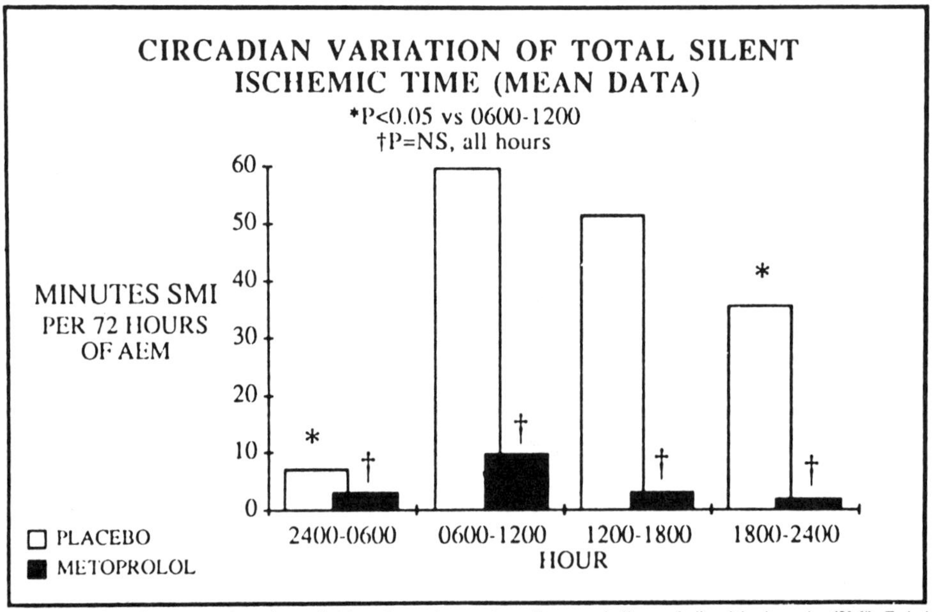

FIGURE 24.2. Influence of metoprolol treatment on circadian variation of silent ischemia (SMI). Total silent ischemic times recorded during four 6-hour time windows for placebo and metoprolol periods. During placebo most silent ischemia occurred in the 0600 to 1200 time window. This was significantly greater than total silent ischemia occurring in the 1800 to 2400 and 2400 to 0600 time windows. During metoprolol therapy compared with placebo, total silent ischemic item was reduced in each time window. Furthermore, no significant difference (NS) was observed in total silent ischemia times occurring in each of these time windows during metoprolol. Thus, metoprolol treatment appeared to eliminate the circadian variation in silent ischemia observed during placebo. (Reproduced with the permission of the authors and the *American Journal of Cardiology*.)

with chronic stable angina and an exercise stress test that was positive for ischemia, the drug increased the time to angina and to the development of 1-mm ST-segment depression. Twenty-four-hour Holter recordings obtained before and during drug therapy and analyzed by the compact analog technique indicated that bepridil significantly reduced the cumulative duration of silent myocardial ischemia per 24 hours. The effects of nifedipine in this setting are discussed in Chapter 24. Schnellbacher et al[20] studied the effects of diltiazem (60 mg three times daily) on silent and symptomatic episodes of myocardial ischemia in 19 patients. Holter monitoring revealed no episodes of ischemia in 7 patients. In the remainder, after the first day of therapy with the calcium-channel blocker, the frequency and duration of ischemic episodes (over 90% silent) were reduced by 65 and 77 percent, respectively, and by 69 and 65 percent, respectively, on the seventh day. Verapamil is likely to exert similar action on silent myocardial ischemic episodes in chronic stable angina, but systematic data are needed from controlled clinical trials.

COMBINED BETA-BLOCKERS AND CALCIUM ANTAGONISTS IN SILENT ISCHEMIA AND CHRONIC STABLE ANGINA

Two controlled studies will be discussed to emphasize the effects of combined beta-blocker and calcium-channel blocker therapy in silent myocardial ischemia in this context.

In the first, Lynch and his colleagues[21] objectively evaluated the antianginal and antiischemic effects of propranolol, nifedipine, and their combination in 16 patients with severe exertional angina. The study was conducted double-blind with multiple end points including parameters of exercise stress tests, subjective features (chest pain, nitroglycerin consumption), and ECG data obtained from 48-hour Holter recordings (the total area and amount of ST-segment depression on the precordial exercise map and the total number of episodes of ST-segment depression). Two doses of each drug were used in the study: nifedipine 30 and 60 mg/day and propranolol 240 and 480 mg/day, each drug being given in three divided doses. Both drugs exerted a beneficial effect on the conventional subjective and objective indexes of angina and ischemia. The effects of combination therapy in general were more striking than the effects of either drug given alone at both doses. The overall data on the effects of the two drugs and their doses and combination are summarized in Figure 24.3. At both doses, nifedipine and propranolol given alone significantly reduced the number of episodes of ST-segment depression per 48 hours (most episodes being silent); propranolol was somewhat more potent in this regard. The combination therapies at both doses were significantly more potent than either drug given alone with evidence of a synergistic effect. Data (not shown) for the effects on exercise induced ST-segment depression during treadmill stress test were also similar.

The second study from our own laboratory[22] was a double-blind study of the an-

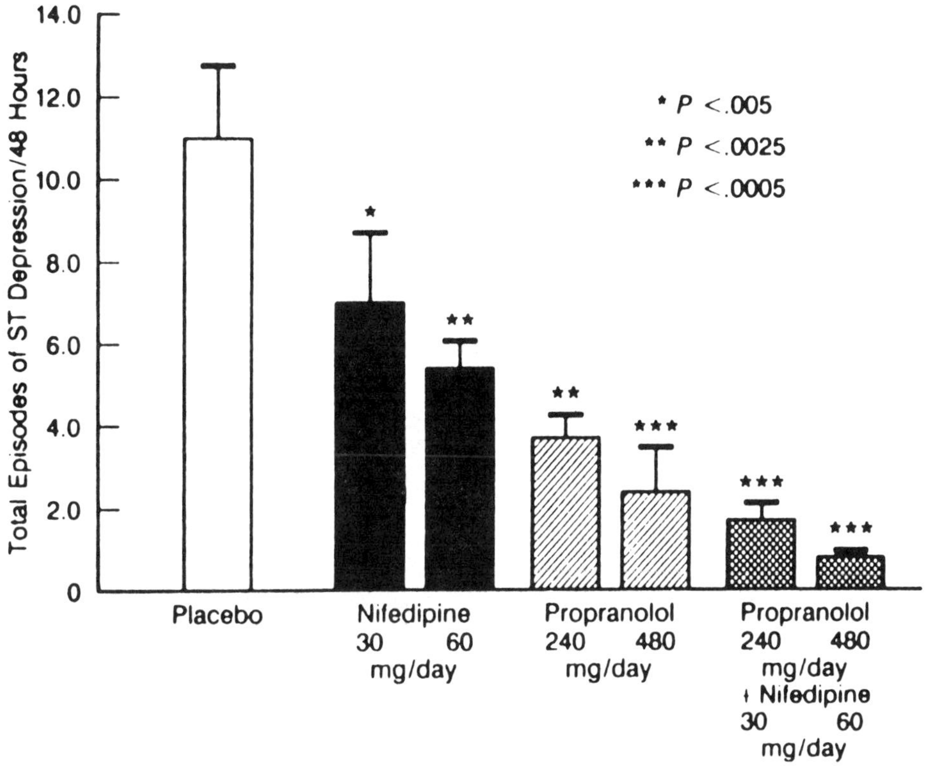

FIGURE 24.3. Effects of propranolol, nifedipine, and their combination in two doses on transient myocardial ischemia with chronic stable angina. Note that the combination of a dihydropyridine and a beta-blocker was the most effective regimen in reducing ischemia documented on Holter recordings. (Reproduced with permission from Lynch et al[21] and the *British Medical Journal*.)

tiischemic effects of propranolol and a new dihydropyridine type of calcium antagonist, nicardipine, and their combination versus placebo using a protocol with an extended latin square design in chronic stable angina. The goal was to evaluate the relative efficacy of these agents in terms of standard clinical parameters and treadmill variables. The major focus was placed on the effects of the two classes of drugs and their combination on episodes of silent myocardial ischemia as determined by ST-segment deviations occurring during ambulatory Holter monitoring in patients with chronic stable angina.

Twenty-one men over the age of 21 years with at least a 3-month history of classical stable angina were enrolled into the study. They all completed the study. Mean data with respect to the conventional subjective and objective parameters of ischemia were similar to those reported for beta-blockers and the dihydropyridine type of calcium antagonists. Only data referable to silent myocardial ischemia will therefore be presented.

The mean data demonstrating the effects of propranolol, nicardipine, and combination therapy on the number of episodes of ischemia (over 80% being silent) per 24 hours documented on ambulatory ECG recordings are shown in Figure 24.4. Although both propranolol (−29%) and nicardipine (−18%) given alone did reduce the number of episodes, the change did not reach statistical significance. In contrast, the combination therapy was effective in significantly ($p < 0.05$) reducing the number of ischemic episodes (−86%) compared with the placebo as well as the beta-blocker and calcium antagonist given alone.

The effects of the various regimens on the duration of ischemia of the longest per episode and the total cumulative duration of ischemia per 24 hours are shown in Figure 24.5. Again, neither propranolol nor nicardipine, given alone, exerted a significant effect on these parameters. The combination regimen reduced the frequency of ischemic episodes by over 90 percent ($p < 0.05$), the maximum duration by 90 percent ($p < 0.05$), and the total duration per 24 hours by 92 percent ($p < 0.05$). The combination therapy had a significantly greater effect than either propranolol or nicardipine given alone.

DISCUSSION AND COMMENTS

The data that have been reviewed in this report clearly indicate that beta-blockers and calcium-channel blockers, in doses at which they reduce anginal frequency and increase the duration of exercise stress testing on the treadmill, also exert a significant suppressant effect on episodes of silent myocardial ischemia documented by Holter recordings in patients with chronic stable angina. Of particular interest is the finding that such an effect on silent myocardial ischemia was more striking when combination regimens of beta-blockers and calcium antagonists were used. These observations raise the issue of the possible synergistic effects of the two classes of drugs in eliminating transient episodes of myocardial ischemia in chronic stable angina. The data are consistent with the differing modes of antiischemic actions of calcium channel-blockers and beta-antagonists.

The observed effects must be interpreted in relation to the perceived mechanisms for transient episodes of silent myocardial ischemia occurring in chronic stable angina. Numerous investigators have found that many episodes of ischemia in this

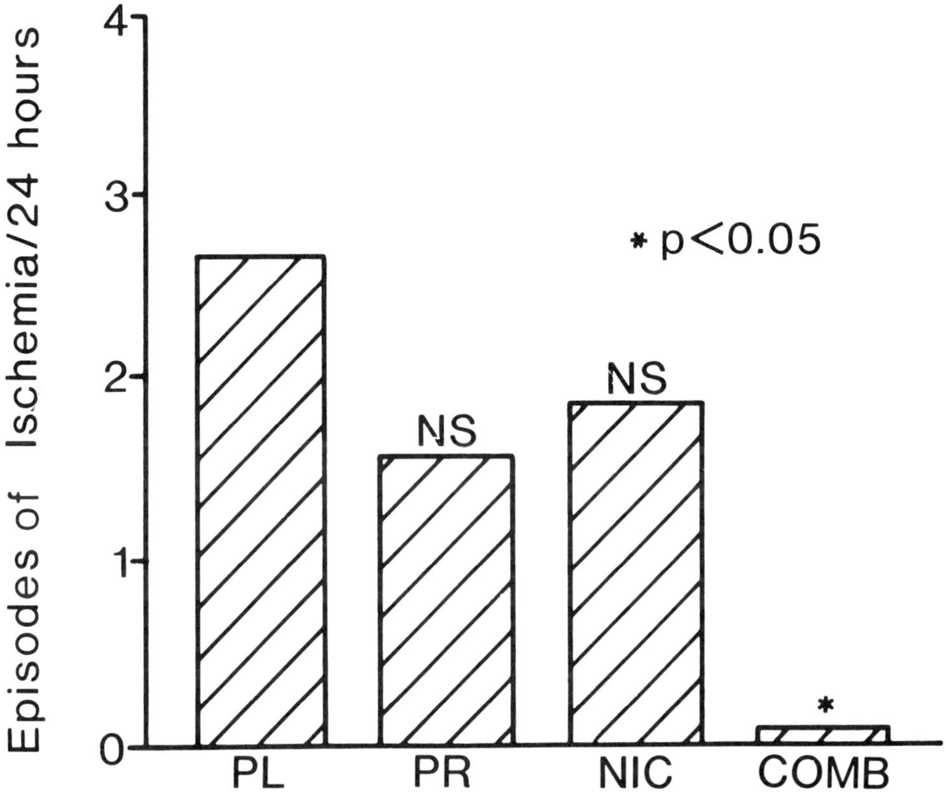

FIGURE 24.4. Effects of propranolol, nicardipine, and their combination on the number of ischemic episodes during continuous ambulatory ECG monitoring in patients with chronic stable angina. Note that although both drugs given alone did reduce the number of ischemic episodes, the difference compared to the placebo period was not significant. The combination therapy produced over 90 percent reduction ($p < 0.05$), a change that was greater than that produced by the summated effects of the two individual agents, indicating a synergistic effect during drug combination.

setting are not triggered by increases in heart rate. It is presumed that such episodes are produced by alterations in vasomotion at the sites of eccentrically located obstructions in the coronary vessels. Thus, coronary vasodilators might be expected to produce their beneficial effect in ischemia by reducing the tendency for vasoconstriction. In contrast, beta-blockers, by attenuating the reflex increases in heart rate and blood pressure induced by ischemia itself, are likely to shorten the duration of individual episodes of ischemia, thereby reducing the total ischemia time over a finite period.[12] It is therefore of interest that Imperi et al[16] found that the beta-blocker metoprolol shortened the duration of ischemic episodes and abbreviated the maximum duration of ischemia per 24 hours. The effects of the so-called rate-lowering calcium antagonists have not been investigated in this manner, but their overall action in some respects might resemble those of weak beta-antagonists. The overall data clearly establish the rationale for the combination therapy of a beta-blocker and a calcium antagonist in the suppression of silent transient episodes of myocardial ischemia. At present the most convincing data for the efficacy of combination therapy are those for propranolol combined with either nifedipine or nicardipine.

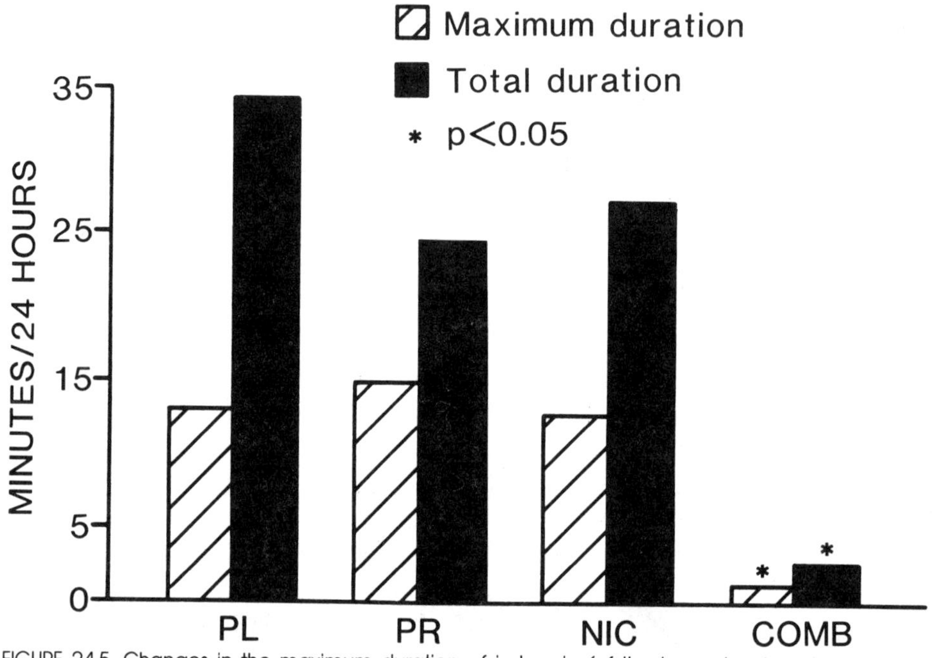

FIGURE 24.5. Changes in the maximum duration of ischemia (of the longest episode) and in the total cumulative duration of ischemia per 24 hours produced by propranolol, nicardipine, and their combination compared to the effects of placebo. Note that only the combination regimen reduced the ischemia indexes significantly. (See text for details.)

RATIONALE FOR COMBINING A BETA-BLOCKER AND A DIHYDROPYRIDINE CALCIUM ANTAGONIST

The hemodynamic effects of the dihydropyridines such as nifedipine and nicardipine establish the basis for combining the drugs with a sympatholytic agent. For example, Lambert et al[23] found that intravenous nicardipine increased heart rate by 19 percent, stroke volume by 13 percent, and myocardial oxygen consumption by 18 percent with a disproportionate increase in coronary flow of 41 percent and a decrease in coronary resistance of 39 percent. They concluded that nicardipine functioned as a coronary and systemic vasodilator while causing reflex tachycardia and an increase in myocardial oxygen demand. These findings, also noted by Josephson et al,[24] indicate that although some indexes of ischemia may be ameliorated by the use of nicardipine alone, others may not because oxygen demand may be increased. The tendency for the oxygen demand to be increased by nicardipine in this setting is likely to be negated by beta-blockade; conversely, the coronary vasoconstrictive propensity of beta-blockade is likely to be reversed by calcium antagonism. The data reported by Lynch et al[21] are in line with these considerations. It is noteworthy that in nearly all parameters tested nifedipine exerted somewhat smaller effects than did propranolol as an antianginal and antiischemic agent when the two compounds were given individually to patients with chronic stable angina. In contrast, a synergistic effect was clearly evident especially during episodes of silent myocardial ischemia when the two drugs were given in combination at two somewhat differing drug doses.

SIGNIFICANCE OF COMBINATION THERAPY

The data reported by Lynch et al[21] and Nademanee et al[22] support the safety and particularly the efficacy of combination therapy with beta-blockade and of nifedipine or nicardipine, respectively. Previously, the combination of various calcium antagonists with beta-blockade revealed beneficial effects on various indexes of ischemia in chronic stable angina,[25–28] but none has examined the effects on silent ischemic episodes. Although the doses of nifedipine and nicardipine used in the two studies just cited produced modest effects on anginal frequency or nitroglycerin consumption, the times to the development of chest pain and ST-segment depression on the treadmill were markedly prolonged. When combined with propranolol, significant improvements occurred in nearly all indexes of ischemia induced by treadmill exercise. It is of interest that the combination therapy was highly effective in reducing the total cumulative duration of ischemia per 24 hours as well as the number of discrete episodes of essentially silent myocardial ischemia. Although these data cannot be extrapolated unreservedly to patients with unstable angina, it is noteworthy that Gottlieb et al[29] recently reported a summated effect of propranolol and nifedipine in reducing spontaneous myocardial ischemia in patients with unstable angina.

THERAPEUTIC IMPLICATIONS AND CONCLUSIONS

The data outlined in this chapter indicate that both beta-blockers and calcium-channel blockers can reduce silent ischemic episodes in patients with chronic stable angina. The fact that the effect is most marked when the two classes of agents are combined might be of therapeutic significance. Such an effect appears to be synergistic rather than simply additive. It may reflect the complementary effects of two classes of antiischemic agents on myocardial oxygen supply as well as demand relative to their differing hemodynamic effects. However, it must be emphasized that the prognostic significance of such silent episodes in chronic stable angina remains uncertain. Recent studies in unstable angina indicate that the persistence of silent ischemia with medical therapy is associated with an adverse short-term clinical outcome.[9,10] Whether this may also hold for chronic stable angina is unknown. If it were demonstrated that reduction or elimination of silent myocardial ischemia by pharmacologic therapy in chronic stable angina did lead to a reduction in the occurrence of morbid events, a combination of a calcium antagonist and a beta-blocker may constitute an effective prophylactic regimen. The resolution of this issue will require stringently controlled clinical trials involving a combination regimen of beta-blockers and calcium-channel blockers in appropriate doses.

REFERENCES

1. Ellrodt G, Chew CYC, Singh BN: Therapeutic implications of slow-channel blockade in cardiocirculatory disorders. *Circulation* 1980;62:669–679.
2. Singh BN, Nademanee K, Baky S: Calcium antagonists: Clinical uses in treating arrhythmias. *Drugs* 1983;25:125–153.
3. Singh BN, Collett JT, Chew CYC: New perspectives in the pharmacologic therapy of cardiac arrhythmaias. *Prog Cardiovasc Dis* 1980;22:243–301.
4. Hamm CW, Opie LH: Protection of infarcting myocardium by slow-channel inhibitors. *Circ Res* 1983 (suppl 1)53:129–138.
5. Leon MB, Rosing DR, Bonow RO, Lipson LC, Epstein SE: Clinical efficacy of vera-

pamil alone and combined with propranolol in treating patients with chronic stable angina pectoris. *Am J Cardiol* 1981;48:131–137.
6. Deanfield JE, Maseri A, Selwyn AP, Ribeiro P, Chierchia S, Krikler S: Myocardial ischemia during daily life in patients with stable angina: Its relation to symptoms and heart rate changes. *Lancet* 1983;2:753–758.
7. Cecchi A, Dovellini EV, Morchi F, Pucci P, Santo-Oro GM, Fazzini PF: Silent myocardial ischemia during ambulatory electrocardiographic monitoring in patients with effort angina. *J Am Coll Cardiol* 1983;1:934–939.
8. Cocco G, Brown G, Strozzi C, Leishman B, Chu B, Rochat N: Asymptomatic myocardial ischemia in patients with stable and typical angina pectoris. *Clin Cardiol* 1982;5:403–408.
9. Gottlieb SO, Weisfeldt ML, Ouyang P, Mellits DE, Gerstenblith G: Silent ischemia as a marker for early unfavorable outcomes in patients with unstable angina. *N Engl J Med* 1986;314:1214–1219.
10. Nademanee K, Intarachot V, Josephson MA, Rieders D, Mody Vaghaiwalla F, Singh BN: Prognostic significance of silent myocardial ischemia in patients with unstable angina. *J Am Coll Cardiol* 1987;10:1–9.
11. Singh BN, Hecht HS, Nademanee K, Chew CYC: Electrophysiologic and hemodynamic effects of slow channel blocking drugs. *Prog Cardiovasc Dis* 1982;23:103–132.
12. Singh BN, Nademanee K: Beta-adrenergic blockade and unstable angina. *Am J Cardiol* 1986;57:992–994.
13. Hossack KF, Brown BG, Stewart DK, Dodge HT: Diltaizem-induced effects on sympathetically mediated constriction of normal and diseased coronary arteries: Lack of epicardial coronary dilatory effect in humans. *Circulation* 1984;70:465–471.
14. Brown BG, Bolson EL, Dodge HT: Dynamic mechanisms in human coronary stenosis. *Circulation* 1984;70:917–922.
15. Singh BN, Chew CYC, Josephson MA: Pharmacologic and hemodynamic mechanisms underlying the antianginal actions of verapamil. *Am J Cardiol* 1982;50:886–892.
16. Imperi GA, Lambert CR, Coy K, Lopez L, Pepine CJ: Effects of titrated beta-blockade (metoprolol) on silent myocardial ischemia in ambulatory patient with coronary artery disease. *Am J Cardiol* 1987;60:579–524.
17. Rocco MB, Barry J, Campbell D, Nabel E, Cook EF, Goldman L, Selwyn AP: Circadian variation of transient myocardial ischemia in patients with coronary artery disease. *Circulation* 1987;75:395–400.
18. Nademanee K, Intarachot V, Josephson MA, Singh BN: Circadian variation in occurrence of transient overt and silent myocardial ischemia in chronic stable angina and comparison with Prinzmetal angina in man. *Am J Cardiol* 1987;7:494–498.
19. Nademanee K, Singh BN, Piontek M, Intarachot V, Yale C: Antianginal efficacy of bepridil, a novel calcium antagonist: Double-blind evaluation by quantitating myocardial ischemia by compact Holter analog technique in chronic stable angina. *J Am Coll Cardiol* 1984;3:551.
20. Schnellbacher K, Drosle C, Roskamm H: Medical and surgical therapy of patients with asymptomatic ischemia, in Arnim TV, Maseri A (eds): *Silent Ischemia*. New York, Springer-Verlag, 1987; pp 154–161.
21. Lynch P, Dargie H, Krikler S, Krikler D: Objective assessment of anti-anginal treatment: A double-blind comparison of propranolol, nifedipine and their combination. *Br Med J* 1980;281:184–187.
22. Nademanee K, Khan S, Robertson H, Intarachot V, Singh BN: Nicardipine-propranolol combination reduces silent myocardial ischemia in chronic stable angina. Submitted for publication, 1988.
23. Lambert CR, Hill JA, Feldman RL, Pepine CJ: Effects of nicardipine on left ventricular function and energetics in man. *Int J Cardiol* 1986;10:237–250.
24. Josephson MA, Coyle-Buffkin C, Singh BN: Effects of intravenous nicardipine on hemodynamics and myocardial ischemic consequences of coronary sinus pacing in patients with coronary artery disease. Submitted for publication, 1988.
25. Usitalo A, Arsitala M, Bae E, Harkonen R, Keyrilainen O, Rytkonen U, Schjelderup-Mathiesen PM, Wendelin H: Metoprolol, nifedipine, and the combination in stable effort angina pectoris. *Am J Cardiol* 1986;57:733–737.

26. Higginbotham M, Morris K, Coleman R, Cobb F: Comparison of nifedipine alone with propranolol alone for stable angina pectoris including hemodynamics at rest and during exercise. *Am J Cardiol* 1986;57:733–737.
27. Leon MG, Rosing DR, Bonow RV, Epstein SE: Clinical efficacy of verapamil alone and combined with propranolol in treating patients with chronic stable angina. *Am J Cardiol* 1981;48:131–138.
28. Hung J, Lamb IH, Connolly SJ: The effects of diltiazem and propranolol alone and in combination on exercise performance and left ventricular function in patients with stable angina: A double-blind, randomized, and placebo-controlled study. *Circulation* 1983;68:560–567.
29. Gottlieb SO, Weisfeldt ML, Ouyang P, Achuff SC, Bauchmann KL, Traill TA, et al: Effect of the addition of propranolol to therapy with nifedipine for unstable angina pectoris: A randomized double-blind, placebo-controlled trial. *Circulation* 1986;73:331–337.

CHAPTER 25

Percutaneous Transluminal Angioplasty and Myocardial Revascularization in the Reduction of Silent Myocardial Ischemia in Coronary Artery Disease

Martin A. Josephson, MD

It is now established that transient episodes of myocardial ischemia occur frequently in patients with coronary artery disease.[1,2] These episodes are usually painless and commonly occur spontaneously during normal daily activity.[1] In addition to these spontaneous episodes, which are usually detected by ambulatory Holter monitor recordings, painless myocardial ischemia may be induced by exercise. Although in some patients all ischemic episodes are clinically silent, most silent ischemic episodes occur in patients who also have symptomatic ischemia. It is therefore not surprising that "silent ischemia" has no single definition, an important consideration in examining the effects of myocardial revascularization on this entity. This chapter will critically review the reported data on the effects of myocardial revascularization by either coronary artery bypass surgery or coronary angioplasty on silent myocardial ischemia. The need to monitor silent ischemia in patients undergoing revascularization techniques and what clinically significant issues need further study will also be discussed.

EFFECTS OF CORONARY ARTERY BYPASS SURGERY

In attempting to clarify the role of monitoring silent ischemia in candidates for myocardial revascularization, several points are important. First, although medical therapy may markedly reduce or eliminate silent ischemia, the quality of life may not be significantly improved in patients in whom myocardial ischemic episodes are completely or predominantly silent. Thus, it is important to know whether the presence of silent myocardial ischemia provides prognostic data on survival in addition to that available from coronary angiography and exercise treadmill testing. In addition to providing a possible indication for revascularization, it is important to define the effects of revascularization on silent ischemia and to determine if monitoring this parameter is useful in assessing the effectiveness of revascularization.

Effects on Exercise-Induced Silent Ischemia

Falcone et al[3] compared the 5-year survival of 269 patients with angina during graded supine bicycle exercise (group I) with that of 204 patients with ischemic ECG changes but no angina during similar exercise (group II). A history of significant angina (Class III-IV) was present in only 12 percent of group II patients versus 60 percent of those in group I. There was no significant difference between the two groups in the extent of coronary artery disease or left ventricular function. Group II patients achieved a higher double product (12%), longer exercise duration (29%) and greater ST-segment depression, and were more likely to develop premature ventricular contractions during exercise than were those in group I. Coronary artery bypass surgery was performed in 45 percent of group I patients and 24 percent of those in group II. No significant difference in 5-year survival was present between the groups for those patients who were treated medically. This study did not actually compare outcomes between symptomatic and asymptomatic patients, because a history of angina was present in both groups of patients and silent ischemia was not quantitated by ambulatory Holter monitoring. It is not surprising, therefore, that patients with more significant angina (group I) were also more likely to undergo coronary bypass surgery. It is interesting, however, that in patients with similar severity of coronary disease and decreased left ventricular function the amount of angina did not appear to be an independent predictor of survival. Similar findings were also reported by Weiner et al[4] who analyzed the outcomes in patients from the data base registry of the CASS study. It was found that although the extent of coronary disease in terms of the number of vessels involved was a powerful predictor of prognosis, the absence of pain during exercise treadmill testing did not influence the clinical outcome over a follow-up of 7 years.

Schnellbacher et al[5] examined the effects of coronary artery bypass surgery on the hemodynamic consequences of ischemia in 22 asymptomatic patients. These patients, with no history of angina, demonstrated significant ST-segment depression and elevation of the pulmonary capillary wedge pressure to a mean of 29 mm Hg during bicycle ergometer exercise. In this group of patients with predominantly multivessel coronary disease, bypass surgery eliminated exercise-induced ischemic ST-segment depression (0.3 to 0.03 mV), decreased the maximal mean pulmonary capillary wedge pressure to 22 mm Hg, and increased maximal exercise tolerance by 49 percent. Thus, revascularization in asymptomatic patients appears to be associated with similar beneficial effects on exercise performance as those seen in symptomatic patients. Although it is not clear why relief of ischemia was associated with an increase in exercise duration, it was likely related to improved hemodynamic status following revascularization.

Effects on Holter-Detected Silent Ischemia

Three studies have examined the effects of myocardial revascularization by coronary artery bypass surgery on silent myocardial ischemia detected by 48-hour ambulatory Holter monitoring.[6–8] Quyyumi et al[6] demonstrated that although coronary bypass graft surgery eliminated or reduced the severity or frequency of angina, persistent myocardial ischemia could still be documented by either exercise stress testing or ambulatory Holter monitoring. Thus, silent ischemia in their study decreased but persisted following bypass surgery. Ribeiro et al[7] demonstrated that bypass surgery eliminated silent myocardial ischemia in 10 of 12 patients and caused a marked reduction in 2 others with documented silent ischemia before surgery (Table 25.1). One of the two patients with silent ischemia after bypass surgery had one of three bypass grafts occluded at repeat angiography. The effects of coronary artery bypass surgery on ischemia were similar whether the ischemia was spontaneous and silent or exercise induced. All 12 patients had positive exercise tests for ischemia before surgery and only three had a positive test after surgery. Both of the patients with ischemia on Holter monitoring had exercise tests that were also positive for ischemia. It is interesting that repeat angiography demonstrated an occluded graft in only one of these two patients, leaving the mechanism of postcoronary bypass surgery ischemia in one patient open for speculation. It is also significant that one other patient with an occluded graft had positive exercise test results for ischemia following surgery, but no silent ischemia was demonstrated during ambulatory monitoring. Whether the mechanism of ischemia following bypass surgery is incomplete surgical revascularization at the time of surgery, graft closure, or coronary vasomotion, it is apparent from this study that patients with silent ischemia following bypass surgery also demonstrate ischemic ECG changes during exercise stress.

Crea et al[8] also demonstrated that surgical myocardial revascularization was effective treatment for Holter monitor-detected silent ischemia (Figure 25.1). This study was designed to determine whether surveillance of myocardial ischemia by Holter monitoring improved the sensitivity of exercise treadmill testing in determining graft patency following bypass graft surgery. Forty-five patients were studied with coronary angiography, exercise treadmill testing, and 48-hour Holter monitoring before and 3 to 5 months after bypass surgery. Twenty-six patients had incomplete revascularization defined as one or more occluded grafts at repeat angiography. Sixteen of these patients demonstrated ischemia on exercise testing, whereas only six demonstrated ischemia on Holter recording. Ten patients with incomplete revasculariza-

Table 25.1. Results of Ambulatory Electrocardiographic Monitoring Before and After Coronary Bypass Surgery*

	Before Coronary Surgery			After Coronary Surgery		
Case No.	No. of Episodes	Total Duration (min)	Heart Rate (beats/min)*	No. of Episodes	Total Duration (min)	Heart Rate (beats/min)*
1	3	16	130	0	—	—
2	14	169	65–80	0	—	—
3	6	33	80–105	0	—	—
4	0	0	0	0	—	—
5	2	24	100	0	—	—
6	8	85	70–95	0	—	—
7	19	396	90–120	0	—	—
8	2	8	90–110	0	—	—
9	—	—	—	—	—	—
10	0	0	0	0	—	—
11	2	14	75–85	0	—	—
12	8	90	115–145	4	18	120–135
13	9	190	80–125	2	8	100–125
14	1	10	100	0	—	—
15	18	245	95–140	0	—	—
Mean	6·6(6·5)	91(118)	91–111	3	13	110–130

* Twelve of the 15 patients had ischemic changes during ambulatory monitoring before surgery. (Reproduced with permission from Ribeiro et al[7] and the *British Heart Journal.*)

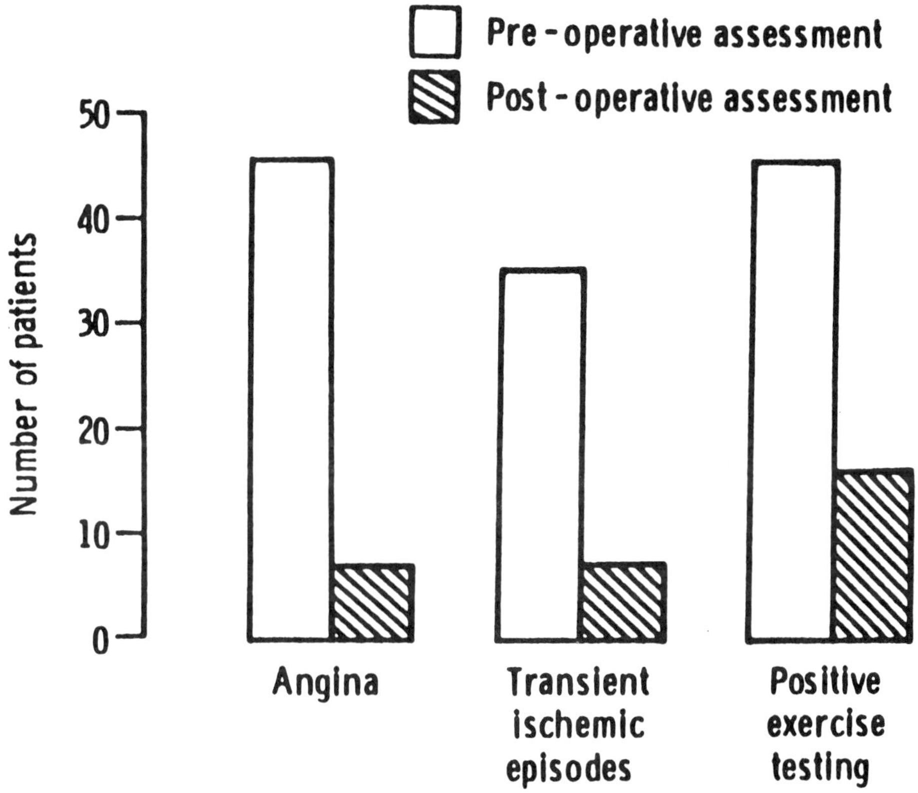

FIGURE 25.1. Incidence of angina and positive results of ambulatory monitoring and exercise testing before and after coronary artery bypass grafting. (Reproduced from Crea et al[8] with the permission of the authors and the *American Journal of Cardiology*.)

tion did not demonstrate ischemia with either method. Of note was the one patient who had evidence of ischemia on Holter monitoring but a negative exercise test result and no graft occlusion. Thus, in agreement with the findings of Ribeiro et al,[7] ambulatory Holter monitoring after bypass surgery did not increase the sensitivity of exercise treadmill testing in detecting postcoronary bypass surgery graft closure. However, the data clearly indicate that after adequate myocardial revascularization, silent ischemia is rarely demonstrated on Holter recordings; this was also noted in patients with unstable angina on medical therapy, requiring coronary artery bypass surgery.[9]

EFFECTS OF PTCA ON SILENT ISCHEMIA

There are even fewer studies on the effects of coronary angioplasty on silent myocardial ischemia. Those that are available also suggest that successful revascularization by angioplasty markedly reduces silent ischemia, whether the episodes are induced by exercise or occur spontaneously.[10–12] Finci et al[10] demonstrated a reduction in ST-segment depression during bicycle exercise and fewer abnormal radionuclide studies (exercise thallium-201 or technetium-99m scintigraphy) after successful angioplasty in 35 patients with significant coronary artery disease but no angina. Höfling et al[11] in a study of 17 asymptomatic patients with thallium-201 SPECT before and after angioplasty, demonstrated a significant reduction in thallium score, indicating improved myocardial perfusion. Both of these studies demonstrated the salient effects of successful angioplasty on exercise-induced ischemia in asymptomatic patients and suggest silent ischemia as an indication for coronary angioplasty in asymptomatic patients who have coronary stenoses suitable for dilatation. Holter monitoring was not performed in either of these studies. Only one study has evaluated the effects of coronary angioplasty on Holter monitor-detected ischemia.[12] In this study, 36 patients were evaluated by exercise treadmill testing and 24-hour Holter monitoring before and after successful coronary angioplasty. Ten of these 36 patients had one or more episodes of myocardial ischemia detected by Holter recording, with 80 percent of these episodes not associated with anginal symptoms (Table 25.2). There were 39 ischemic episodes consisting of 1- to 8-mm ST-segment depression for a total ischemic duration of 398 minutes. After angioplasty no ischemic episodes were detected by Holter monitoring in these 10 patients. An example of portions of the Holter recording from a single patient before and after angioplasty is shown in Figure 25.2. In this study in which 69 percent of patients had single-vessel disease and only a single patient had triple-vessel disease, silent myocardial ischemia was only present in 28 percent of the patients. Because the presence of silent myocardial ischemia correlates with the disease severity, it will likely be more prevalent as increasing numbers of patients with multiple-vessel coronary disease undergo coronary angioplasty. Although there are no data to suggest that Holter recording might be more sensitive or detect restenosis after angioplasty earlier than either exercise treadmill testing or clinical symptoms, extrapolation of data from patients after bypass surgery suggests that this is not likely.

COMMENTS AND CONCLUSIONS

It is likely that a significant number of patients with unstable angina or chronic stable angina undergoing PTCA or surgical myocardial revascularization have episodes of silent myocardial ischemia. At least in unstable angina, residual silent ischemic ep-

Table 25.2. Characteristics of Holter Monitor-Detected Myocardial Ischemia in Relation to Coronary Anatomy in Patients Undergoing Coronary Angioplasty*

		Ischemic Episodes					
		Before Angioplasty			After Angioplasty		
Patient No.	Coronary Stenoses (% diameter reduction)	No.	Duration (min/24 h)	STΔ (mm)	No.	Duration (min/24 h)	STΔ (mm)
1	80 LAD, 85 LCx, 100 RCA	10	144	5–8	0	—	—
2	80 LAD	8	84	1–8	0	—	—
3	80 LAD	6	49	1–3	0	—	—
4	80 LAD	5	45	1	0	—	—
5	80 LAD	4	18	1–3	0	—	—
6	80 LAD, 100 LCx	2	24	1	0	—	—
7	75 LCx, 90 RCA	1	14	1	0	—	—
8	90 RCA	1	12	2	0	—	—
9	85 LAD, 100 RCA	1	5	3	0	—	—
10	90 LAD	1	3	2	0	—	—
		39*	398*	1–8	0	—	—

* Reproduced from Josephson et al[12] with the permission of the authors and the *Journal of the American College of Cardiology*.

A

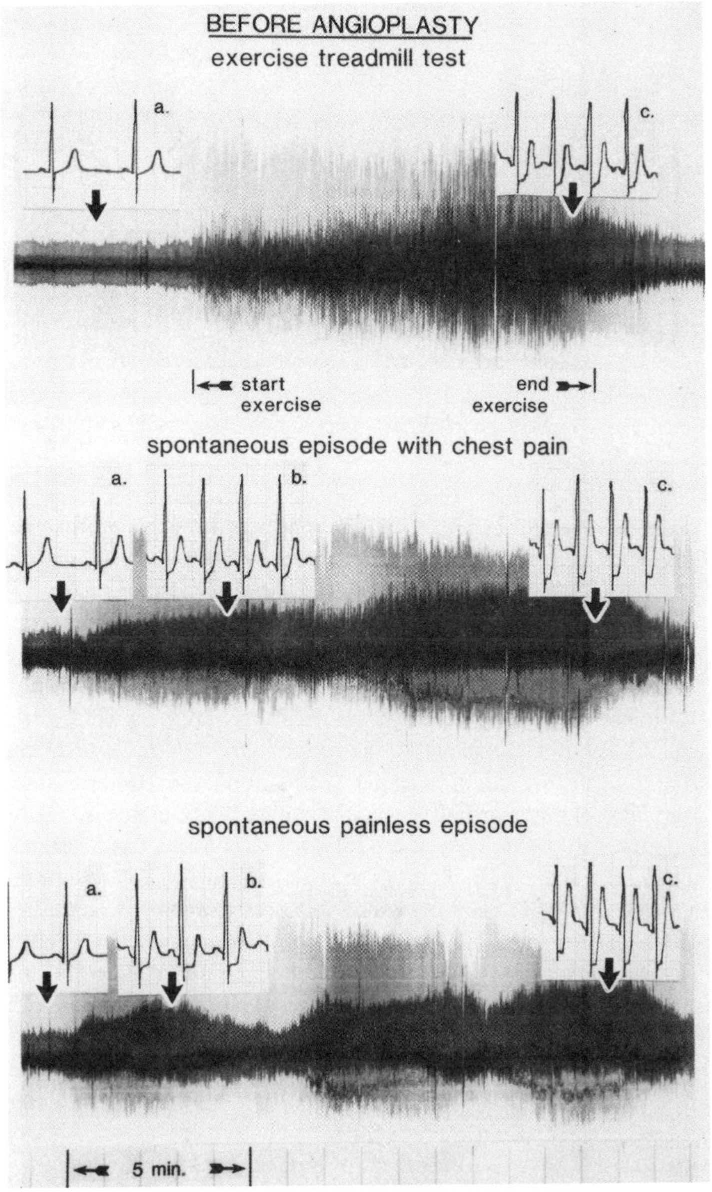

FIGURE 25.2. (A) Selected portions of the 24-hour Holter recording before angioplasty in a patient with 80 percent stenosis of the proximal left anterior descending coronary artery. The *upper panel* was recorded during a treadmill exercise test, the *middle panel* during a spontaneous episode of angina, and the *lower panel* during a spontaneous episode of ischemia without associated chest pain. The inserts of printouts at 25 mm/s paper speed demonstrate the normal QRST complex (a), ST-segment depression at the onset of ischemia (b), and marked ST-segment depression with T-wave augmentation (c). ST-segment depression and T-wave augmentation during spontaneous episodes of ischemia are similar to those induced during exercise. (B) After angioplasty, only T-wave augmentation without ST-segment depression (d) occurred at 13.2 minutes of treadmill exercise. No spontaneous episodes were present on the Holter recording in this patient after angioplasty. (Reproduced from Josephson et al[12] with the permission of the authors and the *Journal of the American College of Cardiology*.)

B

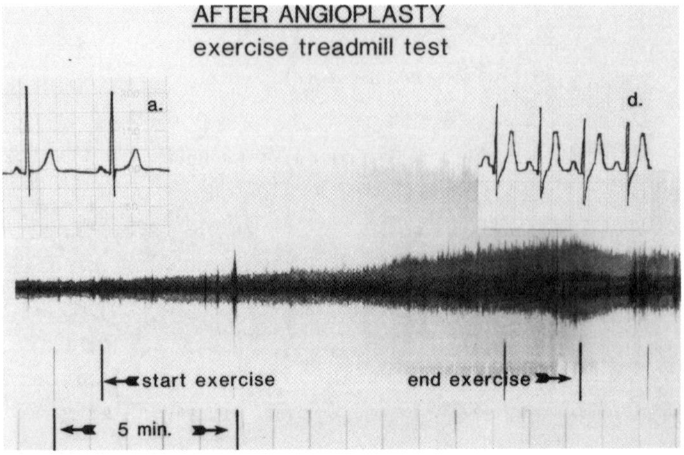

FIGURE 25.2B (continued).

isodes when the symptomatic ones have been eliminated by medical therapy appear to have prognostic significance.[9,13] These patients now generally undergo angiography and myocardial revascularization for indications based largely on anatomic disease rather than ischemic episodes documented on Holter recordings. The available data, albeit from a limited number of patients, show marked efficacy of PTCA and surgical revascularization in eliminating silent ischemic episodes in these patients. It is conceivable that an improvement in morbidity and mortality in certain subsets of patients after surgical revascularization may be linked to the elimination of myocardial ischemia. However, some preliminary data reviewed here indicate that exercise treadmill testing might be superior to ambulatory Holter monitoring in gauging the adequacy of myocardial revascularization. Nevertheless, further studies are needed to define the precise role of ambulatory monitoring assessment of silent myocardial ischemia in these patient subgroups. It is also possible that ambulatory monitoring in silent ischemia may be useful after angioplasty in certain subgroups of patients, such patients who are unable to perform adequate exercise, patients with multivessel coronary disease with incomplete revascularization by angioplasty, patients with only silent ischemia, or patients with unstable angina. The indications for performing elective angioplasty include suitable coronary anatomy and documented ischemia. Patients who have only silent ischemia and negative exercise test results are uncommon, but silent ischemia might become an indication for angioplasty or surgery especially if frequent silent ischemic episodes are shown to correlate with adverse cardiac events. Whether the presence of frequent silent ischemic episodes on Holter monitoring will better define patients who need revascularization for prognostic reasons is unknown at the present time, but it is a subject that clearly merits critical investigation by controlled studies.

REFERENCES

1. Deanfield J, Maseri A, Selwyn AP, Ribeiro P, Chierchia S, Krikler S, Morgan M: Myocardial ischemia during daily life in patients with stable angina: Its relation to symptoms and heart rate changes. *Lancet* 1983;2:753–758.
2. Nademanee K, Intarachot V, Singh PN, Josephson MA, Singh BN: Characteristics and clinical significance of myocardial ischemia in unstable angina. *Am J Cardiol* 1986;58:26B–33B.

3. Falcone C, de Servi S, Poma E, Campana C, Sciré A, Montemartini C, Specchia G: Clinical significance of exercise-induced silent myocardial ischemia in patients with coronary artery disease. *J Am Coll Cardiol* 1987;9:295–299.
4. Weiner DA, Ryan TJ, McCabe CH, Luk S, Chaitman BR, Sheffield T, Tristani F, Fisher LD: Significance of silent myocardial ischemia during exercise testing in patients with coronary artery disease. *Am J Cardiol* 1987;59:725–729.
5. Schnellbacher K, Droste C, Roskamm H: Medical and surgical therapy of patients with asymptomatic ischemia, in Arnim TV, Maseri A (eds): *Silent Ischemia*. Darmstadt, Steinkopff Verlag, 1987, pp 154–161.
6. Quyyumi AA, Wright CA, Mockus LJ, Yacoub M, Fox KM: Effects of myocardial revascularisation in patients with effort angina and those with effort and nocturnal angina. *Br Heart J* 1985;54:557–561.
7. Ribeiro P, Shea M, Deanfield JE, Oakley CM, Sapsford R, Jones T, Walesby R, Selwyn AP: Different mechanisms for the relief of angina after coronary bypass surgery: Physiological versus anatomical assessment. *Br Heart J* 1984;52:502–509.
8. Crea F, Kaski JC, Fragasso G, Hackett D, Stanbridge R, Taylor KM, Maseri A: Usefulness of Holter monitoring to improve the sensitivity of exercise testing in determining the degree of myocardial revascularization after coronary artery bypass grafting for stable angina pectoris. *Am J Cardiol* 1987;60:40–43.
9. Nademanee K, Intarachot V, Josephson MA, Rieders D, Mody FV, Singh BN: Prognostic significance of silent myocardial ischemia in patients with unstable angina. *J Am Coll Cardiol* 1987;10:1–9.
10. Finci L, Meier B, Steffenino G, Righetti A, Bodenmann JJ, Rutishauser W: Coronary angioplasty in silent myocardial ischemia, in Arnim TV, Maseri A. (eds): *Silent Ischemia*. Darmstadt, Steinkopff Verlag, 1987, pp 162–169.
11. Höfling B, Stäblein A, v. Arnim Th: Alleviation of silent ischemia by PTCA, in Arnim TV, Maseri A (eds): *Silent Ischemia*. Darmstadt, Steinkopff Verlag, 1987, pp 170–176.
12. Josephson MA, Nademanee K, Intarachot V, Lewis H, Singh BN: Abolition of Holter monitor-detected silent myocardial ischemia after percutaneous transluminal coronary angioplasty. *J Am Coll Cardiol* 1987;10:499–503.
13. Gottlieb SO, Weisfeldt ML, Ouyang P, Mellits ED, Gerstenblith G: Silent ischemia as a marker for early unfavorable outcomes in patients with unstable angina. *N Engl J Med* 1986;314:1214–1219.

CHAPTER 26

Should Silent Ischemia Be an End Point for Therapeutic Antianginal Treatment?

Shahbudin H. Rahimtoola, MB

In 1984, after reviewing the results of pharmacologic therapy in unstable angina, I concluded that the results were less than satisfactory.[1] Up to that time, therapy had focused on control of pain; however, most episodes of ischemia were demonstrated to be painless,[2] and ischemia rather than pain was the likely precursor of cardiac death and morbidity. Therefore, I suggested that we begin to focus on diagnosing and relieving all episodes of ischemia, not just those associated with pain.[1] Implicitly, there were two important parts to this suggestion or hypothesis: (1) painless ischemia is the cause of untoward cardiac events; and (2) control of painless ischemia will control or reduce untoward cardiac events.

Subsequent studies by Gottlieb et al[3,4] showed that cardiac events in patients with unstable angina correlate with the presence of painless ischemia in the first 48 hours of hospital admission. Importantly, Nademanee et al[5] showed that among patients with unstable angina whose pain was controlled by pharmacologic therapy, subsequent cardiac events occurred mainly in those who continued to have episodes of painless ischemia. However, a direct cause and effect relationship between painless myocardial ischemia and an untoward cardiac event has not been demonstrated by either group in this clinical subset of patients nor has it been shown that control of painless ischemia will lead to a lower rate of cardiac events. Therefore, there currently is no conclusive proof that the control of painless ischemia should be an end point of antianginal treatment in unstable angina. Nevertheless, the important studies of Gottlieb, Nademanee, and their co-workers[3–5] strongly suggest that this proof should be diligently sought.

REASONS WHY PAINLESS ISCHEMIA SHOULD BE AN END POINT OF TREATMENT

There are several important reasons why ischemia, painful and painless, should be eliminated or controlled. The main considerations may be summarized as follows:

1. Ischemia is one of the most important determinants of the outcome in patients with coronary artery disease.[6] The basis for this assertion is summarized in Figure 26.1. Hultgren et al[7] in the VA cooperative study of medically treated chronic stable angina showed that the magnitude of ST-segment depression during ex-

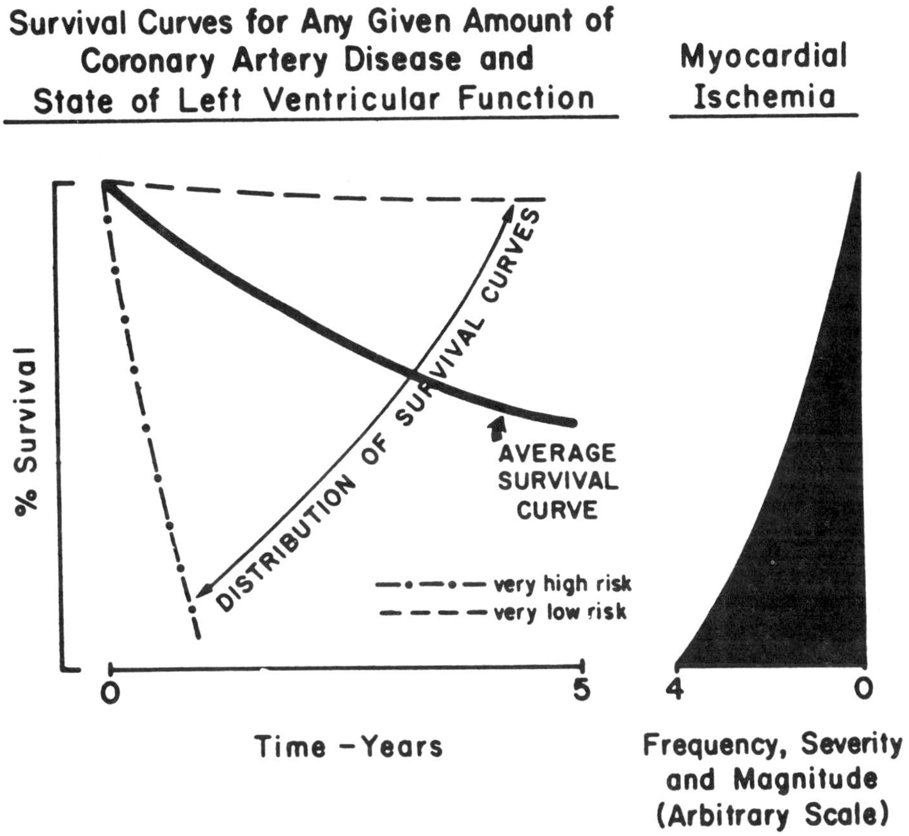

FIGURE 26.1. Diagrammatic representation of the likely spectrum of survival curves and the probable role of myocardial ischemia. The more the amount of myocardial ischemia, the higher the risk category of the patient. (Reproduced with permission from Rahimtoola[6] and *Circulation*.)

ercise was more predictive of mortality than was myocardial oxygen consumption, angina, rate-pressure product, or premature ventricular contractions. As a predictor of mortality, it was independent of impaired left ventricular function and noninvasive terciles. In the European Coronary Surgery Study[8] of chronic stable angina in patients with left ventricular ejection fraction equal to or greater than 50 percent, the major risk factors for mortality in the medical group were:

- ECG abnormalities at rest
- ECG abnormalities provoked by exercise
- Peripheral arterial disease
- Age ≥ 50 years
- Number of diseased vessels
- Left main coronary artery disease
- Proximal LAD (left anterior descending coronary) disease

It is noteworthy that barring the presence of peripheral arterial disease and age, all other features correlated strongly with ischemia.

Table 26.1 shows data from the Coronary Artery Surgery Study (CASS) which indicate that the severity of ischemia as judged by the exercise treadmill test[9] is related to the 7-year mortality in medically treated patients with chronic stable

Table 26.1. Relationship Between ECG Abnormalities on Exercise Stress Test and Subsequent Mortality in Medically Treated Patients with Angina*

	7-Year Mortality in Medically Treated Patients
ST-Segment Depression on Exercise ECG	
<1mm	11%
1–2 mm	16%
>2 mm	21%
Low risk	9%
High risk	28%

NOTE: Low risk = ST-segment depression <1mm *plus* final exercise state >3; high risk = ST-segment depression ≥1mm *plus* final exercise stage ≤1.

* Adapted from Weiner et al[9]: data from coronary artery surgery (non-randomized) study.

angina. Thus, the overall data indicate that ischemia demonstrated by whatever technique is the principal determinant of prognosis in coronary artery disease.

2. The benefits of revascularization (antiischemic therapy) on survival in patients with coronary artery disease are mainly seen in those with myocardial ischemia. Data from three different studies in support of this contention are presented in Tables 26.2 through 26.4. Note the differences between the effects of myocardial revascularization in the group in which ischemia is greater or angina is present on treadmill testing versus those in which there is less ischemia or angina is absent.
3. Many, possibly the majority, of ischemic episodes are painless[2,6] as emphasized repeatedly elsewhere in this monograph. The fact that the symptomatic episodes differ little, if at all, from the asymptomatic ones emphasizes the need for a common approach to treatment.
4. In patients with unstable angina, painless ischemia was shown to be the major determinant of unfavorable cardiac events. This was true in patients who had just started receiving pharmacologic treatment[3,4] and also in patients whose pain had been controlled by pharmacologic treatment.[12] In patients with myocardial infarction, ischemia (painful as well as painless) was shown to be one of the most important predictors of future unfavorable cardiac events.[13,14]
5. The improved survival with revascularization in patients with chronic stable angina is seen in those with severe angina as well as mild angina and also in those

Table 26.2. Relation Between the Effects of Medical and Surgical Therapy on Mortality in Chronic Stable Angina and the Results of Exercise Treadmill Tests*

Exercise-Induced ST ↓	5-Year Mortality			8-Year Mortality		
	Medically Assigned	Surgically Assigned	Value	Medically Assigned	Surgically Assigned	Value
None or <1 mm	10%	5%	>0.20	15%	12%	>0.20
≥ 1 mm	21%	8%	0.0003	23%	10%	0.0003

* Based on European Coronary Surgery Study.[10]

Table 26.3. Impact of Medical versus Surgical Therapy on Long-Term Mortality in Chronic Stable Angina in Relation to the Treadmill Stress Test

Exercise-Induced St ↓	Patient (no)	7-Year Mortality: Medically Assigned	Surgically Assigned	Value
0	94	21%	17%	NS
1 mm	122	28%	30%	NS
>2 mm	95	40%	19%	0.026

*From the VA cooperative study of chronic stable angina.[7]

with no angina provided they have significant myocardial ischemia. For example, in the European Coronary Surgery Study, the conclusions were summarized as follows: "The difference in survival in favor of surgery between the two treatments was significant both in subgroup with Class I and II angina and in the subgroup with Class III angina."[8] In the CASS registry there were 20,137 patients: 1477 with left mainstem coronary artery disease (MCAD) and 53 (3.5%) with asymptomatic MCAD. The 5-year survival of patients receiving medical therapy for symptomatic left MCAD with 58 percent; for asymptomatic left MCAD, 57 percent. Following coronary artery bypass surgery the corresponding figures were 84 percent and 88 percent.[15] Although differences between the effects of medical therapy and those of surgery were significant ($p = 0.02$), the effects of either modality of therapy did not differ in symptomatic versus nonsymptomatic patients.

REASONS WHY SILENT MYOCARDIAL ISCHEMIA SHOULD NOT BE AN END POINT OF TREATMENT

There currently are several important reasons for us to be cautious about using silent ischemia as an end point of therapy:

1. We have documented instances of silent ischemia that led to ventricular tachycardia/fibrillation and death.[16] However, all the other evidence linking painful and painless ischemia to these untoward events is correlative rather than a direct "cause-effect" relationship.
2. There are a variety of techniques to detect silent myocardial ischemia;[10] the most commonly used are transient ST-T wave changes on exercise or at rest. There is a large body of evidence that demonstrates that transient ST-T wave changes are likely the result of myocardial ischemia (Table 26.5). However, there also are many studies that demonstrate that these ST-T wave changes may be nonspecific.[18–25] Thus, it is clear that some ST-T wave changes are not the result of

Table 26.4. Effects of Exercise-Induced Angina on Medical and Surgical Therapy in Patients with Coronary Artery Disease*

Exercise-Induced Angina	7-Year Mortality: Medically Assigned	Surgically Assigned	Value
Absent	29%	21%	0.34
Present	31%	0%	0.0004

* Data based on Coronary Artery Surgery Study (CASS) reported by Ryan et al.[11]

Table 26.5. Transient ST-Segment Shifts with or without T-Wave Changes, with or without Pain, During Exercise or Ambulatory ECG Monitoring is Associated with:

A. Abnormalities of Left Ventricular (LV) Function:
  1. Increases of:
    a. LV end-diastolic pressure
    b. Pulmonary artery wedge and pulmonary artery diastolic pressures
    c. LV end-diastolic and end-systolic volumes
  2. Decreases of:
    a. LV ejection fraction
    b. Positive LV dp/dt
    c. Negative LV dp/dt
  3. Appearances of new LV wall motion abnormalities
B. Abnormalities of Myocardial Blood Flow:
  1. Reduction of:
    a. Cardiac venous 0_2 saturation
    b. Endocardial/epicardial blood flow ratio
    c. Myocardial perfusion
  2. Production of Myocardial Lactate

ischemia; therefore, it may not be possible or necessary to eliminate them, and eliminating them may have no beneficial therapeutic effect.

3. Pharmacolgic treatment of ischemia reduces painful and painless ischemia and eliminates it only in some patients. It is far more successful in patients with mild angina[17] than in those with severe angina.[5]
4. The data of Gottlieb et al[3] showed that in patients with unstable angina, painless ischemia of less than 60 minutes' duration in a 24-hour period was not predictive of subsequent untoward events. Thus, there is uncertainty at the present time as to whether elimination or just reduction is needed in the frequency and severity of painless myocardial ischemia.
5. It has not been shown that eliminating or reducing silent myocardial ischemia will have the desired therapeutic effect; if it does do so, then in which clinical subgroup(s) does the beneficial effect occur?

The expense of diagnosing, treating, and following up persons with painless ischemia is considerable. Therefore, in view of the foregoing it is reasonable that we

Table 26.6. Clinical Subgroups in Which Painless Ischemia is Likely to be Clinically Important

1. Unstable angina
2. Postmyocardial infarction (MI)
   Symptomatic MI: First 3–6 months
   Asymptomatic MI: First 3 years
3. Chronic stable angina
4. Left ventricular dysfunction of unknown etiology
5. Survivors of unexpected cardiac arrest
6. Special subgroups
   Diabetics
   Post-cardiac transplantation
   High-risk professions, eg pilots
   Post-myocardial revascularization
7. People with unrecognized coronary artery disease at risk for sudden, unexpected cardiac events
   Major risk factors: Hypertension, smoking, hyperlipidemia, left ventricular hypertrophy, and peripheral vascular disease
   Particularly in: Men, increasing age, positive family history, and overweight

should be very careful about increasing the cost of health care delivery in most subgroups of patients when there is no proof that the increased cost is of real benefit.

WHAT SHOULD WE DO AT PRESENT?

It seems reasonable that if silent ischemia *is* sought and corrected, then we should direct our attention to those who are at "high risk" of untoward cardiac events. Clinical syndromes in which silent myocardial ischemia is important are listed in Table 26.6. For the present, no specific all-encompassing guidelines can be established because there are limited data on the prognostic significance of silent ischemia in most subsets of patients with coronary disease. It is likely, however, that such guidelines will be forthcoming as our appreciation of the clinical significance of silent ischemia expands.

REFERENCES

1. Rahimtoola SH: Coronary bypass surgery for unstable angina. *Circulation* 1984;69:842.
2. Chierchia S, Lazzari M, Freedman B, Brunelli B, Maseri A: Impairment of myocardial perfusion and function painless myocardial ischemia. *J Am Coll Cardiol* 1983;1:924.
3. Gottlieb SO, Weisfeldt ML, Ouyang P, Mellits ED, Gerstenblith G: Silent ischemia as a marker for early unfavorable outcomes in patients with unstable angina. *N Engl J Med* 1986;314:1214.
4. Gottlieb SO, Weisfeldt ML, Ouyang P, Mellitis ED, Gerstenblith G: Silent ischemia predicts infarction and death during 2 years follow-up of unstable angina. *J Am Coll Cardiol* 1987;10:756.
5. Nademanee K, Intarachot V, Josephson MA, Riediers D, Mody FV, Singh BN: Prognostic significance of silent myocardial ischemia in patients with unstable angina. *J Am Coll Cardiol* 1987;10:1.
6. Rahimtoola SH: A perspective on the three large multicenter randomized clinical trials of coronary bypass surgery for chronic stable angina. *Circulation* 1985;72(Suppl V):V–123.
7. Hultgren HN, Peduzzi P: Prognostic value of ECG exercise tests in stable angina. *Circulation* 1983;68:III–376.
8. Varnauskas E and the European Coronary Surgery Study Group: Survival myocardial infarction, and employment status in a prospective randomized study of coronary bypass surgery. *Circulation* 1985;72:V–90.
9. Weiner DA, McCabe CH, Ryan TJ, Fisher LD, Chaitman BR, Sheffield T, Tristani F: Value of exercise testing in identifying patients with improved survival after coronary bypass surgery (CASS Registry). *Circulation* 1984;70:II–20.
10. European Coronary Surgery Study Group: Longterm results of prospective randomized study of coronary artery bypass surgery in stable angina pectoris. *Lancet* 1982;2:1173.
11. Ryan TJ, Weiner DA, McCabe CH, Davis KB, Sheffield LT, Chaitman BR, Tristani FE, Fisher LD: Exercise testing in the coronary artery surgery study randomized population. *Circulation* 1985;72(Suppl V):V–31.
12. Deanfield JE, Maseri A, Selwyn AP, Ribeiro P, Chierchia S, Krikler S, Morgan M: Myocardial ischemia during daily life in patients with stable angina: Its relation to symptoms and heart rate change. *Lancet* 1983;2:753.
13. Eriksson J, Thaulow E: Follow-up of patients with asymptomatic myocardial ischemia, in Rutishauser W, Roskamm H (eds): *Silent Myocardial Ischemia*. Berlin, Springer-Verlag 1984.
14. Gibson RS: Non-Q-wave myocardial infarction: Diagnosis, prognosis, and management. *Curr Probl in Cardiol* 1988;13:1.
15. Deumite JN, Chaitman BN, Davis KB, Killip TH, Fommer PL, Rogers WJ: Asymtomatic left main coronary artery disease (CASS) (Abstract). *J Am Coll Cardiol* 1985;5:518.
16. Hong RA, Bhandari AK, McKay CR, Au PK, Rahimtoola SH: Life-threatening ven-

tricular tachycardia and fibrillation induced by painless myocardial ischemia during exercise testing. *JAMA* 1987;257:1937.

17. Kawanishi DT, Reid Cl, Simsarian G, Amisola Y, Gonzalez A, Rahimtoola SH: Effect of pharmacolgic therapy on angina frequency, ST segment depression during ambulatory ECG monitoring, and treadmill performance in patients with chronic mild angina. *Am Heart J* 1988;115:220.
18. Stern S, Tzivoni D: Early detection of silent ischemic heart disease by 24-hour ECG monitoring of active subjects. *Br Heart J* 1974;36:467–486.
19. Stern S, Tzivoni D, Stern Z: Diagnostic accuracy of ambulatory ECG monitoring in ischemic heart disease. *Circulation* 1975;52:1045–1049.
20. Crawford MH, Mendoza CA, O'Rourke RA, White DH, Boucher CA, Gorwit J: Limitations of continuous ambulatory electrocardiogram monitoring for detecting coronary artery disease. *Ann Int Med* 1978;89:1–5.
21. Bala Subramanian V, Lahiri A, Green HL, Raftery EB: Ambulatory ST-segment monitoring: Problems, pitfalls, solutions and clinical applications. *Br Heart J* 1980;44:419–425.
22. Armstrong WF, Jordan JW, Morris SN, McHenry PL: Prevalence and magnitude of ST-segment and T-wave abnormalities in normal men during continuous ambulatory electrocardiography. *Am J Cardiol* 1982;49:1638–1642.
23. Quyyumi AS, Wright C, Fox K: Ambulatory electrocardiographic ST-segment changes in healthy volunteers. *Br Heart J* 1983;50:460–464.
24. Quyyumi AS, Mockus L, Wright C, Fox KM: Morphology of ambulatory ST-segment changes in patients with varying severity of coronary artery disease: Investigation of the frequency of nocturnal ischemia and coronary spasm. *Br Heart J* 1985;53:186–193.
25. Kawanishi DT, Reid CL, Simsarian G, Amisola Y, Gonzalez A, Rahimtoola SH: Effect of pharmacological therapy on angina frequency, ST segment depression during ambulatory ECG monitoring, and treadmill performance in patients with chronic stable mild angina, *Am Heart J* 1988;115:220.

Epilogue

Bramah N. Singh, MD, DPhil

Justifiably or unjustifiably, the entity "silent myocardial ischemia" has genuinely caught the imagination of large sections of the medical community. Witness, for example, the exponential growth of the number of symposia and publications on the subject since Rutishauer and Roskamm[1] held the first symposium on the subject in Europe in March 1983, and I presented one in the United States in November 1984.[2] Opinion since then appears to have crystallized into two somewhat extreme ends of a spectrum. One view, perhaps most eloquently championed by William Shell, labels silent myocardial ischemia as the "silent killer";[3] the opposing view is that of George Diamond who, in the present state of knowledge, sums up the issue of treatment as, "Silent ischemia deserves the silent treatment."[4] For most practitioners and clinical scientists, the situation is confusing, but the temptation to make a foray into the polemics of silent myocardial ischemia is reasonably compelling.

This monograph attempts to strike a balanced perspective on the basis of what appears to be reasonably secure data. The findings presented establish a number of features of silent ischemia of potential clinical importance. There now is substantial agreement that in ischemic syndromes such as Prinzmetal's, unstable, and chronic stable angina, over two thirds of ischemic episodes are asymptomatic (silent). Although silent ischemic episodes tend to be shorter in duration and associated with a greater hemodynamic disturbance, there is considerable overlap between silent and symptomatic episodes. Indeed, episodes of ischemia identical in duration and in the degree of associated hemodynamic perturbations may be found in the same patient with or without symptoms. Thus, there is no clear explanation why some ischemic episodes are silent, others painful. Data presented in this monograph raise the role of autonomic dysfunction (eg, diabetes), but this clearly is not the explanation in the majority of patients. It is likely that in some patients an elevated pain threshold may play a role, but the postulated role of endorphins remains to be established.

Other features clearly suggested by the available data should be emphasized. Most spontaneous episodes of ischemia in the various ischemic syndromes (painful or painless) are not preceded by major increases in heart rate (and, by inference, arterial pressure and rate-pressure product), indicating that ischemia in these cases may result from a primary decrease in flow due to focal vasoconstriction (eg, Prinzmetal's angina), normal fluctuations in coronary tone in the context of severe eccentric coronary lesions (eg, chronic stable angina), thrombosis (unstable angina and myocardial infarction), or a combination of both unstable angina and myocardial infarction as demonstrated in some cases of acute infarction.[5] Nevertheless, there is no uniform agreement as to whether or not most episodes of silent ischemia in chronic stable angina are preceded by significant increases in the determinants of oxygen consumption. Further work with careful analysis of the beat-to-beat changes in heart rate and blood pressure will be necessary to provide definitive answers.

Of particular interest is the emphasis placed on the growing appreciation of the potential significance of the circadian variation in the occurrence of silent (and painful) episodes of ischemia. The data on chronic stable angina were clear; few episodes occurred between midnight and 6 AM, the overall pattern being consistent with the circadian variation in catecholamine surges influencing the determinants of oxygen consumption. The circadian pattern in the occurrence of ischemia in unstable angina and Prinzmetal's angina is less well defined. The possibility remains that "activity" of disease in these conditions might not exhibit a circadian periodicity but may have a cyclic variation of ischemic episodes over a wider time span. The issue of a link between the circadian rhythmicity of ischemic episodes and that of myocardial infarction and sudden death was raised. However, as yet there are no data to support the idea that attenuation of the circadian distribution of ischemic episodes (as induced by beta-blockade) might influence morbidity and mortality in coronary artery disease. What has emerged from the data presented, however, is that the greatest number of episodes of silent ischemia occur in patients with known symptomatic coronary disease. As far as Holter monitoring is concerned, if the criteria for detection are strictly defined prospectively, rarely is silent ischemia found in truly "normal" subjects without risk factors for coronary disease. Unfortunately, there are no meaningful studies in completely asymptomatic patients with occult coronary disease with negative or positive exercise stress tests for ischemia. No data were presented to support or deny the possibility that the presence of ischemia documented on Holter monitoring in these patients provides incremental prognostic information that allows the clinician to identify the completely asymptomatic subject at risk of acute infarction and sudden death. However, much prognostic data have been obtained with the exercise treadmill in patients with coronary artery disease and chronic stable angina. A positive test for ischemia in these patients is associated with a clearly augmented risk of a coronary event (infarction, sudden death), whether such patients are symptomatic[6] or completely asymptomatic.[7] Although not discussed specifically in this monograph, it is now well established[4,6] that in patients whose exercise treadmill test is electrocardiographically positive, the prognosis is identical whether such patients develop pain during the stress test or not. These newer data clearly emphasize that it is ischemia (and most likely its extent as reflected by the number of vessels involved and the severity of the stenosis) that is prognostically significant rather than its symptomatic manifestations. At least, in chronic stable angina and in the asymptomatic patient with occult coronary artery disease, it remains entirely uncertain whether ambulatory Holter monitoring will provide incremental prognostic information over that which is available on the basis of exercise testing (and angiographic delineation of coronary stenosis and ventriculographic assessment of myocardial function). Several studies currently in progress might be crucial in establishing the prognostic significance of silent ischemia documented on Holter monitoring in patients with silent myocardial infarction and in those with chronic stable angina. The data reported in this monograph, however, do suggest that in the *diagnosis* of coronary artery disease, Holter monitoring carries a low yield because of a low sensitivity of detection. Whether Holter monitoring might be a useful adjunct in judging the efficacy of medical therapy also remains uncertain and, at the very best, controversial. However, this area needs critical scrutiny by controlled studies.

Of particular interest is the demonstration that in unstable angina, the persistence of silent myocardial ischemia after the symptomatic episodes have been eliminated by medical therapy is highly predictive of an adverse short-term prognosis.[9,10] This observation raises a number of practical questions. For example, does it imply that a more concerted effort should be made to further reduce silent myocardial ischemia by more intensive medical therapy? Or are we already at the top end of the dose-response curve with medical therapy (I suspect we are), and the phenomenon of residual ischemia in this setting is an expression of the fact that drug therapy merely distinguishes responders from nonresponders, the latter having inherently a worse prognosis that is unlikely to be influenced significantly by further aggressive medical therapy? The decisive resolution of this issue is only possible by a stringently controlled clinical trial. Such a trial, however, is unlikely to be undertaken because most patients with unstable angina, at least in the United States, now undergo myocardial revascularization. The issue of a controlled trial may nevertheless be of fundamental importance in chronic stable angina.

The monograph also addresses the issue of silent myocardial infarction in previously asymptomatic patients. The data from the Framingham Study[11] clearly establish that up to 30 percent of patients develop silent myocardial infarction. The subsequent prognosis of these patients is nevertheless identical to that of patients with symptomatic infarcts. The data further emphasize that it is the magnitude or severity of ischemia and myocardial necrosis that is of crucial importance rather than its symptomatic manifestation. Conversely, the relatively low prevalence of asymptomatic coronary artery disease in the population (perhaps 2 to 3%) subject to the disorder, makes the issue of "mass screening" of such a population prohibitive in the absence of major risk factors.

Data were presented on the prevalence of silent ischemia in persons with diabetes and those with hypertension. These reports, however, were based on studies in small patient populations. In both instances, silent ischemia was noted in a subset of these patients, but angiographic and ventriculographic correlations were not obtained. In hypertension, the data are of particular interest in view of the recent finding that left ventricular hypertrophy is associated with an increased incidence of sudden death.[9] It is tempting to speculate that sudden death in these cases may be triggered by myocardial ischemic episodes. This link remains to be established. However, as indicated in this monograph, patients with sudden death from ischemic heart disease do have advanced anatomic multivessel coronary disease, and those who are resuscitated have significant but asymptomatic ischemia induced by exercise stress testing. Whether these patients might also exhibit silent episodes of myocardial ischemia on Holter monitoring has not been systematically studied. Conversely, it is of considerable interest that a reasonably careful analysis of a large number of ECG tapes of patients who died while wearing Holter recorders has shown that less than 12 percent of the patients had significant ST-segment depression preceding the onset of terminal ventricular tachycardia / fibrillation.[12] These observations suggest that although coronary artery disease is the most important substrate for sudden cardiac death, an ischemic episode is not the immediate trigger to the fatal event in most cases. However, the Holter finding does not discount the crucial role of ischemia, because it is entirely possible that a fast ventricular tachycardia initiated by an early extrasystole may worsen the imbalance in oxygen supply and demand in a patient with coronary artery disease; the resulting ischemia may induce ventricular fibrillation by accelerating the rate of ventricular tachycardia. These considerations are relevant to the issue of amelioration of ischemia, silent or symptomatic, as an approach to the prevention of sudden death in patients with coronary artery disease.

Because the focus of this monograph has been silent myocardial ischemia, it is essential to emphasize that the sole reason for treatment is to improve prognosis. Data presented indicate that medical therapy with nitrates, calcium-channel blockers, and beta-antagonists or invasive modalities such as PTCA or surgery are effective in reducing silent myocardial ischemia. However, although pharmacologic therapy, using single agents or combination regimens, is effective in reducing silent ischemic episodes and their duration, it remains uncertain if this will influence prognosis (although theoretic considerations suggest that it might). Neither is it known what degrees of reduction in silent ischemic episodes or their cumulative durations over a finite period may be necessary to effect a favorable change in prognosis. The types of controlled clinical trials that might be necessary to settle these issues and whether Holter-detected ischemic episodes should be treated aggressively (until the results of such controlled studies are known) constituted an integral focus of this monograph on silent myocardial ischemia. It is hoped that this monograph will provide a continuing impetus for further research designed to seek decisive answers on the therapeutic significance of silent ischemia.

REFERENCES

1. Rutishauer W, Roskamm H (Ed): *Silent Myocardial Ischemia*. Berlin, Springer-Verlag, 1984, pp 1–204.
2. Singh BN (Ed): Symposium on silent myocardial ischemia: Detection, quantification and clinical significance in coronary artery disease. *Am J Cardiol* 1986;58(4):1B.
3. Shell WE: Personal communication, 1988.
4. Diamond GA: The silent treatment. *Am J Cardiol* 1987;60(15):1170.
5. Epstein SE, Palmeri ST: Mechanisms contributing to precipitation of unstable angina and acute myocardial infarction: Implications regarding therapy. *Am J Cardiol* 1984;54:1254.
6. Weiner DA, Ryan TJ, McCabe CH, et al: Significance of silent myocardial ischemia during exercise testing in coronary artery disease. *Am J Cardiol* 1987;59:725.
7. Erikssen L, Cohn PF, Thaulow E, Mowinckel P: Silent myocardial ischemia in middle aged men: Long term clinical course, in von Arnim T, Maseri A, (eds): *Silent Ischemia*. New York, Springer-Verlag, 1986;45–51.
8. Falcone C, DeSevi S, Porna E, et al: Clinical significance of exercise induced silent myocardial ischemia in patients with coronary artery disease. *J Am Coll Cardiol* 1987;9:295.
9. Nademanee K, Intarachot V, Josephson MA, et al: Prognostic significance of silent myocardial ischemia in patients with unstable angina. *J Am Coll Cardiol* 1987;10:1.
10. Gottlieb SO, Weisfeldt ML, Ouyang P, et al: Silent ischemia as a market for early unfavorable outcomes in patients with unstable angina. *N Engl J Med* 1986;314:1214.
11. Kannel WB, Cupples LA, D'Agnostino RB: Sudden death risk in overt coronary heart disease: The Framingham Study. *Am Heart J* 1987;113:799.
12. Bayes de Luna A, Guindo M, Ballester D, et al: Sudden death in patients with silent myocardial ischemia. In: Silent Myocardial Ischemia Symposium. Singh BN (ed). *Cardiovasc Rev & Rep* 1988, in press.

Index